WHAT COUNTS

HARNESSING DATA FOR AMERICA'S COMMUNITIES

D0828211

EDITED BY

**Federal Reserve Bank of San Francisco
& the Urban Institute**

FEDERAL RESERVE BANK OF SAN FRANCISCO
101 Market Street
San Francisco, CA 94105

URBAN INSTITUTE
2100 M Street NW
Washington, DC 20037

Senior Editors:
Naomi Cytron
Kathryn L.S. Pettit
G. Thomas Kingsley

Contributing Editors:
David Erickson
Ellen S. Seidman

ISBN 978-0-692-31338-1

Library of Congress Control Number: 2014954968

Printed in the United States of America

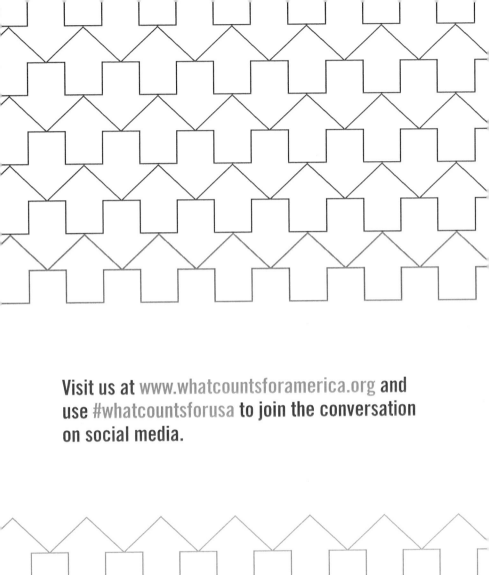

Visit us at www.whatcountsforamerica.org and use #whatcountsforusa to join the conversation on social media.

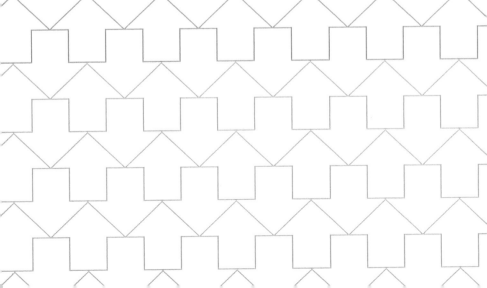

TABLE OF CONTENTS

3   ENHANCING DATA ACCESS AND TRANSPARENCY

4 STRENGTHENING THE VALIDITY AND USE OF DATA

5   ADOPTING MORE STRATEGIC PRACTICES

6 CONCLUSION

ACKNOWLEDGMENTS

This book is a joint project of the Federal Reserve Bank of San Francisco and the Urban Institute. The Robert Wood Johnson Foundation provided the Urban Institute with a grant to cover the costs of staff and research that were essential to this project. We also benefitted from the field-building work on data from Robert Wood Johnson grantees, many of whom are authors in this volume.

Our advisory committee also deserves special acknowledgment. Their perspectives, insights, and deep expertise were critical in shaping this volume. Most of all, we are indebted to our authors; their profound commitment to the idea that data has the potential to improve the policies and programs affecting the lives of low-income people and communities is registered on every page of this book.

Barbara Ray and her team at Hiredpen, Inc. were more than copy editors. Barbara has been a co-creator of this project and for that we are grateful. The cover art and layout were designed by C&G Partners LLC, who created an important visual theme for this work. Burness Communications was invaluable in helping us think through how to take what can often be a dry subject and make it more accessible to a wider audience. And our colleagues at the Urban Institute and the Federal Reserve Bank of San Francisco provided important encouragement and support.

This book builds on an earlier one, *Investing in What Works for America's Communities*. That book started a national conversation on the next generation of community development and anti-poverty work and we are grateful to the Low Income Investment Fund and their sponsor, the Citi Foundation, for keeping this conversation alive, engaged, and productive.

And finally, we want to thank Sarah Wartell, president of the Urban Institute, and John Williams, president of the Federal Reserve Bank of

San Francisco. Sarah was an early architect and advocate of this project and both Sarah and John provided support and enthusiasm as we brought this project to fruition.

Senior Editors

Naomi Cytron
Senior Research Associate, Community Development
Federal Reserve Bank of San Francisco

Kathryn L.S. Pettit
Senior Research Associate, Metropolitan Housing
and Communities Policy Center
Urban Institute

G. Thomas Kingsley
Senior Fellow, Metropolitan Housing and
Communities Policy Center
Urban Institute

Contributing Editors

David Erickson
Director, Center for Community
Development Investment
Federal Reserve Bank of San Francisco

Ellen S. Seidman
Senior Fellow
Urban Institute

Ingrid Gould Ellen
Paulette Goddard Professor of Urban Policy
and Planning, Wagner School of Public Service
and Director, Furman Center for Real Estate
and Urban Policy
New York University

David Fleming
Director and Health Officer
Public Health—Seattle & King County

Ira Goldstein
President of Policy Solutions
The Reinvestment Fund

Josh Guyer
Program Analyst, Office of Economic Resilience
*U.S. Department of Housing and
Urban Development*

Alaina Harkness
Program Officer, Community and
Economic Development
MacArthur Foundation

Ben Hecht
President and CEO
Living Cities

Douglas Jutte
Executive Director
Build Healthy Places Network

David Kindig
Emeritus Professor, Population Health Sciences
*University of Wisconsin, Madison School of
Medicine and Public Health*

Alan Mallach
Senior Fellow
Center for Community Progress

Lisa Nelson
Senior Policy Analyst, Community Development
Federal Reserve Bank of Cleveland

Aaron Wernham
CEO
Montana Healthcare Foundation

FOREWORD

Sarah Rosen Wartell
President, Urban Institute

John C. Williams
President and CEO, Federal Reserve Bank of San Francisco

What Counts is the product of an exciting collaboration between the Urban Institute and the Federal Reserve Bank of San Francisco. It represents our shared interest in the health and strength of America's communities and the importance of evidence-driven policymaking.

What Counts is a follow-up to the 2012 volume Investing in *What Works for America's Communities*, a joint effort by the San Francisco Fed and the Low Income Investment Fund. That book's emphasis on the need for integrated, collaborative solutions to the problems plaguing our nation's communities resonated widely. At the same time, its call for practitioners and policymakers to understand and direct resources to "what works" generated an avalanche of questions about how, exactly, to recognize and evaluate what does indeed work. This book responds to those questions.

The past two decades have seen a profound increase in data that can help us better respond to communities' needs and interests; a burst of technology that has made it possible to more effectively use that data; and a movement to make that data more freely available, so that more people—from the most marginalized neighborhoods to City Hall to Washington DC—can use it to inform their decisions.

There has never been an absence of appetite for transformative change in the world of community development. There has, however, been a dearth of data. *What Counts* brings together authors from a variety of backgrounds to consider new ways of analyzing and collecting information: How to transform disparate sets of data into useful evidence; how to share data across organizations and sectors; and how to arm practitioners and policymakers of all stripes with the skills they need to use data more effectively. It offers advice on overcoming policy pitfalls and guidance on developing, evaluating, and improving programs. And finally, it offers counsel on the best ways to listen to communities, understand their dynamics, and account for their specific needs, constituencies, and characters.

We have made tremendous strides in community development over the past several decades, but there is still a way to go. The best way to get there is to combine the passion of the community development world with the power of data. It is our sincere hope that this book will act as a roadmap for practitioners and policymakers throughout the sector.

That roadmap would not be possible without the contribution of key partners. We would like to offer our sincere thanks to the Robert Wood Johnson Foundation for its generous support. And we could not introduce *What Counts* without recognizing the five people—Naomi Cytron and David Erickson of the San Francisco Fed and Kathy Pettit, Tom Kingsley and Ellen Seidman of the Urban Institute—who conceived of and created this volume. Their dedication and insight make us proud to call them our own. Their work is a model of what we hope this book will accomplish: a cross-organizational collaboration of talented, committed professionals solving problems by bringing the best data to light.

■ ■ ■

SARAH ROSEN WARTELL *became the third president of the Urban Institute in February 2012. A public policy executive and housing markets expert, Ms. Wartell was President Bill Clinton's deputy assistant for economic policy and the deputy director of his National Economic Council. At the Department of Housing and Urban Development from 1993 to 1998, she advised the federal housing commissioner on housing finance, mortgage markets, and consumer protection.*

Ms. Wartell cofounded the Center for American Progress, serving as its first chief operating officer and general counsel. Later, as executive vice president, Ms. Wartell oversaw its policy teams and fellows. Her work focused on the economy and housing markets, and she directed the Mortgage Finance Working Group and "Doing What Works" government performance program. Ms. Wartell practiced law with the Washington, DC, firm of Arnold & Porter and was a consultant to the bipartisan Millennial Housing Commission.

Ms. Wartell has an AB degree with honors in urban affairs from Princeton University's Woodrow Wilson School of Public and International Affairs and holds a JD degree from Yale Law School.

■ ■ ■

JOHN C. WILLIAMS *took office as president and chief executive officer of the Federal Reserve Bank of San Francisco on March 1, 2011. In this role, he serves on the Federal Open Market Committee, bringing the Fed's Twelfth District's perspective to monetary policy discussions in Washington.*

Dr. Williams was previously the executive vice president and director of research for the San Francisco bank, which he joined in 2002. He began his career in 1994 as an economist at the Board of Governors of the Federal Reserve System, following the completion of his PhD in Economics at Stanford University. Dr. Williams' research focuses on topics including: monetary policy under uncertainty; innovation; productivity, and business cycles. He has collaborated with economists from throughout the country and across the globe to examine economic and policy issues from different perspectives, and has published numerous articles in leading research journals.

Prior to completing his doctorate at Stanford, he earned a Master's of Science with distinction in economics from the London School of Economics, and an AB with high distinction from the University of California at Berkeley.

1

INTRODUCTION

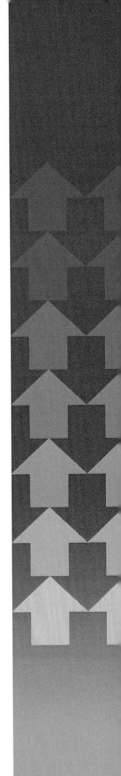

A ROADMAP: HOW TO USE THIS BOOK

This book is a response to the explosive interest in and availability of data, especially for improving America's communities. It is designed to be useful to practitioners, policymakers, funders, and the data intermediaries and other technical experts who help transform all types of data into useful information. Some of the essays—which draw on experts from community development, population health, education, finance, law, and information systems—address high-level systems-change work. Others are immensely practical, and come close to explaining "how to." All discuss the incredibly exciting opportunities and challenges that our ever-increasing ability to access and analyze data provide.

As the book's editors, we of course believe everyone interested in improving outcomes for low-income communities would benefit from reading every essay. But we're also realists, and know the demands of the day-to-day work of advancing opportunity and promoting well-being for disadvantaged populations. With that in mind, we are providing this roadmap to enable readers with different needs to start with the essays most likely to be of interest to them.

For everyone, but especially those who are relatively new to understanding the promise of today's data for communities, the opening essay is a useful summary and primer. Similarly, the final essay provides both a synthesis of the book's primary themes and a focus on the systems challenges ahead.

Section 2, Transforming Data into Policy-Relevant Information, offers a glimpse into the array of data tools and approaches that advocates, planners, investors, developers and others are currently using to inform and shape local and regional processes.

Section 3, Enhancing Data Access and Transparency, should catch the eye of those whose interests are in expanding the range of data that is commonly within reach and finding ways to link data across multiple policy and program domains, all while ensuring that privacy and security are respected.

Section 4, Strengthening the Validity and Use of Data, will be particularly provocative for those concerned about building the capacity of practitioners and policymakers to employ appropriate data for understanding and shaping community change.

The essays in section 5, Adopting More Strategic Practices, examine the roles that practitioners, funders, and policymakers all have in improving the ways we capture the multi-faceted nature of community change, communicate about the outcomes and value of our work, and influence policy at the national level.

There are of course interconnections among the essays in each section. We hope that wherever you start reading, you'll be inspired to dig deeper into the book's enormous richness, and will join us in an ongoing conversation about how to employ the ideas in this volume to advance policy and practice.

Naomi Cytron, Kathryn L.S. Pettit, and G. Thomas Kingsley, Senior Editors
David Erickson and Ellen S. Seidman, Contributing Editors

DATA AND COMMUNITY— FOUNDATION FOR AN AGENDA

G. Thomas Kingsley and Kathryn L.S. Pettit
The Urban Institute

This book explores the use of data to improve conditions in America's communities, with particular attention to low-income communities and the people who live in them. Using data more intensively and creatively in decision-making at the local, metro, state, or federal level in itself will not eliminate poverty, produce healthier lives, or fully address the other major social problems of our time. But data driven decision-making can make a tremendous difference in results that communities and their residents care about.

Today, very few of the institutions that work in America's communities can honestly be characterized as "data driven." However, the past two decades have seen truly remarkable advances in the availability of relevant data and the technical ability to use the information inexpensively and in exciting ways. In the coming decade, these new capacities are likely to spur fundamental changes in how community-oriented institutions operate and how policy is made. The essays in this book examine this potential and promising new practices, as well as barriers to be overcome.

Before we begin talking about the data, however, we need to be clear about scope. This book was motivated by the 2012 volume, *Investing in What Works for America's Communities* and the conversations it generated.[1] That volume endorsed an integrated view of community development, going well beyond the narrow "bricks and mortar" vision the field had settled into, to consider issues such as health, education, jobs, and connectivity. Similarly, although we, too, see community development playing a central role, we recognize the need for all institutions

---

1 Nancy O Andrews and David J. Erickson, eds., *Investing in What Works for America's Communities: Essays on People, Places and Purpose* (San Francisco: Federal Reserve Bank of San Francisco and Low Income Investment Fund, 2012). Available at www.whatworksforamerica.org.

that affect our communities to more effectively use data. These include city and town governments as well as neighborhood groups, regional collaborations, social service providers, housing developers, community development financial institutions (CDFIs), public health agencies, private entrepreneurs, and philanthropy.

It is also important to note upfront that although this book talks most about how institutions can use data, we should not forget individuals and families. Important advances have made it easier for them to directly use data to make personal decisions, such as when to arrive at the bus stop or how to choose a doctor.

This first essay offers background information and framing to put the remaining essays in a broader context. We discuss four main themes:

1 Emergence of the community information field describes how the intersection of new data, technology, and innovative institutions in the early 1990s led to a revolution in community information.

2 Advances in the availability of data describes the sources of community data and new ways data are being transformed into useable information.

3 Advances in the use of data opens with a framework on how community data can be used in decision-making, provides successful examples, and discusses roles of the actors in the process.

4 Challenges—What is holding us back? reviews challenges and barriers to taking advantage of the full potential of community data and offers ideas on how to address them.

This essay is intended as an overview for the reader and cannot do justice to all these themes in this condensed format. For a more in-depth examination of the advances in the community information field during the past 20 years, we refer you to our recent book, *Strengthening Communities with Neighborhood Data*.[2]

---

2   G. Thomas Kingsley, Claudia J. Coulton, and Kathryn L.S. Pettit, *Strengthening Communities with Neighborhood Data* (Washington, DC: Urban Institute, 2014), available at www.urban.org/strengtheningcommunities.

EMERGENCE OF THE COMMUNITY INFORMATION FIELD

Those working to improve America's communities have always wanted factual information on conditions in their neighborhoods, how those conditions were changing, and how they compared with those in other parts of the city, county, or state. As late as the 1980s, however, the only viable source for such information was the U.S. census, which is updated only once a decade. In addition, census data do not cover many issues critical to making communities better: rates of property tax delinquency, crime, teen pregnancy, and housing sales are but a few examples of data the census ignores. Locally funded surveys were theoretically possible but, because they were (and remain) enormously expensive, they were almost never conducted. Transaction-by-transaction data on these topics most often existed on paper, buried somewhere in agency files. But the high cost of pulling the records from filing cabinets and plotting them on a map so that staff could add up thousands of transactions by neighborhood and visualize problems and the impact of efforts to solve them almost always made the task infeasible.

The implications of not having such data, however, were serious. Because they did not know where problems were most severe, those working in neighborhoods had no way to systematically target their services. They also had no viable way to measure how the neighborhoods they worked in were getting better or worse from year to year.

By around 1990, however, technology introduced a solution to this problem. As record-keeping for many local government agencies was automated, transaction records containing a street address or some other geographic identifier were now electronic. In addition, marked improvements in Geographic Information System (GIS) technology meant that data could be linked to a location, summed by neighborhood, and mapped with remarkable speed and efficiency.

Government departments found valuable ways to use these new capacities to analyze their own data; police departments mapping crime patterns is a prime example. Some hospitals began to examine data on the neighborhoods of their patients to better plan education campaigns and outpatient service delivery. Some cities began to release their GIS data on individual properties to the public, eventually over the web.

The GIS data were an enormous time saver for community development corporations (CDCs) and other housing developers who previously had to spend days in city hall basements searching through musty paper records to collect enough information to make competent decisions about land assembly.

The ability to combine data sets was another major advance. It is difficult to learn much about neighborhood conditions and trends by looking at only one agency data set at a time. As a result, institutions in several cities convinced several local agencies to share their administrative data files. They made the commitment to regularly assemble the data across agencies and make the indicators available to a variety of users and the public at large. In these cities, users only had to go to one place to get time series data by neighborhood on a variety of topics (such as health, housing conditions, crime, and public assistance).

The "data intermediaries" who built the cross-agency information systems had different types of institutional homes, including community oriented university research centers, social service providers, and local foundations. Six of them joined together in 1995 to form the National Neighborhood Indicators Partnership (NNIP) to facilitate peer networking, advance methods, and inform social policy more broadly. The authors of this essay have led the team at the Urban Institute that coordinates the NNIP network, and we have noted several of the network's contributions in this essay. As of 2014, nearly three dozen cities have adopted the NNIP model. Most began this work because of a strong interest in community building. These new capacities represented a true revolution at the time: moving from no data to very rich ongoing sources of information in just a few years.

The most important stories, of course, are not about information systems or underlying innovations in data availability and GIS technology. Rather, the most important stories are those about the practical applications they have yielded. These too have grown and are the subjects of many of the essays in this book.

The demand for richer data is now being generated by a much broader array of actors than initially. For example, although community developers in the early 1990s understood how vital data on multiple indicators of neighborhood conditions were, leaders in public health now see these data as essential as well. Their new emphasis on the social determinants of health requires them to understand all the interactions in poor neighborhoods that both positively and negatively affect the health of residents.

ADVANCES IN THE AVAILABILITY OF DATA

Since the mid-1990s, the data landscape for communities has continued to evolve. Our current challenges are too much data to sift through and difficulty in accessing the right data for the decisions at hand. The term "data" has many different meanings, and we first provide an overview of the types of data and recent data trends. The final portion of this section will describe ways that researchers, technologists, and policymakers are enhancing the value of the raw data stream for practitioners through both easier access and integration of data across sources and organizations.

Types of Data

Many types of data can be useful to practitioners. In particular, data can be generated from administrative records, surveys, or qualitative methods. Administrative data are collected as part of an organization's operations, whether to provide services, collect taxes, run the courts, or maintain property records, but the data can be repurposed for other uses. Government agencies generate a wealth of administrative data in operating programs, such as data on school performance, food stamp enrollment, or reported crimes. They also maintain information on property ownership and characteristics, both as a definitive legal record and to assess and collect taxes. Finally, government agencies collect data for national data systems, such as monitoring births and deaths through the Vital Statistics program.[3]

Other sectors also collect administrative data that could be valuable for designing community initiatives or service programs. Businesses maintain administrative records, such as credit data for businesses or individuals or grocery purchases tied to loyalty cards. Nonprofits create data systems that record client characteristics and social services or

---

3 See Claudia J. Coulton, "Catalog of Administrative Data Sources for Neighborhood Indicators" (Washington, DC: Urban Institute, 2008).

property information for housing development. To use administrative data most effectively, community users should understand the original motivation for the data collection, which determines which individuals and properties are included in the data, which fields are likely to be of higher or lower quality, and how often the data are updated.

The second major source of data is surveys. These surveys may be about people and households and can be conducted at many levels, including nationally, such as the American Community Survey from the U.S. Census Bureau, and in a single city, such as the survey conducted to support the Jacksonville Quality of Life study described in Ben Warner's essay. Surveys may also catalog a mix of community assets, such as parks, schools, and churches, or risk factors, such as graffiti, liquor stores or fast food outlets. Finally, property surveys catalog characteristics of residential or commercial properties, documenting vacancy, land use, and building condition. The Detroit Residential Parcel Survey, commissioned by the Detroit Blight Removal Task Force, is one impressive recent example (http://www.timetoendblight. com/). The nonprofit organization Data Driven Detroit partnered with Loveland Technologies, a local technology company, to develop and implement a streamlined data collection and quality control system for collecting information about residential properties. Called the Motor City Mapping Project, a team of 200 people collected information on almost 380,000 properties in just a few weeks. With this common set of information, government agencies, community developers, and neighborhood residents can better strategize about how to address blight and vacancy. Another innovation of the project is that they are exploring how to keep the data updated so they can have contemporaneous information for planning and track progress over time.

The third major source of data comes from qualitative methods. These can be interviews with knowledgeable stakeholders, formal focus groups, or community meetings. These data can provide information about external factors affecting neighborhoods and families and resident perceptions and priorities. Several of the essays in this volume emphasize the importance of including qualitative data to paint a fuller picture of communities. Ira Goldstein, for example, describes the need to "ground-truth"—check the validity of assumptions of—the neighborhood typology assignments derived from quantitative sources, incorporating data from visual surveys. The essays by Meredith Minkler and Patricia Bowie and Moira Inkelas recognize how including the voices of community residents and program clients improves data quality and results in a fuller picture of a program's impacts. Claudia Coulton recommends using interviews and focus groups to understand the nature of mobility in a given neighborhood, including people's motivations and decision process for moving.

New Trends in Data Sources

Data kept in government computers are of only limited use. The open-government data movement, which in the past few years has grown significantly, is about overcoming that problem, and affects governments at all levels. A central premise of open data is that transparency of processes and information enables citizens to hold governments accountable, and technology can improve transparency. Advocates view government data as a public good that should be available to the taxpayers who funded their creation. Open data can also encourage citizen engagement in government decision-making and spur economic growth through private-sector applications. Emily Shaw's essay explains that open data encompasses both practice, as in distributing data through a city open data portal, and policy, formal tenets adopted by governments or organizations. Although the origins of the open data movement are rooted in government responsibilities, more nonprofit organizations are integrating the principles of open data in their work.

The emergence of "big data" is often mentioned along with open data. Big data is defined in many ways, but can be thought of as data with very high volume, velocity, and variety that traditional computational techniques cannot handle. These include data generated from traffic sensors, which may capture data every 20 seconds from hundreds of locations around a region. They also include new types of data that require new ways to analyze, such as posts to Facebook or Twitter or photos from Google StreetMaps.

More important than the specific definition of big data is the need to connect technologists and data scientists who can visualize, manipulate, and find patterns in this wealth of data with the local nonprofits and governments who could benefit from new insights that data can generate about neighborhood conditions, resident sentiment, and human behavior. One example of this convergence is Data Science for Social Good, a University of Chicago summer program for aspiring data scientists to apply data mining and machine learning to projects proposed by governments and nonprofits on topics such as education, health, energy, and transportation. DataKind, a nonprofit organization based in New York City, has a similar mission to bring new skills to benefit community groups. The organization brings nonprofits working on community problems together with data scientists to improve the quality of, access to, and understanding of data in the social sector. DataKind sponsors weekend "Data Dives," arranges technical assistance engagements of up to a few months, and facilitates ongoing local relationships through their five local chapters.

Adding Value to Raw Data

Raw data alone are a little like the ingredients of a cake—necessary, but only useful if put together thoughtfully. Integrated data systems (IDS), for example, link individual-level records over time and across data sets from different programs and agencies, such as school performance, child welfare, birth data, and juvenile justice data.[4] IDS allow us to ask new questions about how various public systems overlap and point to a more holistic approach to helping children and families. Rebecca London and Milbrey McLaughlin share lessons from their experience with the Youth Data Archive, an IDS for several counties in California that is governed by a university-community partnership. The authors describe how the IDS process combined with a shared research agenda can support collaboration and improve youth services. John Petrila's essay discusses the tension between using linked data sets like the Youth Data Archive to inform policy and the privacy and other concerns that emerge from the use of such data. He relates the political, legal, and technical challenges of establishing and using linked data and suggests potential solutions.

Linking data is an approach that extends beyond government-generated data. Robert Avery, Marsha Courchane, and Peter Zorn document the

---

4   For more information about integrated data systems, see the Actionable Intelligence for Social Policy website at http://www.aisp.upenn.edu/

National Mortgage Database (NMDB), which links data for a sample of mortgage loans with credit and property data to gain a better picture of the housing finance market and borrower behavior. The database will break new ground in many ways, primarily by bringing together extensive private data sets on loan performance and borrower credit activity with public data, including property records, and adding occasional surveys. This will enhance understanding of both the workings of the mortgage market and the impact of housing on the broader economy.

Visualization is another way to add value to raw data. Ren Essene and Michael Byrne's essay describes an excellent example of this. The Home Mortgage Disclosure Act (HMDA) dataset on mortgage originations has been available to the public for many years and has served as the basis for many valuable studies. The source data set, however, is large and difficult to manipulate. The work described in the essay made critical elements of HMDA quickly accessible as interactive charts and maps on the website of the Consumer Financial Protection Bureau (CFPB). In addition, the CFPB created a series of tools that make it easy for users with minimal computer skills to download understandable exhibits they can use directly. Code for America is a nonprofit organization committed to expanding user-centered design in local government websites. The organization brings advanced technology into the public sector through their Fellows program, which matches teams of designers and technologists with individual local governments for a year to tackle a proposed problem.

ADVANCES IN THE USE OF DATA

Although access to raw data is essential, using data for decision-making requires transformation, including excerpting selected data from a larger data set and then arranging the selections so they provide information to decision makers at the right time and in the right form. This section begins by framing how community data can be used to support better decisions. It then offers examples of integrated applications and discusses roles of different actors and broader applications.

Using Data to Make Better Decisions

Both the federal government and philanthropic funders have been urging communities to engage in data-driven decision-making. But what does that mean? There are three distinct functions in which data are critical to making good decisions, although in practice, they are often performed jointly:

- Situation analysis: learning more about the problems and opportunities you face and their implications;

- Policy analysis and planning: deciding the course of action to address your situation;

- Performance management and evaluation: tracking and assessing the progress of your selected course of action, and making mid-course corrections based on what you learn.

Situation Analysis: Ben Warner's essay discusses "Community Indicators Projects," in which a group of local stakeholders (in one neighborhood or citywide) get together and select a multi-topic set of indicators they think best reflects their collective well-being. They recurrently collect data on the indicators and look over the results to see where things are getting better or worse, and by how much. Indicator projects are most effective when they lead directly to responsive action. In Warner's community (Jacksonville, Florida), for example, a citizen's committee reviews the recent trends and, depending on whether they are positive or negative, assigns either a "gold star" or a "red flag." Every year, the organization selects one or more of the red flags to "mobilize the community for action through a shared learning engagement and advocacy process."

Using data in this way is key to setting priorities, and it helps keep the focus on actions that are critical to addressing the issues that are most urgent and avoids too much investment in things that are getting better by themselves. For example, suppose that, even though foreclosures have been a hot topic in the last few neighborhood association meetings, new data show the neighborhood actually ranked low on that indicator compared with others and the rate was dropping fast. Alternatively, suppose that although the neighborhood ranked very low on juvenile crime in the prior year, the new data show that it had the second highest increase in the juvenile crime rate since then. Timely data that allow a community to distinguish between such trends are essential to the ability to allocate resources effectively.

Sometimes, the facts uncovered in a situation analysis are enough in themselves to force decision. In Providence, Rhode Island, for example, laws regarding sales of tax-foreclosed properties were revised after solid data demonstrated that the share of these properties purchased by slumlords had been shockingly high for several years.[5]

Policy Analysis and Planning: This function involves using data to design an effective course of action to respond to the findings of the situation analysis. It implies conceptualizing alternative ways of doing things and then assessing and comparing the likely advantages and disadvantages of each. The main uses of data in this function revolve around improving the ability to estimate the likely effects of the alternatives: in what ways and by how much they will change desired outcomes, how much they will cost, what side effects and unintended consequences they might produce, and so forth.

Community development practitioners have done this type of analysis for years when developing real estate: creating financial pro formas on alternative designs and schedules for new housing and other real estate projects and comparing the estimated rates of return. The recent innovations have been in use of data-driven analysis to uncover and quantitatively evaluate a more complicated mix of effects for a more complicated mix of programmatic actions.

So far, we know of no attempts to estimate the effects of all activities in a complex (multi-program) community initiative. But there is evidence that many local institutions are devoting considerably more effort to assembling and analyzing data to back up their planning than they did in the past. For example, the essay by Erika Poethig describes the evolution of Chicago's use of data to enhance the quality of the city's five-year plans for affordable housing. Nancy Andrews and Dan Rinzler describe how the Low Income Investment Fund's innovative Social

---

5   Jake Cowan, *Stories: Using Information in Community Building and Local Policy* (Washington, DC: Urban Institute, 2007) provides accounts of several other cases where bringing community data together in innovative but often quite simple ways has, in itself, led to important changes in laws and policies.

Impact Calculator leverages existing social science research to estimate the dollar value of the social benefits of their investments. Other essays in this volume discussing similar efforts to measure potential and actual program effects include Aaron Wernham's essay on health impact assessments and Ian Galloway's essay on making "impact investment" decisions.

Ira Goldstein's essay describes a tool called Market Value Analysis, which starts by assembling a substantial amount of data on a city's neighborhoods and then uses a statistical procedure (cluster analysis) to sort neighborhoods into several different "types," based mostly on their housing market conditions. The contrasts among the market types are vivid and help city officials and community groups understand both the situations different neighborhoods face (situation analysis) and which mixes of programmatic actions are likely to work best in which types of neighborhoods (policy analysis). Interventions may involve cleaning up vacant lots, intensive code enforcement, stimulating market-based rehabilitation, acquiring and demolishing vacant buildings, or a mixture of strategies.

Foundations are emphasizing another use of data in planning: "evidence-based practice." Do data from other locations show that a program you are considering is effective or not? If so, how did it work? Groups can use data on similar programs' inputs, approaches, and effects (including changes in outcomes, costs, side effects, etc.) to estimate probable program effects. Although not all good solutions have been tried and evaluated, and many solutions that work in one situation are not directly replicable in another, programs whose inputs, outcomes, and impact are well documented can definitely provide practitioners with a better place to start.

Data are also key to flexibility—the ability to make mid-course corrections and multiple iterations as results suggest certain strategies are more or less successful, and as new problems develop. For some urban planners in the past, the idea was make a good plan and try to stick with it. As the world becomes increasingly complex and uncertain, being adaptable may be more effective than consistency. If one can quickly spot an important new trend, it is easier to adjust plans and secure better outcomes. As Patricia Bowie and Moira Inkelas demonstrate, this flexibility enabled by real-time data is important to improving outcomes for individuals as well as communities.

A new data-driven approach will not completely replace the way practitioners design strategies and programs. It will always be important to weigh the probable positives and negatives of different ways of doing things, based on experience, "how the world works," and the facts at hand. Good judgment in this process will always be essential. But data will be used more often as a basis for estimating the effects of alternative strategies, replacing more of the guesswork and intuitive choices, and enhancing the predictability of outcomes.

Performance Management and Evaluation: Pressure to use data to expand the accountability of social programs has grown markedly over the past decade.[6] Whatever the intervention (whether it is a single youth employment program or a full comprehensive community initiative), the implication is that the managers need to select a set of indicators of the results they are trying to achieve. Then, as the work is underway, they regularly collect data on those indicators, hold meetings to review what has happened (good and bad), and design mid-course corrections to program plans as the data may suggest.

Performance management uses data to improve program performance in the short- to medium-term. In contrast, program evaluation attempts to determine whether a program has met its goals over the long term. Performance management is conducted by the program's management team while the program is underway, whereas evaluation is most often conducted by outsiders after the fact. Evaluation has been much more frequently supported by funders than performance management over the past two decades.

Victor Rubin and Michael McAfee's essay explains the requirements for effective performance management in the federal Promise Neighborhood initiative. They describe how a standard data and

---

6 See, e.g., Mario Marino, *Leap of Reason: Managing to Outcomes in an Era of Scarcity* (Washington DC: Venture Philanthropy Partners, 2011), and Mark Friedman, *Trying Hard Is Not Good Enough: How to Produce Measurable Improvements for Customers and Communities* (Victoria, BC: Trafford Publishing, 2005).

technology infrastructure can facilitate performance management. They acknowledge the challenges in cultivating an organizational culture that views data as essential to getting results, but share examples in Hayward and Nashville where data-driven approaches are taking hold. They also demonstrate how a national intermediary can support better practice locally. The essay by Cory Fleming and Randall Reid describes a similar process, "Performance Stat," that has been adopted by a sizable number of state and local government agencies in the past few years.[7] Features seen as key to the success of this approach are insistence on the involvement of high-level officials in the management reviews and holding those reviews frequently and regularly, as well as careful thinking to select the right metrics up front. Review meetings work best, the authors suggest, when they are not mainly about celebrating success or addressing failure, but when they focus on figuring out what worked, what did not, and why, and then revising plans accordingly.

The essays by Susana Vasquez and Patrick Barry, and by Alaina Harkness, consider the application of performance management in nonprofit-managed community development. After-the-fact evaluations will still need to be supported, but Harkness argues that funders should place higher priority on building the data capacities of their grantees so the grantees can better manage their own programs in the short term.

Some communities are using "collective impact" strategies to make improvements. Collective impact is an expanded form of performance management that recognizes that most fundamental societal objectives (such as improving education) cannot be achieved by individual institutions working in a field one-by-one.[8] Rather than each institution employing performance management to improve results in its own narrowly defined silo, collective impact joins all of the relevant actors together in one performance management process, committing to the same overarching goals and using an ongoing system of "shared measurement" to track performance against the goals. To date, the

---

7   For a useful review of these processes, see Robert D. Behn, "The Seven Big Errors of PerformanceStat." Rappaport Institute/Taubman Center Policy Brief. (Cambridge, MA: Harvard University, John F. Kennedy School of Government, February 2008).

8   John Kania and Mark Kramer, "Collective Impact," *Stanford Social Innovation Review* (Winter 2011); Fay Hanleybrown, John Kania, and Mark Kramer, "Channeling Change: Making Collective Impact Work," *Stanford Social Innovation Review* (Winter 2012).

collective impact approach has been applied most often to citywide or regional objectives. The most notable example is the "Strive" initiative, which focuses on education objectives in the Cincinnati area and other cities. However, the approach has now been applied successfully to many other problems and opportunities, including finding jobs for public housing residents (Chicago), reducing violent crime (Memphis), and addressing childhood obesity (Somerville, MA).[9]

It is important to recognize the differences between performance management and program evaluation. Ideally, program evaluations determine the extent to which the program caused the final outcomes that are observed. The only sure way to do that is to construct a plausible counterfactual. For example, if program participants are randomly assigned to either an experimental group that receives the program treatment) or a control group that does not, and the context for each group is the same or very similar, one can typically say that the program caused the differences in outcomes.[10] These randomized controlled trials (RCT) are considered the gold standard, but are extremely difficult to construct for complex efforts such as multi-program community initiatives. A variety of alternative approaches have been proposed that, even though they cannot meet the RCT standard in full, can provide useful information to guide decisions about future investments.[11] In their essay, David Fleming, Hilary Karasz, and Kirsten Wysen wrestle with these issues in evaluating programs that attempt to address the social determinants of health. Raphael Bostic explains why insisting on RCTs as the only standard of evidence may hinder, rather than promote, evidence-based policymaking.

Putting It All Together

So far, we have reviewed the three basic elements of data in community decision-making separately. In reality, however, they are often combined and span one or more institutional environments. And the process of

---

9 Hanleybrown et al., "Channeling Change: Making Collective Impact Work."

10 There is a sizable literature on methods for evaluating social programs in varying circumstances, summarized by Adele V. Harrell et al., *Evaluation Strategies for Human Services Programs: A Guide for Policymakers and Providers.* (Washington, DC: Urban Institute, 1996).

11 See James P. Connel et al., eds., *New Approaches to Evaluating Community Initiatives: Concepts, Methods and Context* (Washington, DC: Aspen Institute, 1995).

decision-making normally does not occur in an orderly sequence; there is a considerable amount of back and forth among the elements. As one example, the essay by Alex Karner and his colleagues at University of California–Davis Center for Regional Change describes their work to help diverse stakeholders in California's San Joaquin Valley prepare sustainable communities strategies that incorporated equity values, in a region characterized by significant inequality. This involved examining and presenting new data on multiple dimensions and using those data to devise collaborative regional planning strategies to advance social equity. Rather than following a pre-determined linear process, the personal relationships, staff capacity, and political climate shaped the ways in which the local advocates and planners incorporated data into regional planning. The next three sections illustrate other approaches used to expand data-driven decision-making by local players.[12]

Sharing Data Within a Place: The Camden Coalition of Healthcare Providers (CCHP) has developed an integrated (shared) data system that includes demographic, diagnosis, and financial information for all admissions and emergency room visits made by city residents to the city's three main hospitals. Analysis showed that just 1 percent of the 100,000 people who used Camden's medical facilities accounted for 30 percent of all costs. Under the leadership of a young physician, Jeffrey Brenner, the new approach focused on identifying and developing trusting relationships with many of these "super-utilizers." Care is provided in home visits or over the phone. It consists of services that emphasize prevention, such as helping patients find a stable residence, ensuring they take their medications on schedule, and addressing their smoking and other substance abuse problems. The data system provided substantial information on each patient, allowing providers to target services sensitively. Results for the first 36 patients were impressive. The average number of hospital and E.R. visits for this group dropped from 62 per month before joining the program to 37. The average hospital bills for the group declined from $1.2 million per month to just over

---

12 Just a few examples are noted here. For more, see *Stories: Using Information in Community Building and Local Policy.*, by Jake Cowan. (Washington, DC: Urban Institute, 2007); Federal Reserve Board of Governors, *Putting Data to Work: Data-Driven Approaches to Strengthening Neighborhoods* (Washington DC: Federal Reserve Board of Governors. December, 2011); and Chapters 5 and 6 of *Strengthening Communities with Neighborhood Data* (by G. Thomas Kingsley, Claudia J. Coulton and Kathryn L. S. Pettit, Washington, DC: Urban Institute Press, 2014).

$500,000. The data were also used to target community-based interventions for diabetes. A *New Yorker* article featured this approach and the coalition is assisting other communities trying to build similar systems.[13]

NEO CANDO (the Northeast Ohio Community and Neighborhood Data for Organizing), developed and maintained by the Center on Urban Poverty and Community Development at Case Western Reserve University, is a property-based information system that illustrates key advances in the field.[14] The system incorporates vast amounts of data from many sources. It incorporates property-level data on topics that are typically in the files of local property tax assessors and recorders of deeds, such as ownership, physical characteristics, tax amounts and arrearage status, sales transactions, and sales prices. It also integrates, and makes available on a real-time basis, records of other city departments (e.g., housing code violations, building and demolition permits) and other data that are normally either unavailable or not integrated with other property records in a usable manner (e.g., vacancy status, foreclosure filings, sheriff's sales, REO status).

The data are used for many purposes. The most notable is to support decisions about what to do with individual properties within neighborhoods. Groups of Cleveland stakeholders (CDCs, other nonprofits, city officials—with support from NEO CANDO staff) meet and jointly to examine recently updated parcel-level maps, tables, and analyses, paying attention to the spatial clustering of conditions as well as the circumstances of individual properties (situation analysis). Fairly sophisticated analyses have been used to support decisions by the Land Bank, CDCs, and others about which buildings warrant demolition or rehabilitation. The data also help the city's code enforcement staff and other special purpose agencies and nonprofits to prioritize their activities. Because the data on individual properties are regularly updated, they show changes in status that can directly serve as a basis for performance

13 Atul Gawande, "The Hot Spotters: Can We Lower Medical Costs by Giving the Neediest Patients Better Care?" *The New Yorker*, January 24, 2011. The CCHP database was developed initially by CamConnect, the NNIP partner in Camden, but it is now operated by CCHP.

14 This account is based on Lisa Nelson, "Cutting Through the Fog: Helping Communities See a Clearer Path to Stabilization." In *Strengthening Communities with Neighborhood Data*, edited by G. Thomas Kingsley, Claudia J. Coulton, and Kathryn L. S. Pettit (Washington, DC: Urban Institute Press, 2014).

management, answering questions such as, what types and how many properties did we address? What happened as a result of our efforts? And how rapidly?

Participants have said that the data and process of using the information in this way have been an important boost for collaboration and influence. That the organizations were all operating from the same data, and that the data were themselves broadly available, promoted broader inclusiveness and diminished controversy. Participants were less likely to disagree because they knew the reasoning and facts behind the choices that had been made.

Sharing Data Across Places: Shared measurement can also be helpful when individual organizations in different cities that belong to a network or industry agree to collect data so that selected indicators can be brought together centrally and the results shared with all participants. The essay by Maggie Grieve offers a useful framing of this approach and describes several examples, including a multi-year joint effort by NeighborWorks America and the Citi Foundation to capture and assess outcome measures for 30 Citi grantees operating financial coaching programs. This essay recognizes that shared measurement systems have special data quality and data consistency challenges, requiring common data standards (or crosswalks) to make them work.

Another valuable example is the emerging Outcomes Intiative described in the essay by Bill Kelly and Fred Karnas. Stewards of Affordable Housing for the Future (SAHF) members will collect consistent data on the outcomes of efforts to holistically improve the well-being of residents of affordable housing developments. The same underlying concept is behind the CoMetrics and HomeKeeper data sets, which facilitate cooperative businesses and community land trusts decisions, respectively, which are described in the essay by Annie Donovan and Rick Jacobus. The Aeris Cloud, which Paige Chapel discusses, allows CDFIs and investors to track a variety of financial and performance metrics against peers. This helps meet the information needs of capital markets while enabling both CDFIs and investors to realize efficiencies through standardized reporting.

The main motivation for these systems is to help improve decision-making by the individual participants. With access to the central system, participants can see how their own characteristics and performance compare with similar organizations on any number of selected metrics, and then adjust their own strategies accordingly. Comparing differences in program approaches against differences in results can yield the greatest benefit as managers think through the factors behind successful performance in a way they never could with internal data alone. An added benefit is that because data can be aggregated across multiple entities in a network, the resulting information informs users of the health and impact of the entire network.

Dashboards: Too much data can be almost as dysfunctional as too little. Thus, a higher priority is now being given to "boiling down" the data to focus on the most important and informative metrics—that is, a collection that will be manageable—and displaying results in ways that enable users to quickly grasp the main messages. One such tool is the "dashboard," normally a one-page summary of key results presented in an easy-to-read (and remember) display. This tool directs focus on a comparatively small number of indicators. This focus does not mean discarding the rest of the data set. In today's best practice, organizations maintain much more data than they put on their dashboards and use the information in supplementary analyses to shed light on the forces at work behind the key results. Bridget Catlin's essay on county health rankings explains both the allure and perils of dashboards and indices and offers a broader assessment of visualizing and communicating information through design and display. Ben Warner's essay also offers useful guidance on dashboards.

Actors, Roles, and Broader Uses

Using data effectively depends on more than the data; it also depends on who is involved, what roles they play, and how they use the data beyond its initial purpose.

Involving the Community: As in other endeavors, many decisions affecting a community can legitimately be made solely by the staff and managers of one "professional" institution, like a Head Start provider deciding how many staff to hire for next year, or a community health center deciding which of two alternative pieces of equipment to buy. In many cases, however, a community's residents and their institutions should be involved in the process, whether they are directly involved in making the decisions or are consulted during the process. This is particularly true for more comprehensive community development initiatives, but it is also true for some decisions about individual programs, including, for example, the overall strategies of the Head Start provider or community health center.

Since 1995, "democratizing information" has been the theme of the local data intermediaries in NNIP. This means in part that, rather than conducting the analysis and writing the report themselves, they take the data to the community. They help the residents and community groups probe the data and structure them to support decisions that will benefit the community. The intention is that at the end of the day, the residents recognize that the decisions that have been made are *their* decisions. They "own" the process and its results, and the data intermediary was only their coach and facilitator. Some of the most valuable experiences have been when a neighborhood group understood a community problem (crime in the neighborhood, for example, is most prevalent near vacant buildings) and saw a solution (focus police resources near the vacant buildings), but the powers in the city paid no attention to them. Yet once the community presented maps that showed the overlay of crimes and vacant buildings at a public forum with the press in attendance, policies began to change.

The essay by Meredith Minkler on community-based participatory research takes the concept a step further, explaining that involving the community in data collection generates more relevant data as well as more effective actions in response—albeit not without potential inconsistency with academic or programmatic standards. The essay by Patricia Bowie and Moira Inkelas discusses the development and use of data in real time by community residents and service providers to enhance health outcomes. In addition to quantitative data, these strategies encourage collection of qualitative data, which can convey understanding of critical topics that are normally impractical (often impossible) to quantify, such as community perspectives, social networks, and community assets. The greatest payoff is when stakeholders can use both qualitative and the quantitative data in mutually reinforcing ways.

Empowerment, Education, and Advocacy: The data that are generated for all phases of community decision-making can be extremely powerful in engaging diverse audiences and changing mindsets. Linking data to a plausible argument can convince neighborhood residents to get involved in an initiative, local philanthropies to provide needed funding, city councils to revise unproductive legislation, and the public to change their vote on an issue of community concern.[15]

Raphael Bostic's essay makes this point in stark terms at the federal level, contrasting the relative budgetary success of programs to counter homelessness and the difficulties housing counseling programs have had getting and retaining funding. The data provide the credibility that is essential to both advocacy and longer-term education. But Bostic argues the data alone are not enough. Successful data-driven decision-making also requires a narrative, a clear story that makes a case that the public and relevant policymakers can understand, and an effective communication vehicle, such as publications, meetings, websites, and other strategies that will reach the relevant audience and convince them to act.

Enhancing Individuals' Decisions: The information revolution is not just about institutions. It is also enabling individuals, including the residents of low-income communities, to access and use data directly. Many of these applications are quite straightforward, such as apps that show city buses' arrival times or street snowplowing in real time, but many are more complex. These include online tools that can help individuals use personal data that may not be easily accessible to them to improve their lives, such as when applying for public benefits, preparing their tax returns, or developing new job skills. For example, expunge.io, a Code for America app built as a collaboration with the Mikva Juvenile Justice Council in Chicago, assists people who were arrested when they were under 18 to determine whether they are eligible to have the records erased (expunged), access their records, and help them apply for the process.

---

15 Many relevant stories can be found on the NNIP website, www.neighborhoodindicators.org.

Amias Gerety and Sophie Raseman's essay introduces My Data, an emerging strategy that allows individuals to access and bring together the electronic records that institutions keep about them (e.g., the records of doctors, schools, employers, utility companies) and use the data themselves for a variety of purposes (such as credibly verifying their situations to third parties such as mortgage lenders or prospective employers). They also discuss "Smart Disclosure," the release of multiple data sets that allow developers to build applications that, for example, help individuals to compare potential college choices, taking into account interest, cost, and likely return.

Supporting Neighborhood Research: More and better use of data in research is essential to the future of low-income communities. City neighborhoods are varied and complex. Thus far, we have little capacity to predict how they will change, or to understand the interaction of forces that produce change and the implications of the changes that do occur. Recent work by Claudia Coulton has documented advances in neighborhood research and trends in work around key questions that remain unanswered.[16] A better understanding of the dynamics of neighborhood change will benefit all institutions engaged in community improvement. And better data will enhance that research.

CHALLENGES—WHAT IS HOLDING US BACK?

The last 25 years have seen impressive advances in the capacity to use data to improve conditions in low-income communities. But much remains to be done before these communities can fully take advantage of this potential. To realize this potential, we must overcome challenges in the availability of good data, tackle privacy and confidentiality issues, and improve our ability to use the data. We also must implement today's best practices in many more places. We urge you to keep these challenges in mind as you read the remaining essays in this volume. The concluding essay in this volume will return to these themes and suggest ways for the field to move forward.

---

16 See Chapter 7 of *Strengthening Communities with Neighborhood Data*, by G. Thomas Kingsley, Claudia J. Coulton and Kathryn L. S. Pettit, (Washington, DC: Urban Institute Press, 2014)

The Availability of Relevant Data

Although progress is being made, we need forceful efforts to address five data-availability problems:

Access. Many relevant government data files are still not released to the public. Local data intermediaries (such as NNIP partners) have succeeded in convincing local agencies to share data broadly in several locales, and the open data movement has motivated sizable data releases online in many localities. Although this still represents a very small share of what should be released, the trend is in the right direction and accelerating. Although focused efforts to get more program managers to share their nonconfidential data externally are still needed, their willingness to do so appears to be expanding.

The challenge is different of course with systems that contain confidential information on individuals and households. The highest standards must be met to ensure that confidential information will not be released to the public. Even in these cases, however, some types of data (often summarized) are becoming more available for use in the public interest. The work discussed earlier on integrated data systems demonstrates that professionals are finding ways to use selected data in such systems for legitimate purposes while rigorously protecting the confidentiality of individual records.[17]

Another serious concern is where public data become proprietary; that is where governments either sell public files directly, or license the data to private firms who then charge often prohibitively high rates to would-be users. The public has already paid for the creation of the original data and should not have to pay a second time to access them. A strong national effort should be mounted to develop effective policy for these situations.

Quality and Timeliness. Many administrative records, especially at the local level, are still replete with errors. One of the most useful steps to reduce errors is to make the commitment to release files to the public. That commitment creates strong pressures on managers, and thereby staff, to improve (or create) strong quality control procedures. Ideally,

---

17 Also see Dennis P. Culhane et al., "Connecting the Dots: The Promise of integrated data systems for Policy Analysis and Systems Reform," *Intelligence for Social Policy* 1 (3) (2010): 1–9.

such procedures would include systematic feedback loops that: (1) share data collected by the line staff back with them, ideally embedded in a process that encourages them to understand data issues and improve day-to-day operations; and (2) make it easy for nongovernment users to share identified errors with the agencies that own the data and have the authority to correct the source files. Timeliness is also critical to the value of data. For some types of decisions, data that are a year old, or even a few weeks old, are useless. Fortunately, this is an area seeing rapid progress. We are moving toward a time when a considerable amount of administrative data will be available to users on a real-time basis. The essay by Patricia Bowie and Moira Inkelas explains how important this is, as does our discussion of Cleveland's property information system (NEO CANDO).

Usability. The open data movement has resulted in a growing number of raw administrative data sets released to the public over the web. Many are complex and can only be used directly by experts. More effort is needed by the originating agency or intermediaries to transform many of these data sets into more accessible sources for a wider range of community stakeholders. The HMDA visualization and query tools described earlier are excellent examples of more accessible data.

Fragmentation. Most administrative data sets released by cities are the products of individual agencies and, because of different standards and protocols, the data sets cannot be used together. Yet, as we have noted, some of the most valuable community applications require the joint use of data from different sources. Data intermediaries (such as the NNIP partners and those developing integrated data systems) have solved this problem at the local level by developing data-sharing agreements across agencies, excerpting relevant data from various files and integrating them to create consistently defined indicators for common geographies. The problem for the field at this point is that such integration is not yet underway in nearly enough places.

Topical Coverage. Administrative data sets are compiled for operational purposes. It is not surprising that they do not contain information on a number of topics that are important to understanding and addressing neighborhood change. Claudia Coulton's essay offers one example.

She points out that it is impossible to understand shifts in some key neighborhood conditions without data on residential mobility, but that these data are hardly ever available in neighborhood indicator systems. However, as more managers of social programs recognize the importance of data about mobility, some programs are considering collecting data on moves of program participants. Similarly, data on characteristics of neighborhood social networks are not available in administrative data sets. There is hope here too, however. It has been suggested that it may ultimately be possible to obtain information on such networks by creative analysis of data from Facebook and/or other social media sites.

However, some concepts important to neighborhoods may never be captured in administrative data sets. In these cases, priority should be given to studies (involving limited surveys, analyzed in conjunction with administrative data) that scientifically identify administrative indicators that serve as good "proxies" for the missing concepts. Where this does not work, surveys and qualitative research remain the only possibilities. Hopefully, expanding the coverage of administrative data into new areas and aggressively searching for proxies will provide information on more community topics we now know little about, freeing up resources for better-focused surveys and qualitative work on key topics still not covered.

Tackling Privacy and Confidentiality

Open, big, and linked data raise the stakes for privacy issues, as it becomes easier to combine sources to identify individuals. One challenge is disclosure practices and norms related to the collection and use of data. Whether sensors are installed in neighborhoods to track pedestrian traffic or health records are consolidated to improve health care delivery, people may question the monitoring and lack of advance notification. In another example, employers may use proprietary data compiled from numerous sources, such as credit agencies, online commerce websites, or social media, to determine eligibility for employment. The applicant may or may not have a chance to review this data or even know that the information is being used in the process.

The nonprofit sector also needs to be concerned with these issues. The sector can play a role in asking governments and private companies to be more transparent in how data are collected, shared, and used in decision-making, but nonprofits should also be concerned about improving their own practices. As we encourage service and community groups to collect and use data about their clients, more training in obtaining permissions and sharing confidential data responsibly will be needed.

Nevertheless, as the successful implementation of integrated data systems in a number of communities and contexts demonstrates, personally identifiable data can be shared in a way that simultaneously protects people's information and creates new understanding to benefit both the individual and the community. Advanced technology can assist in controlling permissions and structuring queries and in implementing analytic approaches like masking and synthetic data. The Data Quality Campaign has developed materials on communicating with the public on privacy issues related to education data, but more work is essential in all topic areas.[18]

Capacity to Use Data Productively

Although the barriers to making more relevant data accessible to community actors remain serious, the more formidable challenges lie in making productive use of data that are already available. We see a chain of reasons for these challenges. The underlying problem is that many of the institutions that work in low-income communities are not yet committed to regularly conducting the systematic management processes that create the demand for good data: situation analyses, policy analysis and planning, and performance management.

Why is that? One issue is the lack of education and training about data and practical approaches to using them for staff in community organizations. Another reason is the comparatively slow pace in the development of automated "decision-support" processes and tools. These aids could dramatically simplify the task of manipulating, structuring, and presenting the right data at the right time in any decision-making process. These tools also encourage the use of standardized data, which enhance effectiveness both across and within organizations.

---

18 Data Quality Campaign's materials on communicating about privacy issues to different types of stakeholders are available at http://www.dataqualitycampaign.org/action-issues/privacy-security-confidentiality/.

But even if the relevant practitioners were adequately trained and motivated to be strong advocates for more systematic and data-driven decision-making in their organizations, the pace would still be very slow. Assembling and applying data to the complex processes that make up a community would still be too much work for most practitioners to handle on their own. Practitioners' energies need to be focused on the already challenging work of community development. They should be responsible for improving their own internal data systems and using them more effectively. Although they will need to learn more about using data if they are going to move into a truly data-driven world, they will need help in the process. Therefore, perhaps the most important barrier is the lack of adequate institutional infrastructure to simplify the work of the front-line organizations in assembling and using data. New intermediary services are needed to help them build or transform their own internal information systems so they work with greater efficiency and are structured to support better decision-making. Intermediaries are also needed to help practitioners acquire and take advantage of data from other sources.

Many of the intermediaries should be local. NNIP partners, who consider their primary mission to be assembling local data and ensuring community institutions use the data, are good examples. But, as noted earlier, this type of organization does not yet exist in many places. Supporting infrastructure for data also needs to be strengthened substantially at the national level.

Notwithstanding these challenges, our overall conclusion about the state of the field is considerably more positive than negative. There is now substantial momentum behind expanding the availability of relevant data to help communities function better for the benefit of their residents. While lagging, efforts to develop tools and processes to help local practitioners put the data to productive use are accelerating as well. We are nearing an important inflection point. The coming decade could well see these new capacities spur fundamental changes in how America's communities function.

■ ■ ■

G. THOMAS KINGSLEY *is a senior fellow at the Urban Institute. His research specializes in housing, urban policy, and governance issues at the Urban Institute. He served for more than a decade as the Director of the Institute's Center for Public Finance and Housing. He has also directed the National Neighborhood Indicators Partnership—an initiative to further the development of advanced data systems for policy analysis and community building in U.S. cities. In recent years, his personal research has focused on neighborhood impacts of the foreclosure crisis, trends in concentrated poverty, and lessons from the HOPE VI program. He previously served as Director of the Rand Corporation's Housing and Urban Policy Program, and as Assistant Administrator of the New York City Housing and Development Administration. He has also taught on the faculties of the graduate urban planning programs at the University of California, Berkeley, and the University of Southern California.*

■ ■ ■

KATHRYN L.S. PETTIT *is a senior research associate in the Metropolitan Housing and Communities Policy Center at the Urban Institute, where her research focuses on measuring and understanding neighborhood change. She directs the National Neighborhood Indicators Partnership, a network of local organizations that collect, organize, and use neighborhood data to inform local advocacy and decision making. Pettit is a recognized expert on small-area data sources and the use of neighborhood data in research and practice. She has conducted research on a wide range of topics, including neighborhood redevelopment and federally assisted housing, and recently co-authored the book Strengthening Communities with Neighborhood Data.*

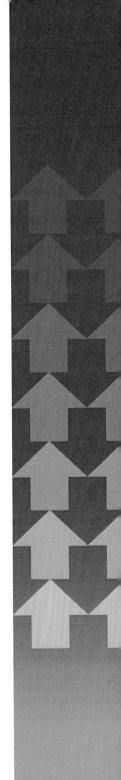

2

TRANSFORMING DATA INTO POLICY-RELEVANT INFORMATION

For the community indicators movement, finding the right measures to use to inform policy and action has been an ongoing effort. This essay looks at how the frameworks used to determine what measures matter—and more recently, who is allowed to take part in deciding what measures matter—influence public decision-making processes, and uses the Jacksonville Quality of Life Progress Report to illustrate how a citizen-driven indicators project can foster inclusive civic debate. It also explores the tensions between aligning indicator projects toward universal measures and encouraging continued local-level experimentation to respond to unique community conditions.

THE FUTURE OF COMMUNITY INDICATOR SYSTEMS

J. Benjamin Warner
Jacksonville Community Council Inc.

Historically, governance decisions have been informed by a range of data, from crop yields to military inventory to population size. As early communities shifted from hunter-gatherer to agrarian societies, the need for data and record-keeping often served as the impetus to create systems of writing, and the systematic use of data allowed for increased complexity in governance. The data practitioner can take pride in the notion that civilization is often built at least in part on measurement.

As our capacity to measure has increased, though, so have information clutter and difficulties in zeroing-in on what matters most for our decision-making processes. Community indicators projects serve a critical public purpose in distilling data into a prioritized set of measures that are chosen to shape action and policy responses.

In creating a community indicators project, participants select a set of data points that describe the well-being of their community. This set can range from a dozen to well over 100 measures that provide a snapshot of the state of the community. The process is repeated on a regular basis, generally annually, as the group reviews both the trend lines and the story the data tell about the community—where progress is being made and where the situation is worsening.

In the last three decades, the rapid development of community indicator systems has accelerated understanding of how to select and use data to generate community change. The creation of different frameworks, and the resulting dialogue from distinct perspectives, adds to the knowledge base as communities search for strong measures to inform policy and action. Two key, interrelated questions have emerged from the debate: Which measures matter, and—perhaps more importantly—who decides which measures matter?

WHAT TO MEASURE: FINDING THE "PERFECT" INDICATORS

That which gets measured has a significant impact on priority-setting, decision-making, and policy. Finding the right metrics has long been a staple of management textbooks and political campaigns. For the indicators movement, finding the right measures has been an ongoing effort. This effort begins with understanding the characteristics of indicators, a collection of data with qualities that distinguish them as more effective than other measures. A single measure outside of a framework is only a statistic. Good indicators are statistics with direction: data whose trend lines tell a story of movement and identify the distance between the actual and the desired. Great indicators add context and allow for projection of future outcomes; by examining anticipated trend lines, policy development and action can be implemented to bend the trend lines. Finding good indicators takes work, but many good indicators exist. Great indicators are much more difficult to hone in on. The community indicators movement is in search of great indicators.

For example, the infant mortality rate for Duval County, at nine per 1000 live births, is a statistic. Adapting that statistic to become a good indicator means situating it in a trend line that can tell a story—for instance, time series data can show that the infant mortality rate in Duval County declined by 25 percent in a four-year period. A great indicator goes beyond trend reporting to create priorities for community action. A great indicator may help identify that the racial disparity in infant mortality rates increased in the same time period, and that African American infants in Duval County are still more than twice as likely to die before their first birthday as white infants. Another approach might place the rate in context with state and national rates to identify whether the county faces geographically-based disparities. A third might look at smaller geographical subsets to identify "hotspots" of negative outcomes. Great indicators can thus highlight specific community needs and challenges, and can point to potential targets for intervention.

Great indicators are responsive to changes and have strong reliability and validity. They are clear in what they measure, filtering out extraneous factors to focus on the issue. They measure an important community condition and are able to be affected by public policy or community action. Moreover, they are powerful storytellers of the community, evoking a response among the public. They are compelling narrators of community conditions and are accessible to a broad range of actors. They anticipate community problems with enough time for action to create tangible outcomes. They spur change and respond with results.

The challenge with indicators is that they are, by nature, descriptive and not prescriptive. They describe what is, but not what needs to be done about what is or how to create what should be. The focus of every indicator project—their reason for existence—is to prompt policy change. Indicators are more than just data curiosities; they are intended to impact policy discussion and action. To be great, then, indicators must both describe a relevant aspect of the community and be linked within a framework that invites a policy response. The difference between interesting and inspiring data may be small, but it is a critical distinction.

WHAT TO MEASURE AND WHO DECIDES?

A common thread among different indicator projects is the desire to find the right measures to influence policy and action. Thousands of indicator sets have been created, and each one reflected a fundamental desire to identify the metrics that would shed light on an important issue and influence the decision-making process of the appropriate governance systems. The questions of what measures matter—and more recently, who is allowed to take part in deciding what measures matter—undergird the community indicators movement. As indicators effectively influence public policy, then those who select the indicators will find themselves with a stronger influence on public policy than those who do not. Indicator frameworks are often designed by people with vastly different community roles. For example, an activist and an academic will differ not only in the decisions they make, but also in their decision-making processes. These differences persist even as projects develop their own "indicator selection guidelines" to inform their decision making. Factors that influence who participates in measurement selection and what measures are selected include the following:

Geography

Some indicator systems take a neutral approach to geography: They measure key factors and report these factors for different geographies for convenience and comparison. The geographic unit does not motivate measure selection. It is not part of who decides what to measure or what is measured. For example, the Annie E. Casey Foundation's KIDS COUNT report is designed to measure the well-being of children, wherever they live in the United States.

Other indicator systems are actively focused on a geographic area (eg. state, metropolitan, or neighborhood level). In these systems, what matters is specific to a particular geography; in these instances, those who make the determination of what to measure are based within that geography, and are both aided by the strengths and constrained by limitations of extensive localized knowledge. The Jacksonville example discussed later falls into this category.

When geography is the driving force, the data system may include rich specificity in localized issues. The trade-off here is that comparing local indicators with other geographies, or placing local trends within the context of broader factors, may be difficult because the localized data may not exist at larger scales. On the other hand, national or global indicator sets may have less applicability to local issues and may be less useful for local decision-making processes.

Framework and Focus

The organizing framework selected often influences what indicators are measured. Since the 1990s, four frameworks have been generally used to determine what mattered most: quality-of-life, sustainability, healthy community, and government benchmarking. Quality-of-life projects described a broad array of issues in the external environment of a city. Sustainability initiatives began with an environmental emphasis, whereas healthy community projects began by looking at health and associated determinants. Government performance benchmarking efforts evaluated the effectiveness and efficiency of public efforts to improve the community.

In the first decade of the 2000s, a fifth framework, centered on subjective well-being, gained momentum. These initiatives focused measures on questions of happiness in a population and sought policy changes to improve public happiness. Noted examples are Bhutan's Gross National Happiness Index, the Organisation for Economic Cooperation and

Development's (OECD) Better Life Initiative, and the United Nations' (UN) World Happiness Report.

The framework of a system drives who is involved in the indicator selection. An indicator system operating from a sustainability framework may engage a number of environmentalists in determining the best measures to describe progress toward sustainability. Another system, developed in a healthy community framework, is more likely to include public health officials in making decisions about what is or is not measured. The same is true for those indicator reports with a focus on economic development, or those framed around social responsibility or racial disparities—the framework influences (and is influenced by) those who share common values.

A primary implication of setting the framework is that indicators that don't align well with the chosen framework may be excluded. In restricting the indicator set's scope, the potential for the indicators to point to innovative or cross-sectoral solutions to issues may be limited. In short, the power of the indicators to illuminate the state of the community and influence changes in programs or policy may be curtailed precisely because the intended policies can be hard-wired into the indicator selection process, leaving little room for unanticipated learning.

Additionally, a strong framework focus can lead to the inclusion of suboptimal indicators to capture particular aspects of a hard-to-measure issue. For example, if the framework suggests that vibrancy in cultural arts is an essential desired quality for the community, but the community lacks effective ways to measure cultural vibrancy, substitute indicators such as "museum attendance" may be shoehorned into the indicator set to plug a perceived hole in the measurement system. This can occur even when the identified indicator is seen as merely a weak approximation of the desired aspect of community life.

Rigor Versus Relevance

Many initiatives often identify indicators in a process tensioned between the ideal and the available, the possible and the practical. In the 1980s, the community indicators movement began by engaging local residents to self-determine the measurements that matter for progress. For initiatives in which decisions are made by citizens, the selection process is generally influenced by a desire for familiar, simple, easily-understood measures. By contrast, academic research in data for improved decision making often points to measures with greater rigor, which may also have increased complexity.

As a result, community-based decisions about what to measure can frustrate a researcher—one famously referred to community indicators as a "folk movement" and argued for increased scientific rigor in their methodologies. The metrics may be seen as too simplistic, or too limited, to answer questions of policy importance, and may not lend themselves to robust policy analysis. Conversely, decisions made by researchers may produce results that are too far removed from the lived experiences of residents, isolating them both from the information presented and the opportunities for policy action. For example, using the Gini coefficient rather than poverty rates has implications for how inequality is understood in a community; the former provides more information but is less accessible to the layperson, whereas the latter has numerous flaws in construction but has the advantage of familiarity.

Many projects have attempted to simplify the complex by using indices, which have the advantage of associating a single number to a concept and allowing a general trend to be understood as easily as a letter grade on a report card. However, as on a report card, a single grade may not provide sufficient information on what specific policy areas need to be addressed—merely that overall performance is unsatisfactory. Unpacking an index into its component parts, on the other hand, may create policy focused on just one piece of a larger puzzle without regard to the interdependencies among multiple factors influencing outcomes.

Politics and Power

Some indicator projects are designed to justify a course of action more than to identify one. The use of data for marketing or advocacy is not a new concept; data a chamber of commerce uses to promote a city is different from the data selected to advocate for unmet social needs in the community. Political pressures to promote the positive and downplay the negative can make public reporting of some information difficult.

The political implications of data reporting can thus shape data selection. If the decisions on what to measure are made by someone attempting to create or preserve a political legacy, the indicators selected may be different from those that might be chosen by someone with a different or competing agenda. This distinction often plays out in national political debates on the state of the economy. For example, the party in power tends to emphasize measures that show positive economic movement, whereas the opposing party emphasizes measures of misery—and the choices of which indicators to measure change with the political tides.

In addition, the availability or quality of information provided can be affected if the data appear to challenge or threaten the institutions responsible for gathering and providing the information. If those in power do not like what the data shows, they might adjust definitional frameworks, limit funding for data collection, restrict access to data, or replace the measures entirely. Data that support institutional values may result in an increased use of that data, even if better data could be made available.

At times, the indicators selected for reporting may reinforce an existing course of action—sometimes referred to as decision-driven data-making. On the other hand, if those with the political power to make policy changes are not involved in the selection of indicators, they may be less inclined to use the data in their decision-making process.

In summary, indicator systems are not neutral collections of statistics. They are shaped by the interests and values of the people and institutions included in making decisions about data selection. This has profound implications both for the utility of these systems for influencing community action and for the inclusion of community in the decision-making process.

CASE STUDY: JACKSONVILLE, FLORIDA

Jacksonville, Florida, has the nation's oldest and longest-running community-based indicator system, the "Quality of Life Progress Report." This project began in 1985 with a group of 94 citizen volunteers attempting to define and measure the quality of life of the

Public high school graduation rate (federal calculation)
Snap recipients per 1,000 people
Percentage of households paying 30 percent or more of their income for housing
Percentage of tributary streams meeting dissolved oxygen standards
Senior suicide rate per 100,000 population
Average police-call response times
Percentage of people without health insurance
Percentage who feel they can influence local government
Daily vehicle miles traveled per person
Serious bicycle accidents per 100,000 people
Total index crime rate
Percentage of vacant housing units

Figure 1. Examples of indicators from the Jacksonville Community Council, Inc. Quality of Life Progress Report.

community, creating an initial indicator set of 83 measures covering topics including the economy, public safety, health, education, natural environment, mobility, government/political environment, social environment, and the cultural/recreational environment. (Figure 1)

The project was motivated by a strong desire for community improvement and began with the assumption that the factors that would be important to community well-being and amenable to improvement through policy or program changes are both measurable and accessible in the external community environment. The committee recognized from the beginning that they could not accurately measure some aspects of community life, owing to existing data limitations. Over time, some (but not all) of these limitations have been addressed; for example, the project has expanded to allow for measurement of how poverty affects access to health care, but it still lacks an adequate measure for religious harmony and cooperation.

At the project's outset, the committee made key decisions that have continued to influence how indicators are selected, maintained, and used:

- The indicators would be selected by citizens in the community, as informed by experts. Every year since 1985, the indicator set has been reviewed by a citizen's committee. This process has directly resulted in improving the usability of the data in to the community. For instance, terms such as "per capita" were changed to "per person" because, as one committee member explained, "If you mean 'per person,' just say so. Don't make it harder for people to understand what you're talking about." Measures such "age-adjusted death rate" or "years of potential life lost" were rejected because they were too technical and took too much effort to explain to laypeople.

- The project was designed to measure Jacksonville's progress over time, and not to compare Jacksonville's progress with other cities. Although regional-, state-, and national-level data are provided for basic context-setting, the focus is on internal progress and change. This means that the project is influenced more by internal trends and needs rather than efforts to find common measures that enable cross-jurisdictional comparison. This has both decreased the capacity for strong comparative data and increased the opportunity for creative, local-specific measures.

- The data set from the first report was explicitly designed to be open to adaptation. In its annual review, both the quality and effectiveness of each of the indicators are up for discussion, and revisions are made quickly as better data become available. For example, in the first report, the data underlying several mobility indicators were generated by having volunteers drive fixed routes and time themselves, and then averaging the results the volunteers obtained to determine changes in commuting times from year to year. As better data have become available, other methods for calculating commuting times have been used.

- The project continues to be shepherded by the Jacksonville Community Council, Inc., an independent, nonpartisan, nonprofit organization. The project has remained outside of the political process, enabling it to survive through multiple changes in local political administrations. The trade-off for independence and sustainability, however, has meant that the project has never been a core initiative of any one political leader, a situation that requires a constant effort to educate and encourage elected officials to embrace and use the data.

- The audience for the project was defined broadly from the beginning to include neighborhood activists, human services planners, media, politicians, students, grant writers, and philanthropists. We recognized that no single presentation format could meet the needs of this wide variety of intended audiences, so we offer multiple presentation options for the indicators, from simple one-page briefings and brochures to more complex, deeper reports, as well as an interactive web-based mapping system.

- The intent of the project was to spur action, not just report trends. In its annual review prior to publication, a citizen's committee assigns "gold stars" to the trend lines moving in a positive direction and "red flags" to trend lines indicating trouble. In any given year, the organization uses one or more of the red flags to mobilize the community for action through a shared learning, engagement, and advocacy process. Meanwhile, organizations that are contributing to positive change are highlighted annually, reinforcing a shared community responsibility for improving the trend lines.

RECENT DEVELOPMENTS

A shared language about measurement is evolving out of two key collaborations among organizations working to improve understanding of measurement systems and their community impact.

Community Indicators Consortium: In 2003, the International Society for Quality of Life Studies sponsored a conference on community indicators, leading practitioners and researchers from various backgrounds, using different frameworks, to recognize the need for a multidisciplinary conversation to advance the science and practice of community indicators. In 2004, organizations and individuals from sustainability, healthy community, quality-of-life, government benchmark, and other perspectives met to create cross-fertilization of ideas and find synergies across efforts. The result was the creation of the Community Indicators Consortium, which continues to sponsor conferences, webinars, training, and research on best practices for community-based measurement and impact.

The Consortium developed a descriptive model on integrating community indicators with government performance measures that encouraged these government benchmarking initiatives to communicate more fully with other frameworks. Government benchmarking initiatives tend to examine internal government processes and practices to determine their effectiveness, whereas community indicators frameworks tend to focus on community outcomes to gauge the success of existing policies. Integrating the two approaches may result in greater effectiveness in community improvement than using a single framework alone.

The Consortium has brought open data and big data proponents into dialogue with community indicator developers to build common understanding of the possibilities and pitfalls of increasing data accessibility and to share lessons learned from community data systems as new actors launch data advocacy efforts. In the process, increased blending among sustainability, healthy community, and quality-of-life frameworks have resulted, as the interconnectivity of metrics has been explored.

Beyond GDP: The limitations of using gross domestic product (GDP) as a sole measure for societal progress has been recognized for decades. Robert Kennedy in 1968 famously said that it "measures everything in short, except that which makes life worthwhile." Building on the many initiatives that have tried to find better measures of well-being that include economic progress as well as societal well-being and environmental sustainability, the Beyond GDP movement started to coalesce in 2007 at the Beyond GDP Conference at the European Parliament.

In 2008, French President Nicolas Sarkozy put together a commission led by economists Joseph Stiglitz, Amartya Sen, and Jean-Paul Fitoussi. The report that resulted continued to drive the debate forward on how to build a new global measure of progress, and initiatives in the OECD and the UN are well underway to find a workable global answer.

In this area, local community indicators systems are serving as laboratories for implementing measures of progress that allow for great creativity and flexibility. As research in understanding new measures of happiness, or internal well-being, continues on the global front, local communities are discovering how to integrate these measures and create new indicator frameworks. The opportunity to share information, from global research to local application and back again, can strengthen both local initiatives and international debate.

CHALLENGES FOR THE FIELD

From inception, the greatest strength of the community indicators movement was perhaps the ability to hyper-localize measures of community well-being. Many early community indicator projects were driven by a desire to democratize data–to make information more available to the general public. The projects were undergirded by the belief that better decision making, public accountability, and community dialogue would result if everyone in the community had access to the same information. Since then, much has changed. The primary challenge today is not making data available to the public. More information is available on the cell phone of the average resident of a community than any organization could hope to publish in the 1980s. The new challenge is sifting through the incredible complexity of available data to discover what is meaningful and what is powerful— the data that shed light on community conditions and inspire action toward improvement.

In addition, the movement has greater information about which indicators have been more effective at creating change than others. There is an increasing demand for standardization of metrics and the creation of a national index of well-being, such as those other countries have developed. This creates a natural (and healthy) tension between local creativity and experimentation in indicators development and national and global accumulation of expertise in effective measurement systems. This also directly impacts the question of who determines what success looks like in communities, and who is involved in selecting the measures to define, report, and hold the community accountable for reaching that success.

The push to create a common index also highlights a tension between the desire for simple measures that aggregate myriad data and the need for granular data that can more accurately reflect complex aspects of communal life. The challenge for the community indicators movement is to advocate for the usability of indicators to create collective impact and influence change, which requires (in most cases) a disaggregation of data to focus public priorities. Greater data availability will allow for more disaggregation across dimensions such as poverty, race and ethnicity, gender, age, and small-scale geography to allow the community to be more precise in targeted interventions and measurement of results. Community indicators at the core are designed to be more than description—they need to compel action.

The likely short-term future for the community indicators movement is increasing diversity of local measurements informed by national and international debates about indicator systems and frameworks. The growth in data literacy, facilitated by easier-to-use tools and clearer data visualization opportunities, allows for local data choices to respond to national and global research about data effectiveness, reliability, and clarity. At the same time, because more people are familiar with and use data in their own organizational decision making, the opportunities for creative data creation strategies are outpacing capacity to analyze effectiveness of these data solutions. In short, more is countable, and more of what is countable can be used to answer local questions about community progress.

A movement that began somewhat idealistically with hope for democratizing data is now focused on the how to use this shared data in public decision making, and increasingly understanding the linkages among sharing information and sharing decision-making power. Once upon a time, the thought was simply that information is power; today, it is perhaps more accurate to say that information, along with the tools to use that information, creates powerful opportunities for change. Indicators, in other words, are a necessary but insufficient portion of a community change model. A primary challenge for the movement is to become intentional about how the indicators fit into a theory of change and create measurable action. Projects that are only reporting information risk irrelevancy if they do not build the collaborative partnerships necessary to ensure targeted use of the data.

The movement is beginning to explore the strengths and challenges of bringing together aspects from different measurement frameworks, and is wrestling with the coordination and tradeoffs that this effort requires. Increased transparency and trust among organizations is needed to work toward a shared vision of community improvement that builds on the values of the community. Integrating subjective and objective measures, as well as externalized community aspects with internal satisfaction measures, are already beginning to happen. A key question that should be at the forefront of these discussions is: How will these measures be used to influence policy?

Over the last 30 years, the community indicators movement has become more widespread and more effective at identifying indicators that are broadly accessible to the public and useful for generating positive change. The next step for the movement is to evaluate and endorse higher-quality indicators that have greater efficacy while encouraging continued local-level experimentation with new measures that will continue to expand the knowledge base of the field.

FOR FURTHER READING

Council of Europe, "Involving Citizens and Communities in Securing Societal Progress for the Well-Being of All: Methodological Guide" (Strasbourg, France: Council of Europe Publishing, 2011).

Jon Hall and Lousie Rickard, "People, Progress and Participation: How Initiatives Measuring Social Progress Yield Benefits Beyond Better Metrics" (Berlin, Germany: Bertlesmann-Siftung Foundation, 2013).

David Swain and Danielle Hollar, "Measuring Progress: Community Indicators and the Quality of Life," *International Journal of Public Administration*, 26 (7) (2003): 789–814

Milan Dluhy and Nicholas Swartz, "Connecting Knowledge and Policy: The Promise of Community Indicators in the United States," *Social Indicators Research*, 79 (1) (2006): 1–23.

J. Benjamin Warner, "The Jacksonville, Florida Experience." In *Community Quality-of-Life Indicators: Best Cases II*, edited by Don Rahtz, David Swain, and M. Joseph Sirgy (Dordrecht, Netherlands: Springer, 2006).

■ ■ ■

BEN WARNER *is the president & CEO of Jacksonville Community Council Inc. (JCCI). He was inaugural president of the international Community Indicators Consortium and a past president of the National Association of Planning Councils (NAPC), receiving from NAPC their Distinguished Service Award. He has consulted on the development of numerous indicators initiatives around the world.*

The County Health Rankings & Roadmaps is a program dedicated to helping communities become healthier places to live, learn, work, and play. Annually, U.S. counties are ranked within each state according to a model where health outcomes are influenced by health behaviors, social and economic factors, clinical care, and the physical environment. The Rankings are constructed and presented in a way to spark action towards improving community health. This essay discusses key decision points, the allures and perils of ranking, and lessons learned from this collaborative effort by the Robert Wood Johnson Foundation and the University of Wisconsin Population Health Institute.

THE COUNTY HEALTH RANKINGS: "A TREASURE TROVE OF DATA"

Bridget Catlin

University of Wisconsin, Madison

Helping communities become healthier places to live, learn, work, and play means attending to many interrelated factors. These include health factors such as access to clinical care and improvements in healthy behaviors, such as diet and exercise, but also social and economic factors, such as neighborhood safety, employment, housing, and transit. By monitoring these factors, we can identify avenues to create and implement evidence-informed policies and programs that improve community well-being and health.

The County Health Rankings, a collaboration between the Robert Wood Johnson Foundation and the University of Wisconsin Population Health Institute (UWPHI), aim to do just this. The rankings are unique in their ability to measure the overall health of each county in all 50 states on the multiple factors that influence health. The rankings provide communities with insights on a variety of factors that affect health, such as high school graduation rates, access to healthy foods, air pollution levels, income, and rates of smoking, obesity, and teen births. The model underlying the rankings underscores that much of what affects health occurs outside of the doctor's office, and stresses that factors such as education, employment, income, the environment play critical roles in determining health and life expectancy.

The goal of the rankings is to help stakeholders understand the many influences on health and vitality and inspire community-level change. My colleagues and I at UWPHI determine the rankings using measures from several publicly available, national data sources. We standardize and combine the measures leading to two overall rankings:

1 Health outcomes: how healthy a county is now.

2 Health factors: how healthy a county will be in the future.

In this essay, I discuss the key lessons we've learned during the past decade about how to effectively design, display, and use rankings to mobilize data-driven action to address the multiple determinants of health.

BACKGROUND

The County Health Rankings has its origins in America's Health Rankings, which since 1990 have ranked states on health indicators. Curious about why their state's rankings rose and fell over time, researchers Paul Peppard, David Kindig, and Patrick Remington at UWPHI wondered if health, like politics, is local. They delved into measuring the health of Wisconsin's counties and released the first Wisconsin County Health Rankings in 2003. During the next few years, leaders in other states became interested in using UWPHI's approach, and in 2009, with funding from Robert Wood Johnson Foundation (RWJF), we began our work to expand the rankings to other states. The following year, RWJF and UWPHI released the first national County Health Rankings, which led to widespread media coverage. Wanting to help communities move from data to action, a year after the initial release of the rankings, RWJF funded a series of activities known as Roadmaps to Health to help communities use the data from the rankings and engage stakeholders from multiple sectors in setting priorities and implementing strategies to improve health.

The 2014 rankings are based on 34 measures, with an additional 40 measures reported to provide context. Combined with the underlying data supporting the current rankings and all the data from prior years, this "treasure trove of data"[1] now contains more than 1 million data points. This data, along with detailed documentation about calculation methods, are easily accessible and downloadable at www.countyhealthrankings.org. RWJF and UWPHI plan to produce rankings for at least four more years.

---

1 M. Beck, "How Healthy Is Your County? A New Data Trove Can Tell You" (*Wall Street Journal*, April 3, 2012, available at http://blogs.wsj.com/health/2012/04/03/ how-healthy-is-your-county-a-new-data-trove-can-tell-you/?mod=WSJBlog.

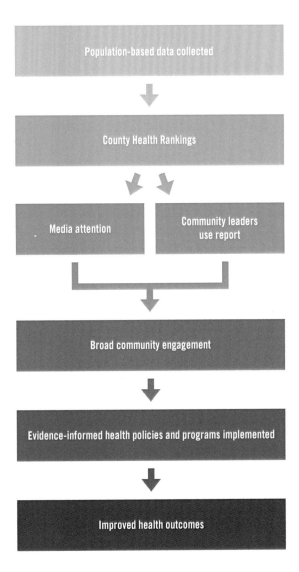

Figure 1. The County Health Rankings Logic Model. The Rankings provide a starting point for change in communities.

Why has RWJF committed to producing annual rankings of the health of every county in the nation? The rankings support RWJF's goal to build a culture of health by raising awareness of the multiple factors that influence health and stimulating and supporting local action to improve health by addressing these factors (Figure 1).

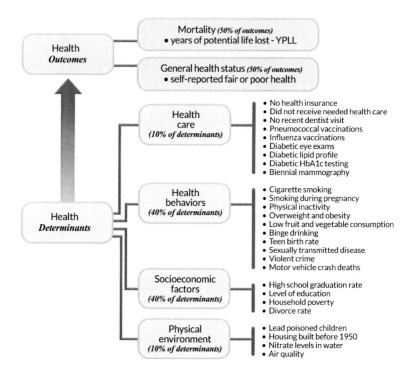

Figure 2a. 2005 County Health Rankings model

DESIGNING THE COUNTY HEALTH RANKINGS MODEL

The UWPHI team determined that to best educate lay users about how the rankings capture population health, a graphic model was needed to clearly depict both the types of measures included and how they are calculated. The design has evolved over time. Figure 2a shows an earlier version depicting health outcomes and health determinants, and Figure 2b shows the latest version. The design of the model has evolved over time to help emphasize the role that factors such as education, jobs, income, and environment play in how healthy people are and how long they live. One notable change was in terminology, from using the term *health determinants* to *health factors* to make it more intuitively understandable. The newer model also conveys that policies and programs fundamentally influence a variety of health factors, which in turn shape community health outcomes.

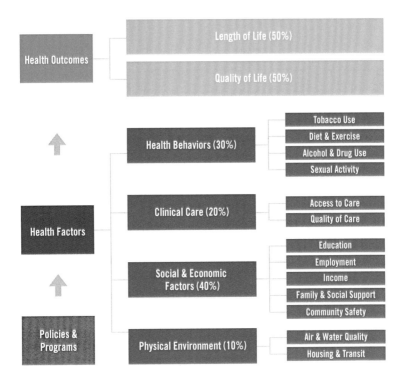

Figure 2b. 2014 County Health Rankings model

The right sides of both models delineate health outcomes and health factors. But the newer model moves away from listing specific measures and, instead, combines the individual factors under broader headings (e.g., diet and exercise now encompass physical inactivity and fruit and vegetable consumption, etc.). This allows the model to remain relatively consistent from year to year even while improvements are made to the underlying measures. Another distinction is the new color scheme. Throughout the County Health Rankings website, health outcomes (frequently described as "today's health") are depicted in green and health factors (referred to "tomorrow's health") are depicted in blue. Such design changes may seem minor but can be important in improving communication about a complicated set of measures.

The adage "a picture is worth thousand words" rings true for the County Health Rankings model. The model does double duty by both providing a high-level overview of how the rankings are constructed and by illustrating that many community factors contribute to health outcomes. For this reason, UWPHI makes this image available for download with no restrictions on its use, other than citing the source.

ALLURE AND PERILS OF RANKINGS

A ranking is appealing because it simplifies complex data into an easily understood measure. Because it is headline-grabbing—and appeals to people's competitive nature and desire to do better—a ranking can generate attention toward specific issues and prompt action by community leaders, politicians, funders, and community residents.

But the simplification comes with a cost—the loss of information. This can mean that the true differences in health standings between counties can be hard to gauge. For example, the top-ranked county may be significantly healthier than the county ranked second, whereas the county ranked second could be barely different from the county ranked third. The County Health Rankings tries to overcome this issue by assigning each county to one of four quartiles, communicating that differences among counties in the same quartile are generally less important than differences between the four main clusters of counties. (There are of course exceptions, as counties at the very bottom of a quartile may be similar to those at the very top of the next.)

Because the rankings cannot, by design, tell the complete story, people are encouraged to use the rankings as a starting point only. Rankings, for example, are relative, not absolute, and are thus not necessarily a reliable way to measure progress. A county's ranking reflects not only its own performance, but also that of every other county in a state relative to it. If one county's health improves at the same rate as every other county in the state, its rank will stay the same, masking the real progress the county is making. In addition, place-based rankings can be unstable for areas with smaller populations, meaning that some variation in ranking from year to year can be anticipated due to the lower reliability of estimates when numbers are small. In 2014, the team added a new tool to help communities measure progress using specific metrics, such as those on which the rankings are based, or measures from other data sources that better lend themselves to tracking over time.[2]

Another potential danger of rankings is that those counties that rank highly within their state may not feel the imperative to improve. To offset possible complacency, for most measures the tool reports the value of "Top Performers," the point at which only 10 percent of counties in the nation are performing at or above. Few counties are at or above this value across all measures, so this helps communities realize that even highly ranked counties have room to improve.

On the flip side, counties ranked low can feel like "losers." Our experience in Wisconsin showed that a common first reaction to low rankings is a mix of denial and anger. We've seen leaders in public health and health care sectors question the veracity of the data or feel that they were being blamed for things beyond their control. However, when provided with an explanation about the source of the data and engaged in a discussion about the many factors and stakeholders contributing to health, many community leaders reframe the results as a call to action.

Another peril is that rankings can perpetuate existing problems if decision makers choose to reward the best performers and penalize the worst. One of the challenges of producing any reporting system is that people will use data to suit a variety of purposes. We urge decision makers to use data from the county rankings to help allot resources to needier places and to recognize that improvements in health can come by investing resources in a variety of settings (i.e., not only in health care).

CONSTRUCTING RANKINGS

There is no one right way to either choose measures or combine them into a set of rankings, and we had to make several key decisions in constructing the rankings. First, we decided to rank counties within states rather than ranking all U.S. counties against one another. Because we want to spark local action, it is far more helpful for a county to see its ranking within its state than be ranked as one among 3,143 counties

---

2   The Measuring Progress tool is available at available at http://www.countyhealthrankings.org/measuring-progress.

in the nation. In addition, some measures are context-dependent and not comparable across state borders, making ranking among states ill-advised.

Second, we determined which measures to include in the rankings and how to weight them.[3] We first looked for measures that are valid and reliable, available at the county-level, preferably updated annually, and available at no or low cost. The five measures used to construct the health outcomes rankings (premature death, poor or fair health, physically and mentally unhealthy days, and low birth weight) are based on the most current data available that can be used to characterize the overall health of counties. Because we wanted the rankings to prompt policy and behavior change, an additional criterion is that the measures of health factors must be actionable. Although genetics clearly influence health, there is no policy change that can affect genetics. Therefore, there is nothing in the rankings reflecting this factor.

Our final guiding principle for selecting measure was that less is more. One of the purposes of the County Health Rankings is to engage people who do not traditionally consider themselves public health (or data) experts. We've learned from experience that too much data can be off-putting and confusing for users.

After the first year we had to decide to either leave the measures unchanged or encourage communities to explore new or additional factors. Leaving the metrics unchanged allows users to compile and track trends. However, allowing changes can offer new insights to communities when new or improved measures become available. The UWPHI team settled on a strategy of keeping the same measures for health outcomes but revising those for health factors as we identified better measures. We likened this decision to the educational metric of a grade point average, which provides a standard, overall metric

---

3 The process of establishing weights for each component of the model was guided by historical perspective, a review of the literature on the effect of various factors on health outcomes, weights used by other rankings, our own analysis, and pragmatic issues involving communications and stakeholder engagement. See Bridget Booske et al., "Different Perspectives for Assigning Weights to Determinants of Health." Working paper. (University of Wisconsin, Population Health Institute, 2010), available at www.countyhealthrankings.org/sites/default/files/differentPerspectivesForAssigningWeightsToDeterminantsOfHealth.pdf.

but—in doing so—can be based on grades from previous, current, and future courses.

Finally, we had to decide how often to update the rankings. We ultimately decided to update the rankings annually even though some of the measures do not change significantly from year to year. Our rationale is that producing data on a regular basis facilitates widespread media attention and enables more people to hear the call to action each year.

On the whole, we attempt to make our decisions as transparent as possible and encourage discussion of the issues underlying our process. In this way, users will understand not only their rankings but also the underlying data and methods. However, we must continually balance the need for simplicity with the need for detailed explanation.

VISUALIZING RANKINGS AND UNDERLYING DATA

Visualization tools help users with different levels of data skills find meaning in the data. The visualization approach used in the County Health Rankings builds on the organizational structure in Figure 2b. The County Health Rankings website relies heavily on tabular display of data. In many of the tables, users can sort data in different ways, and most tables are layered so users can delve deeper than the initial overview data display. A pull-down menu allows users to access data from prior years. Not surprisingly, fewer visits are made to the more detailed data pages on the website, but all the details and associated documentation are available for those who are interested.

Even with the layered structure, more than 70 measures for all 3,100 counties can quickly become overwhelming. Charts and maps help make the data more accessible. Graphs are useful for highlighting trends for individual measures. An interactive map draws users into the data. Maps add context well beyond what a data table provides. See, for example, the two maps in Figure 3. The health outcomes map (green) shows the location of the healthiest and least healthy Alabama counties in 2014, with the counties divided into quartiles, and a similar map (blue) shows where the counties are based on the factors that influence health. These maps show the strong association between health outcomes and the factors that determine health (lighter colored counties

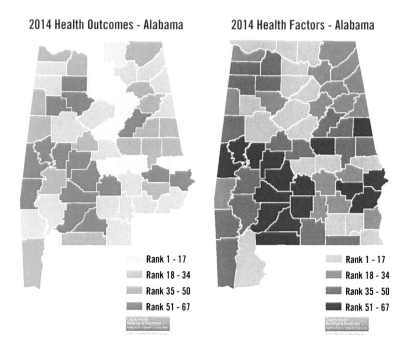

2014 Health Outcomes - Alabama

2014 Health Factors - Alabama

Rank 1 - 17
Rank 18 - 34
Rank 35 - 50
Rank 51 - 67

Rank 1 - 17
Rank 18 - 34
Rank 35 - 50
Rank 51 - 67

Figure 3. Maps from County Health Rankings, 2014. Maps help illustrate the relationship between health factors and health outcomes.

are the healthiest in terms of both outcomes and factors). In addition, the maps show that place matters, even in states known to be less healthy than others.

RWJF has also created add-ons, such as a Facebook application (Figure 4), that can organize data in a more visually appealing manner.

We have also wrestled with the question of how extensively we should use design elements to help users draw inferences from the data versus letting users themselves interpret the rankings data and identify concerns. We strike a balance by providing a guide that walks users through the data and features and that provides suggestions for how to interpret the data. In addition, users can turn on the "Areas to Explore" feature. This feature highlights the measures in a particular county that are significantly different from state or national averages.

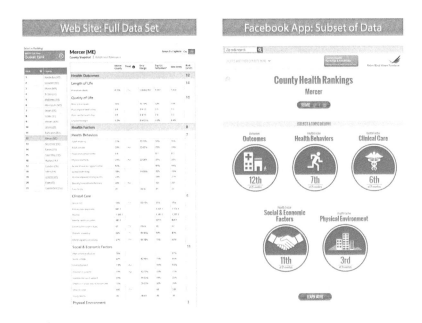

Figure 4. Alternative Data Visualization Efforts. The rankings and underlying data are available in multiple formats to help users with varying technical skills access and share information.

COMMUNICATIONS

As we expanded our efforts to all counties in all states, RWJF helped us think through our goals and develop a strategic communications plan to get our messages into the media. With the assistance of RWJF, its communications team, and County Health Rankings contacts in each state, we develop targeted press releases each year, including national, state, and local releases in some states. Because counties are ranked within states and not on a national basis, the County Health Rankings are best suited for state and local coverage, but national media outlets often press us to compare counties across states to create a national ranking of counties. Although not doing so has cost us some national coverage, the strength of state and local coverage makes up for it. We have also learned that, however creatively we display data visually, we must discuss our data in a clear and compelling manner. We work closely with communications experts to develop messages for different audiences, focusing particularly on nontechnical audiences.

This sometimes requires less focus on scientific precision and more on accessibility and comprehension.

MOVING FROM AWARENESS TO ACTION

Data alone do not spark action to improve community health. People need help determining their next steps and often want access to customized help. To respond to these needs, RWJF added the Roadmaps to Health in 2011. The roadmaps help users identify actions that can improve health. The Roadmaps to Health Action Center provides guidance and tools to support community health improvement. Users can access detailed guides that correspond to each of the steps in the outer circle of Figure 5 and information about specific steps that the entities identified in the middle of the circle can take.

Furthermore, because action to improve our nation's health cannot be automated, the Action Center is staffed by full-time community coaches who provide guidance via e-mail or phone, in addition to in-person visits to communities that have indicated a readiness to collaborate in improving community health. The coaches work with individuals and teams in communities that are at various stages in their journey toward improved health. Coaches also teach community members how to use the rankings to raise awareness of the multiple factors that influence health, identify areas for improvement, and demonstrate how to investigate other data sources for a more detailed understanding of problems within their communities. Then, coaches engage with community members to select priority areas (based on data and other considerations), choose evidence-informed policies and programs, implement these strategies, and evaluate the success of their efforts.

Communities large and small are working to make their citizens healthier, increasingly focusing their efforts on the social and economic determinants of health. For example, the first release of the County Health Rankings in 2010 prompted rural Mason County, Washington, to focus on improving education pathways for its young people. "Mason Matters" and its partners are implementing career and college-readiness programs targeted to youth in Grade 4–8.

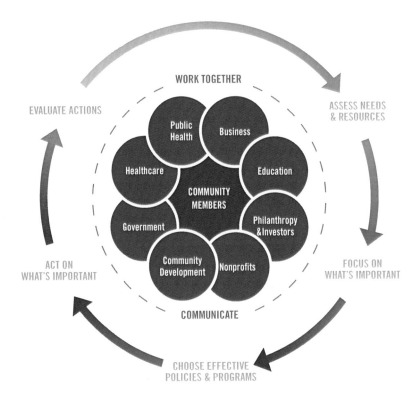

Figure 5. Roadmaps to Health Take Action Cycle. Roadmaps offers guides and coaching for each of the players who can engage in taking action to make communities healthier.

Roadmaps has also included grants to coalitions working to improve the health of people in their communities; grants to national organizations that are mobilizing local leaders and affiliates; and the RWJF Culture of Health Prize, a program to recognize communities whose promising efforts will likely lead to better health. Organizations such as United Way Worldwide and the National Association of Counties are using the rankings to inform their work.

Starting with data but now focusing on action, the County Health Rankings and Roadmaps program is helping communities create new pathways to better health. Representatives from local schools, churches, law enforcement, business, hospitals, government, nonprofit organizations, and ordinary citizens are coming together to improve health and develop innovative approaches to reduce smoking, expand access to healthy foods, increase high school graduation, develop more bike- and pedestrian-friendly neighborhoods, and much more.

LESSONS LEARNED

Our work has taught us several key lessons. First and foremost, keen attention to communications and visualization strategies is required to effectively transform data into usable information. Many data analysts are not attuned to strategic communications planning, but this process was pivotal in helping us articulate what we wanted to accomplish through the ranking, and how to reach and motivate key audiences toward action. In addition, we learned a data tool is not a "Field of Dreams"—even if you build it, users will not automatically come. A compelling "hook" is essential to draw in users. In our case, the hook is rankings; other hooks may be appropriate in other situations.

A layered approach that allows users to choose the level of detail that best suits their needs is also critical for enabling users to navigate the data. Clear and accurate documentation is also important; users want and need to know the source of the data and how the data were collected, as well as more detailed information about time frames, sample sizes, and other details. We strive to help all our users—whether advocates, policymakers, or practitioners—unpack the rankings by offering the underlying data, additional tools, and guidance needed to move from data to action.

Additionally, the perfect must not be the enemy of the good; no perfect measures of health or its determinants exist. Instead, we strive to report the highest-quality data that we can obtain while acknowledging and reporting the limitations of our data.

Finally, compiling and presenting data in interesting ways are still insufficient to generate action; effective dissemination and customer service are essential. Developing appropriate messages and engaging the media (broadcast, print, online, social, etc.) are key components of a successful strategic communications plan. It is also important to prioritize responsiveness to media requests.

Going forward, a new Scientific Advisory Group of national experts representing key stakeholders will help guide the work over the next four years. One area for further exploration will be helping communities drill down from county-level data to more local data about neighborhoods and different subgroups of the population to identify and address disparities within counties. Ongoing improvements to the website and to the Roadmaps to Health program will ensure that communities can effectively translate available data into evidence-informed strategies to improve health and well-being.

■ ■ ■

BRIDGET CATLIN *directs the Mobilizing Action Toward Community Health (MATCH) group in the University of Wisconsin Population Health Institute (UWPHI) in Madison, WI. Since joining UWPHI in 2005, her work has focused on research and development to support community health improvement. She is the co-director of the County Health Rankings & Roadmaps program funded by the Robert Wood Johnson Foundation. She also spent 15 years at UW's Center for Health Systems Research and Analysis, leading consumer information and performance measurement projects funded by federal and state government. Bridget received a PhD in Health Systems Engineering from the University of Wisconsin–Madison, a MHSA from the University of Michigan School of Public Health, and a BA from Clark University in Worcester, MA.*

Government, the for-profit, and the not-for-profit sectors increasingly face mounting housing and community development resource challenges. One strategy for dealing with this has been to incorporate objective and rigorously analyzed market-based data into the decision-making process. This essay examines the Market Value Analysis (MVA), an approach used by many cities to incorporate a geographically-refined analysis of administrative data reflecting the local real estate market into their investment and program deployment strategies. The Reinvestment Fund's 12+ years of experience with the MVA in cities around the country suggests that organized data can support organized people to develop effective strategies and make productive evidence-based decisions.

MAKING SENSE OF MARKETS: USING DATA TO GUIDE REINVESTMENT STRATEGIES

Ira Goldstein
The Reinvestment Fund

During the last several decades, the combination of growing challenges and declining resources has forced many cities and towns to become more strategic in their approaches toward revitalization. Many have turned to data-based approaches to understanding market conditions and determining appropriate expenditures and investments. These data and analytic efforts have frequently served as the basis for attracting nonprofit and for-profit partners in support of neighborhood and municipal change. The Reinvestment Fund's (TRF's) Market Value Analysis (MVA) is one such effort.

Key questions arise in considering how to target limited resources for city revitalization. Which areas should a city prioritize for cleaning up vacant lots, removing abandoned cars, or intensive code enforcement? How should the mix between public acquisition and demolition, and incentivizing private rehabilitation and new construction, vary by market type? Where are "brick-and-mortar" public actions and subsidies generally unnecessary because the market is moving along well on its own? The MVA helps make objective, rigorously analyzed, contemporary market data available to help answer these questions and inform decisions. It starts by assembling a substantial amount of data on an entire city. It then uses a statistical procedure to sort a city's census block groups into categories or types based on their housing market conditions and offers guidance on the mix of public actions appropriate for each market type. Ultimately, the MVA provides an analytic basis for allocating and prioritizing public, private, and philanthropic resources in service of positive change.

BACKGROUND

The MVA was first introduced in TRF's hometown of Philadelphia. Like many older cities with an industrial past, Philadelphia's population and manufacturing sector peaked decades ago, leaving behind vast expanses of vacant and abandoned homes and factories. Philadelphia's population in 1950 exceeded 2 million residents but by 1990, the population had declined 25 percent to 1.58 million. At a postwar peak in the 1950s, Philadelphia had more than 350,000 manufacturing jobs; by 1990, that number was fewer than 85,000. The loss of manufacturing jobs was severe and greater than the national decline in the manufacturing sector. Jobs in the service sector replaced the manufacturing jobs but did not match the wages or benefits. Add decades of "machine politics" and poor political decisions to this trend, and Philadelphia was brought to its knees in 1990 because of financial woes. With municipal bond ratings hovering near junk status and a potential bankruptcy hanging over the city, the state legislature created an oversight and financial vehicle that would save the city from bankruptcy and create a structure to begin to repair its finances.

Newly elected mayor Ed Rendell effectively used that tool and others to stabilize Philadelphia's financial condition and ultimately to begin to turn the corner on decline. However, notwithstanding some extraordinary achievements—particularly in downtown Philadelphia—the neighborhoods of Philadelphia continued to suffer. Citywide, population declined further—albeit at a reduced rate—to 1.52 million in 2000, and those who left took their middle-class incomes with them. Mayor Rendell's downtown successes helped stabilize Philadelphia economically, but life in Philadelphia's neighborhoods was not appreciably better outside of the downtown. After two terms as mayor, Ed Rendell went on to serve two terms as governor of Pennsylvania and John Street was elected mayor of Philadelphia. As a long-time district councilperson and the president of city council, Mayor Street had represented a part of Philadelphia that was predominantly African American and had struggled with high levels of poverty, abandonment, and concentrated public housing. Mayor Street's electoral promise to Philadelphia was that he would work to inject the nascent vitality of the downtown core deeper into the city's many neighborhoods.

Mayor Street began to develop the Neighborhood Transformation Initiative (NTI), stressing that the effort had to be citywide, market oriented, and data driven in order to systematically address the range of blighting influences resulting from long-term neighborhood disinvestment. He turned to TRF to help build out the plan and devise a data-based framework to guide decision-making within the initiative. NTI ultimately grew into a $290 million effort designed to significantly reduce the number of vacant and dangerous buildings (a number that swelled to more than 25,000) and vacant lots (by 2001, there were an estimated 31,000 vacant lots in the city). TRF was a natural partner because, as a Philadelphia-based community development financial institution (CDFI), it had a long and successful history of investing in Philadelphia. Furthermore, TRF had highly respected leadership and public policy expertise along with capacity to develop action-oriented data analysis tools.[1]

In April 2001, the City of Philadelphia released the first MVA prepared by TRF to a large and receptive gathering at a historic theater in downtown Philadelphia. The theater was packed with investors, politicians, media, and stakeholders ranging from community development corporations (CDCs) to private-sector practitioners. In describing every MVA market type, presenters also offered a set of activities and resources that would be in service of the market type and its residents. A little more than a year later, the city council would support the mayor, voting 16:1 to allocate the NTI funds based on the analysis the MVA provided. Thus, the NTI was born.

TRF'S MVA

TRF's MVA is a data-based approach to analyzing real estate markets. It is designed using five underlying assumptions, based in the original principles of NTI:

- Public subsidy is scarce and should be treated as a resource to catalyze a market, or clear a path for private investment, but in general subsidy cannot create a market where there is none;

---

1 To contextualize the significance of this effort, compare NTI with the federal Neighborhood Stabilization Program (NSP), which uses funds allocated by Congress and distributed by HUD from two stimulus bills. Philadelphia received two NSP awards in 2009 and 2010, totaling slightly more than $60 million dollars. NTI, in 2009 dollars, is valued in excess of $360 million.

- "Build from strength"—in distressed markets, those investments built on nodes of strength are most likely to be successful;

- All parts of a city (not just downtowns, midtowns, or those parts that are highly distressed) and its residents are "customers" for the programs, services, and resources of that city, and the challenge is to customize investments to the particular needs and capacities that vary across neighborhoods;

- Decisions to invest public, private, or philanthropic funds should be based on objective and rigorous analysis of market data—as should evaluation of the impact of those investments. Accordingly, all MVAs cover an entire jurisdiction, not a particular parcel or neighborhood. MVAs are designed to uncover the full dimensions of both market challenge and market strength;

- MVAs should rely on market data that reflect actual market activity (e.g., residential sales, mortgage foreclosures, new units permitted).

Since 2001, TRF has completed more than 30 MVAs in cities of all sizes across the country. The cities are on different growth trajectories (growing cities such as San Antonio or contracting cities such as Detroit), or are working to reinvent themselves from their industrial past (e.g., Philadelphia, Baltimore, or St. Louis). In several cities (e.g., Baltimore, Pittsburgh, Philadelphia), TRF has created multiple MVAs on a cycle of approximately three years. Each MVA offers a lesson in how to improve the MVA and ensure greater local engagement.

Typically, the MVA relies on a set of indicators obtained from local jurisdictions (i.e., administrative data). In general, an MVA uses (1) real estate sales transactions; (2) variability in the value of those transactions; (3) mortgage foreclosures; (4) owner occupancy; (5) mixture of commercial and residential land uses; (6) vacant land/buildings; (7) new construction/substantial rehabilitation; and (8) subsidized rental stock. Over time, and with the experience of working in various cities, TRF settled on this set of indicators because it symbolizes the sort of market data an investor might consider when evaluating an investment. These indicators are also generally available because they represent the sorts of data cities often track. Last, the field validation of the data demonstrates that, combined into the MVA, the data are effective in creating both quantitative and qualitative market separation. Although these are the indicators typically used in the MVA, we have found in some cities that additional indicators were necessary to properly distinguish markets (e.g., in St. Louis we included bank and investor sales of real estate as an indicator; in Detroit, we incorporated an indicator of sheriff sales resulting from property tax delinquency).

Most of these indicators are acquired at an address level and then aggregated to the census block group. In our experience, the census block group is the correct geographic level because it is large enough to ensure that the data are reasonably stable yet small enough to ensure that the mosaic of a place is revealed; larger geographies (e.g., census tract, neighborhood, ZIP code) obfuscate meaningful differences. The MVA uses administrative data rather than secondary data sources (e.g., census data) for a few reasons. First, administrative data tend to be more up-to-date. Markets can change rapidly. Although the recent waves of the American Community Survey (ACS) conducted by the Census Bureau represent a substantial improvement from the decennial census long-form data of previous decades, the block group level ACS samples are small and subject to large statistical errors. ACS data are also at least 18 months old and as many as six years old when released in the five-year waves. Second, administrative data are preferred because they represent actual conditions, not an estimation (e.g., home value according to the census) or recollection of a condition at a prior time. Third, because the data are mostly at an address level, we are able to generate measures of central tendency (e.g., mean or median) and variability (e.g., coefficient of variance of sale prices) for each block group. Finally, several critical indicators are not available from secondary data sources (e.g., the mixture of commercial and residential land uses, permits for substantial rehabilitation).

Once acquired, we clean and validate each database with two parallel processes. We validate data first by review with local subject-matter experts and then through fieldwork. The latter involves reviewing the data while driving through the streets of a city with a GPS locator. Validation will typically take us through at least 50 percent of the block groups in a city. In most cities where we have worked, local experts accompany us. Those experts could be from a planning or code enforcement department or even a nonprofit community-based organization. Field validation is a critical part of the MVA process and is one of the things that distinguish the MVA from out-of-the-box market analyses. Aside from the aspect of local engagement, which is itself valuable, we uncover data issues that could impede accurate conclusions. For example, in one city we found unusually low-value sales in an area; however, validation revealed the sales were vacant lots not identified as such in the database. In another city, the vacancy measure turned out to be a more accurate depiction of units that were vacant but could be occupied—as opposed to vacant and abandoned (which is what we thought we were measuring). Once we have faith that the data are correct, they are aggregated to census block groups, mapped, and subject to additional validation.

We use a cluster analysis to combine cases (i.e., block groups) based on all of the measured indicators into categories so that cases within categories are more similar with one another than they are with cases in other categories. Stated differently, within each category, block groups are very similar, but each category is very different. We then map and validate the results of the cluster analysis using a similar process as described earlier. (Figure 1) Cluster analysis is a mix of art and science and, therefore, field validation is again important. For example, it is important that the groups be statistically different from one another. The art emerges when inspecting a section of a city to observe whether differences seen on the ground match those on the map.

Once the MVA is complete, TRF works with local stakeholders to identify a subset of indicators to update on a regular basis. For example, many cities have ready access to sale transactions and foreclosures. These indicators can be updated quarterly or annually, giving those stakeholders the ability to understand how an area is changing along these critical dimensions. We have found that stakeholders seeking to evaluate broad market changes related to investment or programmatic activity may need the MVA to be completely reconstructed periodically to accurately capture new data as it is made available.

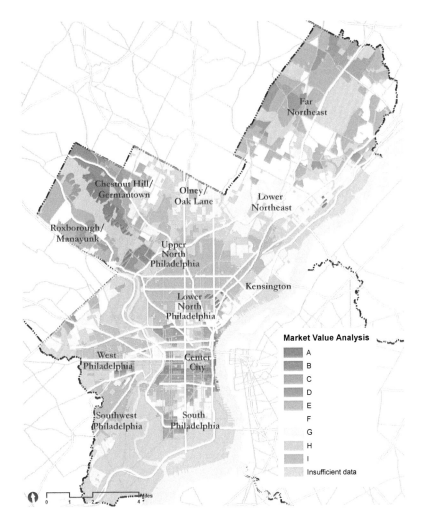

Market Value Analysis

- A
- B
- C
- D
- E
- F
- G
- H
- I
- Insufficient data

Figure 1. Sample MVA map. Each color corresponds to a particular market category identified through cluster analysis.

MVAS IN PRACTICE

A variety of organizations—including local governments, state agencies, the federal government (through technical assistance contract intermediaries), and philanthropy—have funded the creation of MVAs. Our recent experience in Milwaukee stands out as an example of an MVA funded by various sources: government, philanthropy, investors and community advocates. Each of the stakeholders engaged in constructing and validating the MVA brought their own perspective to the process, which contributed to the development of collaborative and coordinated evidence-based actions based on the MVA.

Typically, organizations use the MVA to guide key decisions about allocations of programs and resources. Baltimore, Philadelphia, and St. Louis have used the MVA to inform consolidated and comprehensive planning efforts, while Pittsburgh and Houston have used it to decide which projects to support with local, state, or federal incentives. Baltimore used its MVA to target code enforcement, and Milwaukee used its to coordinate funding from government and philanthropic sources. In Detroit, the MVA has been used in a number of ways, from helping the city target the proceeds from a federal civil rights settlement so that the funds could be maximally effective and consistent with the prescriptions of the settlement, to guiding infrastructure investments, to revising the boundaries of previously approved Neighborhood Stabilization Program (NSP) target areas. Pennsylvania and New Jersey used MVAs to help guide NSP plans for nonentitlement communities. Philadelphia and other cities with land banks are developing acquisition and disposition strategies based, at least in part, on the MVA. Finally, TRF uses the MVA on an ongoing basis in cities where we both invest in and develop affordable housing to target our efforts and assess change.

Figure 2 represents a prototypical template for an MVA implementation exercise that clients and stakeholders can use to think about a variety of programs, activities, and resources and how they might be prioritized and coordinated among different markets (represented as types A through I on the top of the chart). The suite of "activities" on the left side of Figure 2 will vary by the resources and programs a particular set of engaged stakeholders wish to prioritize using the MVA. In essence, the MVA facilitates the creation of a logic around matching the objective condition of various market types to the activities that might have the most potential for generating positive outcomes there. When resources contract, a guiding logic that can help diverse participants reach agreement on how to organize and target programs and activities is not an option but an imperative.

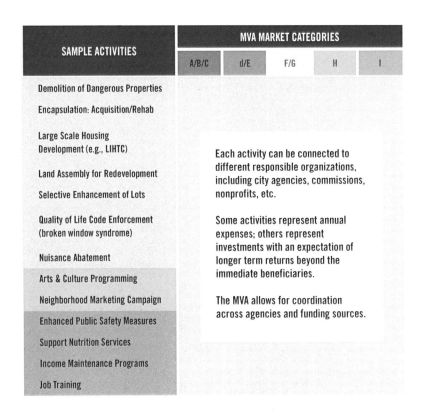

SAMPLE ACTIVITIES	MVA MARKET CATEGORIES				
	A/B/C	d/E	F/G	H	I
Demolition of Dangerous Properties					
Encapsulation: Acquisition/Rehab					
Large Scale Housing Development (e.g., LIHTC)					
Land Assembly for Redevelopment					
Selective Enhancement of Lots					
Quality of Life Code Enforcement (broken window syndrome)					
Nuisance Abatement					
Arts & Culture Programming					
Neighborhood Marketing Campaign					
Enhanced Public Safety Measures					
Support Nutrition Services					
Income Maintenance Programs					
Job Training					

Each activity can be connected to different responsible organizations, including city agencies, commissions, nonprofits, etc.

Some activities represent annual expenses; others represent investments with an expectation of longer term returns beyond the immediate beneficiaries.

The MVA allows for coordination across agencies and funding sources.

Figure 2. Template for establishing activity priorities in different market categories.

Most cities have been open about their MVA and post it publicly on sites they created (e.g., St. Louis, Baltimore, or New Orleans) or on TRF's PolicyMap (e.g., Philadelphia, Milwaukee, Reading).[2] By whatever means the data and analysis are conveyed to the public, revealing the analysis to a broad public audience lends itself to a more transparent process of decision-making, something we encourage.

---

2 For St. Louis, see City of St. Louis, Missouri, "Residential Market Analysis" (2014), available at http://dynamic.stlouis-mo.gov/mva/. For Baltimore, see City of Baltimore, Maryland, "Planning/ Master Plans, Maps & Publications/Housing Market Typology" (2010), available at http://archive. baltimorecity.gov/government/agenciesdepartments/planning/masterplansmapspublications/hous-ingmarkettypology.aspx. For New Orleans, see New Orleans Market Value Analyses 2009–2012," available at http://nolagis.maps.arcgis.com/apps/OnePane/basicviewer/index.html?appid=623139ce8 d3c4f83ade962b79e797164. For TRF, see The Reinvestment Fund, "TRF Policy Map" (Philadelphia, PA: TRF, 2014), available at www.policymap.com.

CHALLENGES IN DEVELOPING AND USING AN MVA

Having conducted many MVAs in a variety of circumstances, we found a limited number of challenges that are similar from place to place. The following challenges fall into three categories: technical, political, and financial. Each category reflects difficulties in implementing data-driven decision-making, but our experiences demonstrate that all can be addressed successfully:

Access to administrative data can be a challenge

Cities have unequal capacity to supply the requisite data. Moreover, administrative offices are sometimes run by elected officials who may not report to a mayor. Therefore, they may not have the same interest in making "their" data available because they believe the MVA will not be relevant to them. This issue has never scuttled an MVA, but it has made the task more difficult.

Data visualization and labels

The MVA map distinguishes markets by shading block groups by color; sometimes those markets are given names. For example, in the original Philadelphia MVA, market types were labeled "regional choice," "high-value appreciating," "steady," "transitional," "distressed," and "reclamation." Although the labels are only meant to serve as shorthand, clients can be reluctant to label a market "distressed," for example. Similarly, color can evoke emotion rooted in the history of many U.S. cities (e.g., red may be associated with the practice of redlining and coloring an area red may give the impression that resources will not flow to the area). We have dealt with these issues by having the recipients and stakeholders choose labels and colors that minimize potential discomfort. In the end, although clients or other stakeholders may contest the name or the color of a market on a map, they do not contest the way the data describe their area. As John Adams once declared, "Facts are stubborn things."

Targeting vs. even distribution of resources

A tension recurs between strategies that emphasize an even (and frequently thin) distribution of programs/resources and those in which resources are pegged to eligibility, need, opportunity, and market characteristics. Consider a city with 10 local legislative districts, and the city has historically distributed to each district 10 percent of the community development resources—as scarce as they may be. Now, change that so districts receive an amount commensurate with what the data suggest about needs and opportunities. Even with an effective argument, the political reality is that not all local legislators command the same amount of dollars they did before. Evidence-based targeting of resources to markets, as opposed to an even distribution, is a bitter but necessary pill that can sometimes be easier to swallow if there is acceptance of the analysis and buy-in to the connection of objective data about a place and the resources that are appropriate to address issues in that place.

Generating action

Sometimes stakeholders fail to take action on the findings presented in a completed MVA. This is most common in locations where TRF prepared the MVA without a champion in local government and a broad base of stakeholders who use the MVA as an organizing vehicle for change. Broad stakeholder support is certainly not a guarantee for success, but it can help. We have had particular success in, for example, Baltimore, Pittsburgh, and Milwaukee, where the MVA was funded by multiple sources and was developed with ongoing input from a set of stakeholders from every relevant sector.

Funding

MVAs are high-touch pieces of work that involve organizing people, organizing data, and a substantial amount of fieldwork. All levels of government experience the squeeze of declining resources, and philanthropy is not always comfortable with funding government activities. However, the value proposition of tackling an MVA in a city succeeds when the city and its stakeholders change behavior and make catalytic and effective investments that transform places.

FUTURE USES OF THE MVA

Data-based analyses and the resulting tools, such as the MVA, have application beyond simply measuring the real estate market to prioritize housing investment. There is, for example, an increasing awareness of the social determinants of health and how place-based organizing around economic stability, health care, education, social context, and the built environment can enhance the physical and psychological well-being of a community's residents.[3] The MVA incorporates several of the more frequently cited social determinant measures, in particular economic stability and the built environment. The MVA can help drive investment that will not only enhance the physical environment but also improve the prospects for healthy people and communities.

Social context is often represented by the extent to which there is free and open choice of housing without regard to race, color, or national origin. To that end, there is renewed public and governmental interest in the Affirmatively Furthering Fair Housing (AFFH) provisions of the federal Fair Housing Act (Act). AFFH requires all executive branch agencies to ensure programs are written and executed in a manner that will support the congressionally mandated purposes of the Act. At a minimum, we understand the "purposes of the Act" to include overcoming the legacies of segregation and concentration of racial/ethnic or low-income populations, ensuring equal access to community assets, and addressing people- and placed-based housing needs and disparities. The MVA and the data on which it relies can serve as a resource to facilitate AFFH efforts. When viewed through the additional lenses of racial/ethnic and economic segregation, the MVA points to places of opportunity and inequity where investment can not only transform a place but also address conditions adversely affecting racial and economic equity.

Finally, interest in understanding middle market areas is growing. The MVA is a tool to identify the location and conditions in a city's middle-market places. Because these areas are not home to large concentrations of very poor people or rampant deterioration of the housing stock, many cities have not directed resources to these places in the past. The middle-market areas are a remarkably important part of the economic and social fabric of any city, and neglecting these places and their residents can have dire effects on the future prospects of cities. As Philadelphia State Senator Dwight Evans said in his remarks supporting NTI, "A neighborhood shouldn't have to go through the process of becoming completely blighted before it can get help."[4] Market-based,

---

3   See, for example, HealthyPeople.gov, "2020 Topics and Objectives, Social Determinants of Health," available at www.healthypeople.gov/2020/topicsobjectives2020/overview.aspx?topicid=39#two.

4   Philadelphia Daily News, April 19, 2001, p. 12.

data-driven analyses, such as the MVA, can help direct attention and provide the market justification for a set of public, private, and philanthropic investments necessary to sustain middle-market areas.

In sum, data are powerful, particularly when they are transparent, ground-truthed, and used as an organizing vehicle for community engagement. With objective, rigorously validated and analyzed data, we can encourage a robust discussion about a future for a place and its people.

■ ■ ■

IRA GOLDSTEIN, *PhD, president of policy solutions at The Reinvestment Fund (TRF), designs and conducts studies used by government and other investors to make evidence-based decisions around resource allocation and policy impacting a broad array of community development issues. He also conducts studies of mortgage foreclosures and abusive lending practices in support of both policy and civil rights enforcement efforts. Prior to joining TRF, Goldstein was a director of Fair Housing and Equal Opportunity for HUD. He is a former member of the Fed's Consumer Advisory Council and currently serves on multiple boards and advisory panels including HUD's Cityscape Advisory Board. For more than 25 years, Goldstein has been a lecturer for the University of Pennsylvania's Urban Studies program.*

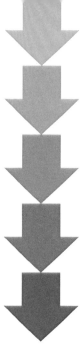

THE LOW INCOME INVESTMENT FUND'S SOCIAL IMPACT CALCULATOR

Nancy O. Andrews and Dan Rinzler
LIIF

Like any investor, we at the Low Income Investment Fund (LIIF) use financial return and other commonly accepted output metrics as key indicators of our performance. We are proud of having invested $1.5 billion in community projects that have served 1.7 million people over our 30-year history, as well as of our track record of financial sustainability and growth. Over the past decade alone, we have doubled our invested capital and tripled the number of people served. These metrics are part of a common language that allows us to easily communicate our performance to a wide range of audiences, such as other investors, policymakers, and programmatic partners.

But LIIF is not just any investor. As a mission-oriented community development financial institution (CDFI), we support projects that aim to generate profound and sustained improvements for disadvantaged children, families, and communities. We also aim to catalyze systems-level changes that deliver more resources to high-impact projects and organizations. In order to achieve our mission, we need to be able to both understand and express the *social value* of our investments, and not just their financial value. Put differently, we want to measure social impact in addition to financial return, as a way to gain a deeper understanding of how well we are achieving our social objectives. This means pushing ourselves beyond measuring outputs—such as child care spaces created, or number of patients served per year in a health clinic—to measuring factors like *income boosts* to families and individuals; *health value* associated with improved health and reduced medical expenditures; and *societal benefits*, mostly in the form of reduced government expenditures.

The current fiscal and policy climate is also pushing us to develop this capacity. Like other organizations in our sector, we must be able to describe exactly *why* and *how* our work is important in order to unlock new sources of capital, form new partnerships—such as with health institutions and transit agencies—and channel public and private investment to the most impactful strategies.

For these reasons and more, we developed a new tool called the **Social Impact Calculator** ("the Calculator") that monetizes—puts a dollar value on—the social value of the projects that we support. In creating the Calculator, our goal was to develop a tool that could powerfully express our impact, but also be easy to use and leverage existing evidence. We do not claim to have developed the single best approach to impact assessment for our sector, but we hope that the tool helps advance a broader discussion about the value of social investments. In this spirit, we developed it as an "open source" online tool for the public to use, learn about its method-ology, offer feedback, and download a customizable version at no cost.[1]

The Calculator's approach and mechanics are straightforward: using an "impact by proxy" design, we leverage high-quality social science research to translate project-level output data that we collect over the normal course of our business into monetized impact estimates. We limit the Calculator to indicators that are central to our mission of poverty alleviation, and which relate to our "impact pathways" or program areas: affordable housing, early care and education, K-12 education, health, and equitable transit-oriented development. At the portfolio level, we believe it generates directionally accurate monetary impact estimates for the projects we finance.

For instance, we estimate the monetary societal impact of the early child-hood education centers that we support using return-on-investment figures that researchers have developed using longitudinal data from randomized control trials—evidence whose statistical power we could never produce ourselves, and which we are happy to leave to academic experts. Another example is our estimate of medical cost savings from weight loss generated

---

1   Social Impact Calculator website: www.liifund.org/calculator.

by LIIF-supported affordable housing developments near transit stations—where, as studies have shown, residents are more likely to commute via public transportation and thus have higher levels of physical activity. Figure 1 shows the historical impact of projects LIIF has financed in each of the Calculator's ten sections.

There are several advantages to the Calculator's approach. First, leveraging existing evidence makes sense given LIIF's capacity and institutional context. As a CDFI, we are not in the position to conduct the analysis to answer the counterfactual question of what would have happened "but for" the intervention that LIIF supported. But high-quality social science research exists that can help us address many of these questions, and we believe it is up to us to take advantage of it. The Calculator also makes use of "lying around" output data that we can easily collect, reducing strain on both LIIF and our customers. Beyond our own constraints, we cannot expect overburdened nonprofit borrowers to take on the added task of developing sophisticated social outcome-tracking systems without grant support, which we are rarely able to offer.

We also recognize that the Calculator has limitations. First, its outputs are not precise enough for it to be used as decision-making tool to distinguish between the merits of one project versus another. And for the moment, most of its monetary estimates do not account for the time value of money. Most critically, very few studies meet all criteria that would make them applicable to the Calculator. The research we use to generate our estimates must be rigorous, using randomized control trials or other longitudinal analyses with large datasets; they must relate to the LIIF impact pathways, and apply across a sizable portion of our portfolio; they must fit output data that is easily available to us; and must show a way to monetize impact. Our strict criteria mean that many stones are left unturned. For example, we do not have the evidence base that tells us the efficacy of cross-sector and comprehensive community development work—an increasingly popular model that LIIF and other partners have supported in recent years. Finally, we recognize that we depend on many partners—other CDFIs, public subsidies, private capital—to support the projects we invest in. Rarely or never is there a project that is accomplished solely through the efforts of one investor or one subsidy source. In its present form, the calculator does not try to estimate the field-wide social value of the entire community

IMPACT CATEGORY	MONETIZED SOCIAL VALUE (billions, as of August 2014)
INCOME BOOSTS	
Increased discretionary income from affordable housing *	$8.40
Lifetime earnings increases from high-performing schools**	$2.00
Subtotal	$10.40
HEALTH VALUE	
Diabetes and extreme obesity improvements from affordable housing in healthy locations**	$0.40
Increased food expenditures from affordable housing	$2.80
Health improvements from permanent supportive housing for the homeless**	$1.30
Weight loss and increased physical activity from equitable transit-oriented development**	$0.01
Improvements in adult health from early childhood education	$0.07
Economic value of community health centers	$1.10
Subtotal	$5.70
SOCIETAL BENEFITS	
Early childhood education	$13.20
High-performing schools**	$0.80
Subtotal	$14.00
Grand Total	$30.10

* $2.8 billion in food expenditures generated by income boosts from affordable housing included in Health Value category
** Category does not include pre-2005 data

Figure 1. Impact of Projects LIIF Has Financed

development sector in the United States, and adjust for the overlap and interdependence of our collective efforts. Rather, the calculator only estimates the social value of the projects supported by the entity using it.

Although we are still in an exploratory phase of using the Calculator, it has already helped us engage with new partners—especially from other sectors—while also revealing industry-wide commonalities that we would not have otherwise discovered. We are committed to learning from and with others as we refine the tool, and are excited to continue to engage partners in advancing our efforts to measure social impact.

■ ■ ■

NANCY O. ANDREWS *is president and CEO at the Low Income Investment Fund, an $800 million community development financial institution. Ms. Andrews' 30 years in community development include positions as deputy director of the Ford Foundation's Office of Program Related Investments and Chief Financial Officer of the International Water Management Institute, a World Bank-supported development organization. Ms. Andrews also consulted for the U.S. Department of Housing and Urban Development and the Department of Treasury during the Clinton administration.*

■ ■ ■

DAN RINZLER *is special projects coordinator at the Low Income Investment Fund. Mr. Rinzler manages a variety of strategic initiatives at LIIF, such as the Social Impact Calculator and internal infrastructure to support development of new and innovative programs and capital products. Prior to LIIF, Mr. Rinzler helped design and manage low-income housing programs at the municipal and state level, and worked as an urban planning consultant.*

This essay explores how community developers can partner with public health professionals in using health impact assessments (HIAs) to improve living conditions and economic opportunities in low-income communities. HIAs bring together scientific data, public health expertise, business acumen, and stakeholder input to identify opportunities for maximizing health and community benefits when making decisions on policies and projects that would not otherwise focus on health. By using HIAs, community developers can more effectively address serious problems like substandard and unaffordable housing and lack of access to health foods while making a profound contribution to the health of low-income communities.

HEALTH IMPACT ASSESSMENTS: IMPROVING PUBLIC HEALTH THROUGH COMMUNITY DEVELOPMENT

Aaron Wernham[1]
The Health Impact Project

In 2007, a community developer in Oakland, California, made minor modifications to a planned low-income senior housing complex that benefited residents' health, generated support from local neighborhood leadership, and garnered recognition for the developer as an innovative company committed to creating healthy neighborhoods. Small design changes opened the door to a healthier living space and, on a larger scale, a new way of thinking about the role that developers can play in a community's well-being.

The tools used to make these changes went beyond the usual hammers, nails, plans, and building permits. Rather, a small group of public health experts worked with the developer to apply a new planning tool: a health impact assessment, or HIA. HIAs bring together scientific data, public health expertise, business acumen, and stakeholder input to identify opportunities for maximizing health and community benefits when making decisions on policies and projects that would not otherwise focus on health. Examples include land use and transportation plans, educational policies, or—as in the Oakland case—plans for a housing development. Moreover, HIAs identify metrics for health and health-related impacts as a new project or plan is implemented.

A growing body of research shows that the major illnesses facing our nation—such as obesity, asthma, heart disease, diabetes, and injury—are

---

1 Dr. Aaron Wernham wrote this essay during his tenure as the founder and director of the Health Impact Project. He recently left the Health Impact Project to become the CEO of the Montana Healthcare Foundation.

shaped by the conditions in the places where we live and work, and by the policies that shape these conditions. For example, well-designed and properly maintained housing can help prevent asthma and injuries from falls.[2] Transportation projects and land use plans that include safe routes for pedestrians and bicycles can minimize the risk of traffic injuries and allow people to be more active, thereby lowering the risk of obesity and many other illnesses.[3] In addition, education policies that improve academic performance among students lead to higher income, better jobs, and—in turn—longer, healthier lives.[4] Large and untapped opportunities exist for improving health among Americans and addressing skyrocketing medical costs. These opportunities involve bringing attention to health-related concerns when making decisions that shape the world outside the doctor's office.

The Oakland HIA demonstrated that minor facility modifications could potentially yield significant health improvements. By relocating the main entrance away from the neighboring freeway, for example, noise exposure among residents was reduced—a significant concern for health. Changing the design of windows facing the freeway and installing air filtration lowered the risk of air pollution exacerbating lung and heart problems.

Community developers seek to improve living conditions and economic opportunities in low-income communities, and public health data offer new metrics to measure and demonstrate the value of this work. Conversely, collaborating with developers provides a pathway for public health professionals to effectively address many root causes of illness. The Federal Reserve and the Robert Wood Johnson Foundation's Healthy Communities Initiative has highlighted the tremendous opportunity for greater collaboration between these fields. Further highlighting the potential, in January 2014, the Commission to Build a

---

2 D. Jacobs, A. Baeder, et al. "Housing Interventions and Health: A Review of the Evidence." (Washington, DC: National Center for Healthy Housing, 2009).

3 T. Litman, "Transportation and Public Health." *Annual Review of Public Health.* 2013, 34: 217–34. Also see M. Trowbridge , T. Schmid. "Built Environment and Physical Activity Promotion: Place-Based Obesity Prevention Strategies." *Journal of Medicine, Law, and Ethics. Supplement, Winter 2013: Weight of the Nation.* Pages 46–51.

4 A. Klebenoff Cohen, L. Syme. "Education: A Missed Opportunity for Public Health Intervention." *American Journal of Public Health.* 2013, 103(6): 997–1001.

Healthier America, a national, nonpartisan commission of public and private sector leaders, recommended that the two fields "fundamentally change how [they] revitalize neighborhoods, fully integrating health into community development."

Community developers face several important challenges in realizing these opportunities, such as financing, technical and design constraints, and permit requirements. Public health professionals will need to learn how to work within these constraints and offer analysis that is not only rigorous but also timely, in addition to recommendations that are not only based on sound evidence but are realistic and feasible. Moreover, public health analysis can be time-consuming and costly, and with the considerable challenges they already face, developers may be reluctant to add work with the potential to significantly increase costs or create delays. For these reasons, understanding each other's objectives and constraints, metrics of measurement, and simple analytic tools assessing readily available data sources are essential for widespread collaboration.

This essay explores HIAs as a practical tool to help community developers factor health into their initiatives, catalyze new partnerships between the two fields, and create metrics that measure the value of community development efforts.

COMMUNITY DEVELOPMENT AND HEALTH OF AMERICANS

Poverty is one of the most important predictors of poor health among Americans. A recent meta-analysis found that 133,000 U.S. deaths per year could be attributed to living below the poverty line, with an additional 39,000 deaths attributed to living in a neighborhood with high poverty rates.[5] Many serious illnesses are more common among low-income Americans including diabetes, coronary artery disease and heart attacks, strokes, asthma, and many types of cancer. Children living below the federal poverty line are seven times more likely to be in poor or fair health—and have higher rates of asthma and many other illnesses—than children in families earning above 400 percent

5   S. Galea et al."Estimated Deaths Attributable to Social Factors in the United States. *American Journal of Public Health.* 2010, 101(8): 1456–65.

of the federal poverty line.[6] These statistics simply reflect the outcome of economic hardships that low-income Americans face—hardships that community developers work to alleviate every day. As early as the 1800s, physicians recognized that poor-quality and overcrowded housing, insufficient heating in the winter, dangerous work, hunger, and malnutrition contributed to higher rates of illness and death among the poor. Today, low-income families are more likely to live in substandard housing, which exposes them to problems such as pest infestations, mold, poor ventilation, and other hazards that increase their risk of asthma, depression, burns, falls, and other health problems. Furthermore, lacking the money to pay for basic necessities often leads to situations that compromise health: going without prescribed medications, skipping meals, eating unhealthy foods because they are more affordable, or making-do with inadequate home heating or cooling.

As a primary care physician who spent many years working with low-income communities in major cities and in rural Alaska, I learned about these challenges firsthand. I would give my diabetic patients advice about eating more nutritious diets, only to find that the nearest grocery store required an hour-long trip by bus. Furthermore, as I encouraged people to walk more, I learned about the barriers that prevent many people from doing so, including high neighborhood crime rates and six-lane roads with no sidewalks.

By addressing problems such as substandard and unaffordable housing, lack of access to healthy foods, and unmet needs for basic services, community developers in the United States are making a profound yet largely unmeasured and unrecognized contribution to reducing health risks and, quite possibly, the associated medical costs.

HEALTH IMPACT ASSESSMENTS

The last 30 years have produced a growing body of public health research on the roots of illness in problems such as poverty, poor education, and substandard housing. These data highlight the need for more attention to health in public policy. In many countries, HIAs have

---

6   P.Braveman, S. Egerter, C. Barclay. "Issue Brief 4: Income, Wealth, and Health." *Exploring the Social Determinants of Health.* (*Robert Wood Johnson Foundation, 2011*) Available at: http://www.rwjf. org/content/dam/farm/reports/issue_briefs/2011/rwjf70448.

become one of the most commonly used tools to assess these concerns. HIAs are used by government agencies; the private sector, such as oil, gas, and mining companies; and by lenders that finance international development projects, including the World Bank and International Finance Corporation. HIAs first emerged in the United States in 1999, and they have gained considerable momentum in the last decade. In 2007, only 27 HIAs had been undertaken in the United States; by 2013, more than 275 HIAs had been completed or were underway.

HIAs assess the baseline health status of the population that will be affected by a policy proposal. Data obtained from HIAs can be used to better understand the needs and vulnerabilities in the neighborhoods developers serve. To create a profile of baseline health status, HIAs draw on a mix of publicly available data, which are sometimes augmented by surveys. Stakeholder engagement—through community meetings, focus groups, or advisory committees—helps identify the issues of greatest importance to the health of the affected population and aims to facilitate consensus among those with diverse and sometimes conflicting perspectives.

To explore the potential health effects of a proposal, HIAs review available research and employ both qualitative and quantitative methods. Most commonly, the predictions are qualitative: Literature reviews and stakeholder input are evaluated to provide insights on the potential connections between health outcomes and project-related changes, such as housing quality, traffic patterns, and pedestrian infrastructure. Most important, HIAs focus on solutions: They provide evidence-based, practical recommendations for optimizing the effects on health.

In practice, HIAs are typically carried out in six steps: (1) screening, (2) scoping, (3) assessment, (4) recommendations, (5) reporting, and (6) monitoring and evaluation. This framework is routinely adapted to accommodate the available resources and decision timeline. A larger-scale "comprehensive" HIA—undertaken for a new, major oil and gas project, for example—might take longer than a year to complete and may involve multiple analysts. Smaller-scale HIAs are often accomplished with far less time and fewer resources, some in as little as four to six weeks. One county government in Maryland has developed a standardized HIA–based approach in which the health department conducts reviews of new planning proposals with only a few hours of staff time.

HIAs AT WORK

The following case examples illustrate how HIAs can be applied to the types of initiatives in which community developers often play a leading role.

Planning a Mixed-Income Housing Development

In Colorado, the Denver Housing Authority and its partners are replacing an older, distressed, 250-unit public housing complex with nearly 900 new mixed-income units in the La Alma/Lincoln Park neighborhood near downtown Denver. The Denver Housing Authority and its master planning team created the Mariposa Healthy Living Initiative in 2009, which established physical, mental, and community health as variables for measuring how redevelopment would change the quality of life among residents. The initiative's responsive and rigorous planning framework advanced broad objectives, including the availability of healthy housing, stewardship of the environment, sustainable and safe transportation, opportunities for social interaction, and a community structure that supports a healthy economy. This extensive framework served as the basis for designers, developers, and practitioners to execute the HIA concept.

The HIA examined the baseline needs and health issues important to current residents. Then, as an integral element of the master planning for the development, the HIA team assessed the health implications of elements of the proposed plan such as building design, road and transit modifications, and pedestrian and cycling infrastructure. The team evaluated the HIA's options by using a customized version of the "Healthy Development Measurement Tool"—an HIA–based set of health indicators related to elements of the built environment, such as proximity to public transportation, health care, and nutritious food. The tool confirmed that the housing authority's plan would offer substantial health benefits for Mariposa residents. The HIA also allowed the housing authority to identify specific measures—such as traffic calming at high-volume intersections, safer and more attractive stairways in buildings, and acoustic modifications for housing nearest to the neighboring railway—that would optimize these health benefits. The final design will help to increase physical activity through improved pedestrian and bike opportunities, increase mobility and traffic safety, improve access to healthy foods, increase safety and security, and improve access to health care.

Since the master plan was adopted four years ago, the first phase of construction has been completed and two other sites are now under construction. The housing authority notes that crime rates in the neighborhood have already dropped from 246 per 1,000 people in 2005 to 157 per 1,000 people in 2011.

In 2012, the housing authority launched a new effort to further integrate health into every aspect of implementation by monitoring progress, refining recommendations, and developing implementation plans. An initial progress report updates and refines the previously used health indicators and tracks health-focused initiatives that have been completed. The report informed the further prioritization of new initiatives, focusing on what is important for the health of residents today.

Urban Greenway Design

A nonprofit developer in California used an HIA to develop plans for a new urban greenway with walking and biking trails along an urban transit line. The HIA identified many health benefits. First, a safe place to exercise would fill a critical need in the struggle against rising diabetes and obesity rates. Next, the space would create the opportunity for community members to interact and get to know one another, thereby improving community safety. In addition, less motor vehicle use could improve air quality and health problems among residents such as asthma. Stakeholder engagement during the HIA also identified challenges: Community members were worried about safety along the high-crime sections of the corridor—a concern that the HIA team recognized might decrease the use of the new path. With local residents, the team developed a series of recommendations including improving lighting, controlling access points, and creating a citizen watch group.

The HIA contributed to a plan that was instrumental in the Alameda County Transportation Authority's decision to grant the developer funds to complete the required environmental impact report. Widely recognized for excellence, the plan received an award in 2009 from the American Planning Association.

Neighborhood-Scale Planning

In 2009, a multidisciplinary team conducted an HIA to inform planning for the redevelopment of the Page Avenue corridor, an economically distressed neighborhood in St. Louis, Missouri. The HIA was led by Washington University faculty in public health, urban design, public policy, and economic development, and involved extensive engagement of the project's lead developer; community members; and city, county and state decision makers. The Page Avenue project envisioned a new grocery store, homes, and businesses, in addition to renovated streets, sidewalks, vacant lots, and intersections. The HIA team conducted literature reviews; mapped important neighborhood concerns and assets such as streets, sidewalks, bus stops, and food stores; and spoke with stakeholders through focus groups, resident surveys, and interviews with 20 key city and county decision makers. The team incorporated this information into an assessment of how the proposed redevelopment would affect health through its predicted effects on jobs, housing, recreation, access to goods and services (including nutritious food), pedestrian infrastructure, and neighborhood safety. The team then developed recommendations based on the findings.

In the short term, the HIA resulted in several important outcomes. It raised awareness of the plan's implications for health among community members and key decision makers including the developer, mayor, and planning and transportation officials. Officials made verbal commitments to improve sidewalks near transit stops, and the mayor and county health department committed to participating on a post-HIA task force. A city initiative to revive fruit orchards and gardens sought to improve local nutrition.

The implementation of the Page Avenue revitalization plan will take place over several years. The HIA has established a starting point for effective collaboration as the project evolves, and it has already contributed to a new culture of health among the stakeholders in which ideas and initiatives to optimize the health benefits of the revitalization have become a priority.

Regional Land Use and Transit Planning

Atlanta was successful in using an HIA as part of planning the BeltLine, a major light-rail system that will link with parks and open space in a ring around the city. The BeltLine involves a complex, multiyear planning effort and coordination among city, county, state, federal, and private sector partners. In 2005, Georgia Tech's Center for Quality Growth and Regional Development conducted an HIA that continues to benefit the planning process and the area's residents.

At baseline, the HIA identified higher rates of diabetes, heart disease, cancer, motor vehicle injury, and other health problems in the low-income neighborhoods in the study area. The HIA found major health benefits were likely to result from constructing the BeltLine as initially proposed, but it also identified important areas for improvement in the project. For example, the plan's focus on transit and trails would increase physical activity (lowering the risk of many illnesses), but the need for these benefits was particularly high in the lower-income southwest neighborhood. Therefore, the HIA proposed adding more acres of parks and better access to trails and sidewalks in this area. The plan would also improve connectivity and thereby increase general access to schools, parks, grocery stores, hospitals, and other amenities that benefit health. To maximize these benefits for the lower-income neighborhoods that had particularly poor access to these amenities, the HIA offered a series of recommendations for location of transit stops and improved connectivity with the regional transit system.

The effects of this HIA continue to evolve as BeltLine planning and implementation progress. Effects to date include a commitment by the mayor to complete the project as quickly as possible given its benefits for health; federal and private sector decisions to award $7 million in grants to clean brownfields and construct green space and trails in low-income neighborhoods; an affordable housing policy for the BeltLine; the addition of health metrics to evaluate BeltLine proposals; and the addition of a public health professional to the advisory committee for the Tax Allocation District that issues bonds to fund BeltLine capital expenditures.

USING HIAs TO ADVANCE THE COLLABORATION BETWEEN HEALTH AND COMMUNITY DEVELOPMENT

The Health Impact Project—a collaboration of the Robert Wood Johnson Foundation and The Pew Charitable Trusts—supports using HIAs to integrate health considerations into new plans, projects, and policies. In the area of community development, the project is funding three pilot HIAs and a simultaneous evaluation to adapt and streamline this approach for easier use in community development initiatives. These assessments address decisions that range from local planning to state-level policies:

- Community Solutions, a nonprofit organization dedicated to strengthening communities and ending homelessness, is working with an art, design, and planning studio to include health considerations in a neighborhood revitalization and sustainability plan for Hartford, Connecticut's northeast neighborhood. This plan will offer a blueprint to inform revitalization efforts, which may include improvements to land use, utilities, housing conditions, open space, and access to transportation and healthy food. The HIA will examine how these changes will influence health, and it will provide recommendations to optimize positive health effects.

- Health Resources in Action, a nonprofit public health institute, is working with the Massachusetts Department of Public Health and Metropolitan Area Planning Commission on an HIA to inform new rules that will guide future funding for community development corporations under the state's Community Investment Tax Credit Grant Program. The HIA will offer ideas for health-oriented criteria that the agency can use to screen projects.

- The Georgia Health Policy Center is conducting an HIA to examine the 2015 Georgia Qualified Allocation Plan for Low Income Housing Tax Credits. The annual plan is required by the Internal Revenue Service to allocate housing tax credits to state agencies, which then award credits to developers. The project will engage the Georgia

Department of Community Affairs, real estate developers, state regional commissions, community representatives, and relevant federal agencies to ensure that all stakeholder perspectives are well represented in the final recommendations.

This community development initiative will create a toolkit to assist developers with integrating health considerations into their initiatives. The toolkit will identify a set of health effects that are commonly encountered, catalogue available sources of health data, provide simple analytic tools, and offer health-based metrics that developers can readily apply to their own initiatives. Using health-based metrics to measure the impact of their work will also help developers better demonstrate the medical cost savings that could accrue from the health benefits produced by their initiatives. The final HIA report and toolkit are expected in fall 2015.

CONCLUSION

For primary health care providers in low-income communities, the connection between neighborhood and health presents a daily challenge. Too often, we find ourselves needing to add more medications to a patient's regimen to control asthma or diabetes, when what is really needed is better housing; readily available access to fresh fruits and vegetables; or a safe, pleasant place to exercise. For public health professionals, collaboration with community developers holds promise as a new means to fill a "prescription" for better health. Public health offers a new way to help developers improve the lives and health of the communities they serve and, equally important, a new way to measure the results of their work. With medical care costs now consuming nearly 20 percent of all the goods and services in the United States, finding ways to contain costs is critical. Demonstrating the health-related value of community development initiatives can contribute to a foundation for a more evidence-based conversation about the most effective ways to invest in improving health among Americans.

Realizing the full potential of this partnership will require hands-on experience gained by close collaboration on specific initiatives. At the second national HIA meeting in 2013, councilmember Joe Cimperman of Cleveland, Ohio, told attendees that HIAs "help me win" by ensuring that important concerns have been addressed early-on in developing new policy, and by providing solid data to support new proposals. The examples in this chapter validate the notion that good stakeholder engagement and an eye to improving health can enhance the planning process and build support for new proposals. Moreover, collaboration on an HIA can be an effective way for developers and public health professionals to gain a working knowledge of each other's fields, identify metrics to measure the health benefits of a well-planned project, and develop actionable recommendations that are both feasible for the developer and good for health.

FOR FURTHER READING

National Research Council of the National Academies: Improving Health in the United States: The Role of Health Impact Assessment. www.iom.edu/~/media/Files/Activity%20Files/Environment/EnvironmentalHealthRT/2011-Nov-RT/132291.pdf.

The Health Impact Project Web site, www.healthimpactproject.org, offers many resources, including a searchable map, for finding practitioners and funders in a particular area or sector.

Health Affairs, "Health Impact Assessments Are Needed in Decision Making about Environmental and Land-Use Policy." http://content.healthaffairs.org/content/30/5/947.abstract.

■ ■ ■

DR. AARON WERNHAM *is CEO of the Montana Healthcare Foundation and the founder and former director of the Health Impact Project, a collaboration of the Robert Wood Johnson Foundation and The Pew Charitable Trusts established to promote and support the use of Health Impact Assessment (HIA) in the United States. Dr. Wernham is a family physician and leader in public health policy who has served on several National Academies committees, and advised multiple government agencies and community-based organizations on HIAs and healthy public policy. Previously, Dr. Wernham provided primary care for rural Alaska Native communities, and led Alaska's efforts to establish a collaborative tribal-state-federal HIA program.*

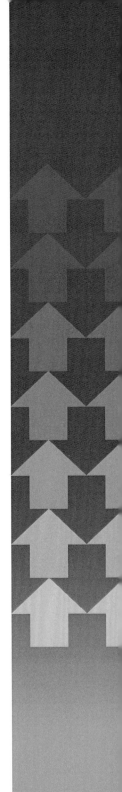

3

ENHANCING DATA
ACCESS AND
TRANSPARENCY

We've recently seen a number of state and local governments work to achieve public goals through openly publishing data. However, we're also seeing that the power and value of this data can be realized only by engaging data users and taking stock of their interests. It is therefore important both for government actors to know the range of approaches that exist for opening data, and for those outside of government to take advantage of the opportunity to shape government open data practices. This essay describes how governments can open data, why this is so useful, and how nongovernmental actors can help the process along.

MAKING THE MOST OF OPEN DATA

Emily Shaw
Sunlight Foundation

In the past six years, we've seen significant growth in state and local governments' approaches to open data as they realize they can achieve many goals by openly publishing the data they collect. They're recognizing the importance of publishing data in formats easily accessed by "civic hackers" and app developers. They're also discovering cost savings by publishing data online rather than waiting for individual citizens' requests. Finally, they're finding that their departments can cooperate better when they share data using a common platform.

The aim of open government data—to open the storehouses of government data to the world in order for the data to have maximum use and effectiveness—is a bold one. Open data initiatives reposition governments as suppliers of data and also anticipate the participation of additional parties in using those data. Those parties, whether other members of government, members of the public, or individuals with a specific professional or technical interest in the data, are the "demand" side of the equation, and are vital partners in using the data to solve key problems or make progress toward goals.

This essay describes how governments may choose to open data, the benefits of doing so, and how nongovernmental actors can interact with the process. It also argues that governments should recognize that the power and value of their data holdings can be realized only by engaging data users and taking stock of their interests—and that it is critical that actors outside of government recognize and make use of the opportunity to shape open data policy and practice.

WHAT IS "OPEN DATA"?

The meaning of *open data* is rooted in the principles outlined in the 2005 Open Definition, which states that data are "open" when they are available to everyone, free for use and reuse, and when data sets have a minimalist form of licensing that, at its most stringent, requires author attribution and the obligation to "make subsequent derivative works similarly open."[1] The Open Knowledge Foundation, which uses advocacy, technology, and training to open data, offers three criteria for "open": 1) legal openness and freedom from restrictive licensing terms; 2) social openness (making information easily available for collaboration); and 3) technological openness (making information available in machine-readable and nonproprietary data formats).[2] The concept has evolved to encompass the idea that information should be available online, from a primary source, timely and complete, and published in machine-readable formats that promote maximal use and reuse.[3]

Open "data" can be more than numeric data. Information such as the text of legislative bills or laws (e.g., data sets used by the Sunlight Foundation's Open States project or the OpenGov Foundation's America Decoded project) can fall under a more expansive definition of open data.[4] Text-based data become open data when data-holders eliminate legal restrictions on its use, publish data online for public access, and structure data in a way that improves search and text analysis, such as by implementing a consistent data format.

---

1 Open Knowledge Foundation, "The Open Knowledge Definition" (Cambridge, UK: Open Knowledge Foundation, 2005), available at https://web.archive.org/web/20060819043123/http://www.okfn.org/okd/definition.html. The Open Knowledge Foundation credits the open source coding movement, and specifically the 1997 "Debian Free Software Guidelines," for providing roots for the broader "open definition." See Open Knowledge Foundation, "The Open Source Definition" (Cambridge, UK: Open Knowledge Foundation, 2005), available at https://web.archive.org/web/20060924131931/http://www.opensource.org/docs/definition.php. See also opendefinition.org.

2 Open Knowledge Foundation, "The Three Meanings of Open" (Cambridge, UK: Open Knowledge Foundation, 2005), available at https://web.archive.org/web/20060113133743/http://www.okfn.org/three_meanings_of_open.html.

3 These additional qualities were first described in a document called "The Eight Principles of Open Government Data," created by a collection of open government advocates in 2007, available at http://opengovdata.org/.

4 See Open States project at http://openstates.org/ and America Decoded project at http://americadecoded.org/.

Arriving at a common understanding of open data matters for individual open data initiatives: A narrow definition of open data limits what the government is expected to produce and what people are expected to use the data for, whereas a more comprehensive definition may entail higher costs for government and higher expectations that the data-using community will produce real public benefits from the data. The public has a compelling interest in open government data because the data were created and gathered under public authority.

OPEN DATA EXAMPLES

Governments have taken two main approaches to opening government data. They either publish data on a website or they develop a legal structure to undergird a more complex and ongoing process of open data release. The first method is by far the more common. The next section describes the second method: establishing an open data policy. This method is more difficult and less common, but it has the advantage of laying the groundwork for improving continuity of access to data, creating a better understanding of government data holdings, and ensuring access to specific types of data negotiated through the policy.

Simply publishing open data on a website—for example, by creating a new open data portal—is the more familiar approach for governmental data managers. If we understand all information to be a form of data, government websites have always been synonymous with data release. Even early descriptions of the goals for government websites anticipated that they would allow citizens to perform a wide variety of tasks and that information systems within and between governments would be effectively integrated online.[5] The introduction of open data as a separate concept to specifically enable greater public use and reuse of government data is built on the foundation that governments serve their citizens not only in the traditional sense but also through an online presence.

The concept of making data available and reusable also has roots in existing government practice. Most notably, the U.S. Census makes

---

5 K. Lange and J. Lee, "Developing Fully Functional E-Government: A Four Stage Model," *Government Information Quarterly* 18 (2001): 122–136.

"published census statistics... available to anyone who needs them."[6] The U.S. Government Printing Office has published the daily activities of Congress online in the Congressional Record since 1994, and the U.S. Congress created the THOMAS website to open legislative data to public oversight the following year.[7] At the state level, Florida and Hawaii were early adopters of online campaign finance disclosures, maintaining publicly accessible campaign finance websites by 1997.[8] In general, making records available by computer tape, disk, or dial-up servers provided an intermediate step between paper copies and the advent of government websites to provide the public with free access to government data.[9]

Although aspects of government actions during the 1990s and early 2000s resembled ideals of open data, governments began using the term *open data* to describe such efforts only later in the process. Nongovernment groups such as the Open House Project[10] and the Open Government Working Group[11] advocated for aligning the established principles of open government with open, machine-readable, license-free, and online access to government data. In January 2009, the U.S. government provided the most visible legitimation of these principles. President Obama's "Memorandum on Transparency and Open Government" identified online publication of government data as a method to improve government transparency and also implied that technology could be used to improve civic participation and

---

6   U.S. Census Bureau, "Fact Finder for the Nation" (Washington, DC: US Census Bureau, 2000), available at www.census.gov/history/pdf/cff4.pdf.

7   Joshua Tauberer, *Open Government Data* (self-published, 2012), available at http://opengov-data.io/#chapter_1.

8   Christi Parsons, "State Campaign-funding Data Hasn't Found A Home On Web," *Chicago Tribune*, February 26, 1997, available at http://trib.in/1omVOmx.

9   For an example of the widespread nature of this intermediate step to online data sharing, see the variation in public access to campaign finance disclosure in Elizabeth Hedlund and Lisa Rosenberg, *Plugging In the Public: A Model for Campaign Finance Disclosure* (Washington, DC: Center for Responsive Politics, 1996).

10 See the Open House Project, available at http://www.theopenhouseproject.com/.

11 The Open Government Working Group was a group convened to create a list of shared principles, available here: http://opengovdata.org/.

collaboration.[12] Later that year, the White House and executive agencies used the term *open data* to refer to methods of releasing the data in their open government plans.[13]

In the course of these developments, local government began sharing many data sets, and private companies began to provide platforms for open formats, later called "open data portals." In 2006, Washington, DC, was among the first local governments to create a website featuring a wide range of government data with the specific purpose of "streaming data that the agencies gather through normal operations" to the public.[14] Soon after, Seattle-based Socrata opened its doors with the intention of providing "open government data, readily accessible over the internet, in a form that maximizes comprehension, interactivity, participation, and sharing."[15] The earliest commercial provider of open data platforms, Socrata was selected to power a number of new federal, state, and local open data sites by 2010. (Since this time, a number of other of commercial and free open data platforms, e.g. CKAN, have also come into routine use.)

Many U.S. state and local governments have continued to build on this trend. Governments currently post a wide range of data sets from both internal and external sources. Unfortunately, because of the sheer number of state and local government sites and the varying methods and naming conventions, it has proved challenging to aggregate a comprehensive list of sites. Nonetheless, efforts such as the federal government's Data.gov, informal collaborative efforts such as Datacatalogs.org, or simple iterative web searches demonstrate that US federal agencies, states, and localities share government data using hundreds of sites.

12 Executive Office of the President of the United States, "Memorandum for Heads of Department and Agencies" (Washington, DC: Executive Office of the President of the United States, 2009). http://www.whitehouse.gov/sites/default/files/omb/assets/memoranda_fy2009/m09-12.pdf.

13 See, e.g., the Open Energy Information plan at www.whitehouse.gov/open/innovations/OpenEnergyInformation or the Presidential Open Government Report at www.whitehouse.gov/sites/default/files/microsites/ogi-progress-report-american-people.pdf.

14 Robert Bobb, "Streaming of DCStat Data to www.dc.gov." Memorandum (Washington, DC: Executive Office of the Mayor, 2006). http://www.scribd.com/fullscreen/26442622?access_key=key-20rfsh26eu0ob66xlbmu.

15 Socrata, "Opening Government One Dataset at a Time" (Seattle, WA: Socrata, 2010), available at https://web.archive.org/web/20100208173200/http://www.socrata.com/about.

DEVELOPING OPEN DATA POLICY

Opening data can be a relatively straightforward process. Open data advocate Waldo Jaquith has pointed out that governments can create an open data site by running a search for CSV, XLS, and XML files that already exist on their network of public sites and posting them on the same page.[16] However, providing lasting access to the same data requires the additional step of legally codifying public access to data.

As was the case with the development of open data portals, the development of open data policies began without the open data label. For example, the 2006 memorandum from a Washington, DC, city administrator contains many of the elements of the later open data policy. It mandates a rationale for streaming data online, describes a timeline for specific data release, mandates specific agency responsibilities, and describes the need to maintain quality and review.[17] After the 2009 White House memorandum, additional local governments began to develop policies that explicitly used the language of "open data." The city council of Portland, Oregon, for example, passed a resolution to "mobilize and expand the regional technology community…by promoting open and transparent government, open data, and partnership opportunities."[18] The mayor of San Francisco issued an executive directive to "enhance open government, transparency, and accountability by improving access to City data that adheres to privacy and security policies."[19]

The Portland and San Francisco examples also demonstrate the two primary paths to developing state and local open data policy: the legislative and executive approaches to mandating government data release. Since 2009, several states and cities have chosen to follow one of these paths. The Sunlight Foundation has documented more than 30 formal state and local open data policies; approximately two-thirds of these

---

16 Waldo Jaquith, public presentation at Open Data NJ Summit, May 16, 2014, Montclair, NJ.

17 Robert Bobb, "Streaming of DCStat Data."

18 City of Portland, Resolution No. 36735 (City of Portland, 2009), p1, available at www.portlandonline.com/shared/cfm/image.cfm?id=275696.

19 City and County of San Francisco, Office of the Mayor, Executive Directive 09-06 (San Francisco, CA: Office of the Mayor, 2009), available at http://sfmayor.org/ftp/archive/209.126.225.7/executive-directive-09-06-open-data/index.html.

policies were established through legislative means (by law, resolution, or ordinance) and approximately one-third were created through executive means (by memo or directive). In at least one case (San Francisco), an open data policy originally established by the executive was later superseded by legislative policy.

The pace of development of open data policies on a local level has only increased. The Sunlight Foundation identified eight policies new policies in 2010–2011 and six new policies in 2012. Fifteen were enacted in 2013 and eight were enacted in the first four months of 2014.[20] Open data policies have been enacted in the most populous American municipalities—Los Angeles, New York City, and Chicago—in several midsized cities, and in places as small as Williamsville, New York, a village of 5,277 residents. As of mid-2014, eight states—Texas, Illinois, Utah, New York, Hawaii, New Hampshire, Connecticut, and Maryland—had passed open data policies, while an additional seven state-level open data bills had been introduced for consideration.[21]

Because it involves political processes, achieving an open data policy is more complicated than publishing government data on a website. However, the value of the open data policy is that it offers the public a far better guarantee of access to specific data sets in specific formats and of specific quality. Without a formal policy, the public may lose access to posted data if the government website is revised or if department staff change. Individuals who posted those data sets may or may not choose to keep them current. They may or may not choose to make the data sets available in formats that are easy to use and reuse. Moreover, open data policies usually describe a specific rationale for making government data available to the public, and this formal statement provides people who interact with government data an opportunity to make a case for access to existing or new data.

The two methods for implementing open data—releasing open data and creating an open data policy—are not mutually exclusive. In many cases, governments begin by publishing open data online and

20 Several locations developed multiple policies during these years; San Francisco, e.g., developed four increasingly ambitious policy approaches to open data between 2009 and 2013.

21 The Sunlight Foundation maintains a map and database of enacted and pending open data legislation at http://sunlightfoundation.com/policy/opendatamap.

then develop a formal policy about their practice. Individuals who are interested in enjoying more access to government data may gain the necessary backing for a broader-scale policy by building gradually toward it, by both building political support and demonstrating the value of existing government data releases.

It is unclear whether the pace of open data policy enactment will continue—or whether a majority of governments will adopt open data as a formal policy—but if the practice continues to spread, we may achieve the same outcome even without an official policy.

BENEFITS AND STAKEHOLDERS OF OPEN DATA

Regardless of how governments choose to open data, the success of the data release relies on people connecting with those data. To capture the attention of additional users, governments will need to understand the various motivations for using the data and stakeholder preferences about which data are most important to achieve their goals. Recognizing the range of potential benefits and stakeholders allows governments to craft an open data initiative tailored to the interests of their local actors.

From community activists, to small businesses, to civic technologists, open data can help groups of people achieve their goals, and those goals can be quite different.

The Sunlight Foundation collected examples of how open data were used to accomplish several objectives.[22] In reviewing the collection, the foundation found:

- Governments and nongovernmental actors can use open data to increase transparency by linking government revenue and expenditure details to a publicly accessible tool for exploring government finances. The New York City comptroller office's Checkbook NYC 2.0 does this with open-source software that other cities can mimic.

- Open campaign finance and government spending data—including contracts, grants, and subsidies—have allowed watchdogs and

---

22 Sunlight Foundation, "Impacts of Open Data" (Washington, DC: Sunlight Foundation, 2013), available at http://bit.ly/1wwpoQL.

journalists to improve political accountability by highlighting improper and publicly-discoverable behavior. For example, WAMU, the community radio station in Washington, DC, used the district's open spending and campaign finance records to document the connection between real estate developers' campaign contributions and their receipt of public development subsidies.

- Some local governments, such as New York City and Chicago, are using open data to increase interdepartmental cooperation and increase efficiencies within government. Several nongovernmental organizations are also using open government data to identify potential areas for cost savings, including DataKind's project to identify optimal public tree maintenance schedules and Data Science for Social Good's documentation of the relationship between crime and extended streetlight outages.

- Open data can point to issues of service quality and enable advocacy for improvement by increasing transparency about existing services. For example, The *Los Angeles Times* used public municipal emergency response data to map neighborhood experiences of emergency response time. SeeClickFix deployments in several municipalities allowed citizens to register 311 complaints about nonemergency municipal service concerns.

- Finally, open data can enhance citizens' participation by providing new opportunities to communicate with governments. 596 Acres, a group of advocates fighting blight, used data to map vacant lots and facilitate public-private agreements on temporary land use solutions, for example. This effort created new avenues for government-public interaction. Others, such as Philadelphia's OpenDataRace—a contest where individuals and organizations were encouraged to nominate new datasets for public release—provide a format for government outreach to increase local citizens' interest in and use of government data.

Individuals and organizations outside government are using open data with a variety of motivations. For example, organizations that focus on using open data to find technological solutions to governance problems, typified by Code for America brigades and other civic hackers, are seeking improved trust and collaboration between governments and citizens.[23] Other organizations are seeking business opportunities. The new US node of the UK-based Open Data Institute, for example, plans "to identify valuable, unreleased data sets, identify the audience for those data sets, and then identify the business proposition that makes that data set valuable and its use sustainable."[24]

Other organizations promote more community-focused benefits. Data intermediaries, such as the members of the National Neighborhood Indicators Partnership, are using open data in targeted ways to tackle social issues. Bob Gradeck of the University of Pittsburgh's Center for Social and Urban Research describes the variety of data "consumers" who benefit from the work his organization does to collect, clean, prepare, and present open data on property and community conditions. Beneficiaries include students, university faculty, community-based organizations, social service organizations, journalists, residents, home buyers, local journalists, and government agencies, as well as civic hackers.[25] The Baltimore Neighborhood Indicators Alliance aims "to show how using city and state data can help communities reduce crime rates, improve public transit, and help students perform better in school"[26] and "to strengthen Baltimore neighborhoods by providing meaningful, accurate, and open data at the community level."[27]

Rufus Pollock of the Open Knowledge Foundation described open data initiatives as functioning like an ecosystem, with "data cycles" in which data come from a government source and pass through "infomediaries" who work with, clean, and "wrangle" the data for improving their

23 Bob Sofman, "Here Are Our Values" (San Francisco, CA: Code for America, March 27, 2014), available at www.codeforamerica.org/blog/2014/03/27/here-are-our-values/.

24 Open Data Institute, "USA Node News: January 2014" (London, UK: Open Data Institute, January 2014). http://theodi.org/usa-node-news-2014.

25 Bob Gradeck, "OpenGov Voices: The Role of Information Intermediaries in Open Data" (Washington, DC: Sunlight Foundation, March 28, 2014), available at http://bit.ly/1iLhXva.

26 Andrew Zaleski, "Baltimore Data Day Puts Big Data in Communities' Hands" (Baltimore, MD: Technical.ly Baltimore, July 13, 2012), available at http://bit.ly/1qJn9km.

27 Baltimore Neighborhood Indicators Alliance, "About Us" (Baltimore, MD: Baltimore Neighborhood Indicators Alliance, 2014), available at http://bniajfi.org/.

utility and quality before returning them to the original data source.[28] The governments that provide the source data, the players that analyze and repackage the data, and the ultimate users of the derived products are all part of the "open data ecosystem." This perspective acknowledges the interdependence between government data and nongovernment data producers and users in achieving the goals associated with open data. It highlights the need for robust feedback between data producers and data users and anticipates data flowing not only in one direction from a government to a nongovernment user, but in complex cycles that feed back into government data use and production.

The multidirectional nature of current open data flows is well illustrated by the growing set of government websites hosting open data that have been collected by specialized community actors. The federal open data site Data.gov, for example, now allows community organizations to post information on their website. At the municipal level, Baltimore. gov similarly hosts community data gathered by the Baltimore National Indicators Alliance. Nongovernment actors can benefit by using the government data site as a platform for sharing their information, and governments benefit by maintaining a broader open data collection for their constituents.

CREATING A SUCCESSFUL OPEN DATA INITIATIVE

The Sunlight Foundation recommends that governments and open data advocates starting or improving an open data initiative engage with a broad range of stakeholders to identify core values and goals that their community (and community-based data users) collectively supports. The goals and values that result from these discussions should help shape decisions as the system develops. This process also offers an opportunity for potential individual and organizational users to articulate their own goals and build relationships with others who have similar aims.

The Sunlight Foundation's Open Data Guidelines help communities answer the next question about what data should be made public. Open data initiatives are about gaining access to more quality government data for free use and reuse, but these initiatives are not intrinsically

---

28 Rufus Pollock, "The Present: A One-Way Street" (Cambridge, UK: Open Knowledge Foundation, March 31, 2011), available at http://blog.okfn.org/2011/03/31/building-the-open-data-ecosystem/.

connected to access to any particular data set. To know what data are available, the Sunlight Foundation recommends that governments provide a public list of all data sets they maintain, including descriptions of those they believe cannot yet be released because of privacy concerns. Governments and open data advocates should then work together to explore which data sets should receive priority attention for release. The data sets selected depends on both existing public records laws, explicit stakeholder goals, and the public interest. The Sunlight Foundation advocates that governments consider public input in a number of ways when deciding what to release first, including thorough review of past Freedom of Information requests, other inquiries from internal or external actors, or data used in public hearings and public law-making. The guidelines also advise how to make data public, which include specifying formatting, documentation, and technology platforms. Although this is generally the government's purview, decisions should be made in light of the values and goals outlined for the initiative.

Finally, communities will need to grapple with how to implement the open data policy. Sunlight's guidelines recommend providing regular opportunities for public feedback, both formally and informally. Informally, governments can collect comments through the open data portal or Twitter, or through interactions at community events. Nongovernment actors may also participate in open data policy implementation in a formal oversight role. Governments may choose to create open data working groups that include seats for nongovernment members to oversee the implementation of an open data initiative. Maryland's development of an Open Data Working Group through state statute provides one example of this. New York City officials regularly meet with the local Transparency Working Group, a less formal relationship but one that nonetheless plays an important consultative role and illuminates additional information or datasets needed by stakeholders.[29]

CONCLUSION

It makes a difference who is involved in advocating for open data because different actors are motivated by different goals, and the mix of

---

29 See New York City Transparency Working Group, at http://nyctwg.org/.

goals pursued will produce different outcomes for the initiative, at least in the short term. What motivates governments to create an open data initiative may differ from the goals that citizens' groups, community service organizations, journalists, academics, or civic hackers may have in using open data. These different motivations will influence which data sets are made available and maintained. Therefore, wide participation in the early stages of an initiative will help to shape it to the community's preferences. Being aware of the range of options, methods, and roles in open data initiatives eases the process of figuring out how different user groups can get what they need from open data. All stakeholders may begin by identifying their own role within the open data ecosystem.

For government agencies, beginning an open data initiative can be as simple as discovering which data sets are publicly available online, collecting them together on a single page, and conducting outreach to increase awareness and gather feedback about the holdings. They can inform the public that the data can be used without restriction, and they can make the data available in formats that facilitate that use. If governments are ready to consider a more comprehensive process, they can begin by identifying their primary goals for the open data initiative, meet with relevant stakeholders, and explore the Sunlight Foundation's resources for open data policy development.

Nongovernment organizations—whether community-serving groups, research institutions, associations of journalists, or citizens' groups—can help lead change by opening up their own data. They can also participate by advocating for their local governments to develop or improve an open data initiative. Where collaboration with government is more challenging, it is possible to create a community open data portal with partner organizations. Asking for input from local civic technologists, such as local Code for America brigades or civic hacker MeetUp groups, may help groups more quickly use open data to achieve organizational goals.

Open data initiatives are still relatively new, but through persistent and positive interaction between government agencies and citizens, this new government function can achieve many important public interest goals. Resources developed by the Sunlight Foundation and other national groups, as well as highlights and lessons from emerging initiatives, can motivate new localities to launch their own open data practice and promote continuous improvement of existing efforts. By sharing our experiences, we can advance the state of practice and achieve the maximum social and economic benefits from opening up government data.

■   ■   ■

EMILY SHAW *oversees state and local policy work for the Sunlight Foundation in Washington, DC. She holds a PhD in political science from the University of California, Berkeley and a BA from Brown University. Before coming to the Sunlight Foundation she taught political science and worked for a variety of civil and human rights organizations. In all of her work she is a regular and enthusiastic user of open government data.*

A thoughtful analysis of the factors that contributed to the collapse of mortgage markets was hampered by the lack of a dataset that included information on borrowers along with information on mortgage underwriting, pricing and performance. This essay describes the process and challenges of creating the National Mortgage Database (NMDB), which, when complete, will combine these data from many sources. Creation of such a database requires navigation of homeowner, business, and public policy interests. Among other things, the NMDB will lead to a better understanding of the recent financial crisis and, perhaps, why mortgages perform as they do.

THE CREATION OF THE NATIONAL MORTGAGE DATABASE

Robert Avery
Federal Housing Finance Agency

Marsha J. Courchane
Charles River Associates

Peter Zorn
Freddie Mac

Public policy, regulatory agendas and the growing enthusiasm with big data have sparked an interest in the creation of comprehensive data sets to better monitor and understand financial markets. In this chapter, we use the experiences gained in constructing the National Mortgage Database (NMDB) to offer insights into the process and challenges of dataset creation. When complete, the NMDB, a joint effort of the Federal Housing Finance Agency (FHFA), the Consumer Financial Protection Bureau (CFPB), and Freddie Mac, will be a comprehensive database of loan-level information combined with information on associated properties and borrowers, starting with mortgages outstanding in 1998.

The NMDB will, among other things, help us to better understand the recent financial crisis and, as the market evolves, how and, perhaps, why mortgages perform as they do. With this knowledge, we can develop better mortgage products that meet the needs of a changing population, and far more effectively supervise and monitor the players in the housing finance market—perhaps avoiding or mitigating any future crises. The creation of the NMDB has been and continues to be an enormously challenging task. It requires bringing together multiple data sets, each developed for a specific purpose, covering different time periods and universes, and owned or operated by several public and private parties. This essay describes how the dataset is being built.

THE INTENT OF THE DATA

The first stage in any data creation exercise considers the purpose of the dataset's usage. From its inception, the NMDB was intended to be used to address a wide variety of economic and policy related questions. For example, the NMDB is designed to provide more accuracy in order to:

- Satisfy statutory report mandates such as those required under the Homeownership Economic Recovery Act of 2008 (HERA) for the FHFA, or under the Dodd-Frank Act for the CFPB and the Department of Housing and Urban Development (HUD).

- Measure trends in delinquencies for first and associated second lien mortgages overall and for many subpopulations (such as by previous mortgage status, credit score, race/ethnicity, geography and others).

- Analyze the effectiveness of actions to reduce delinquencies and examine changes in indebtedness and credit scores over time.

- Benchmark performance for regulatory oversight and enable regulators to monitor and set targets for the affordable housing performance of Fannie Mae and Freddie Mac (the GSEs) and institutions subject to the Community Reinvestment Act (CRA). In particular, performance of mortgages in targeted programs, such as the Federal Housing Administration (FHA), and those meeting the standards of the GSEs, can be compared to performance of a market-wide portfolio of comparable mortgages matched by date of origination, geography, loan size, borrower credit score and other factors.

- Evaluate the efficacy and potential impact of counseling programs on mortgage performance, as well as counseling's potential impact on "distressed" borrowers.

- Using the NMDB's survey and performance components, analyze the suitability of borrowers' mortgage choices and their ability to sustain the mortgage, which will allow for the assessment of proposals to limit unfair or abusive lending activities.

- Determine the contributions to and causes of the recent subprime crisis (both the boom and bust phases), as well as assess methods that may reduce the likelihood of its recurrence, using either the mortgage or borrower as the unit of analysis.

- Allow limited conceptual analysis of broad fair lending issues on a national and market (although not lender) basis, using key information on mortgage terms and conditions, as well as borrowers' credit worthiness and wealth.

- Enable policymakers, researchers and regulators to improve their prepayment and default modeling and to implement "stress-test" scenarios for the entire U.S. mortgage market or for a subset of mortgages, incorporating assumptions about house prices, default and prepayment.

These potential uses determined the following key design requirements for the NMDB:

Representativeness: The purpose of the NMDB is to make inferences about the market. It is absolutely critical, therefore, that the NMDB be representative of the entire mortgage market.

Comprehensiveness: The NMDB is designed to address a wide variety of issues. This requires an equally wide variety of data, including detailed information about the mortgage, associated borrowers, and the underlying property. It also requires loan level data to conduct detailed analyses.

Timeliness: The intended regulatory and policy demands of the NMDB require that data on mortgage originations and mortgage performance be made available in relatively short order.

Usefulness: The intended public policy focus of the NMDB means that the data must be accessible to a wide variety of researchers, analysts, and housing and mortgage market advocates and practitioners in a form they can easily use but that balances privacy and competitive concerns.

COMPARISON OF DESIGN CRITERIA
WITH EXISTING DATA SOURCES

Based on these design criteria, existing databases were examined to determine the extent to which they already met the requirements and to assess their utility in constructing the NMDB. The primary sources explored were the Home Mortgage Disclosure Act (HMDA), the Federal Reserve Bank of New York's Equifax Consumer Credit Panel, and the servicing databases owned by CoreLogic and LPS McDash. We also looked at public survey databases, including the American Housing Survey (AHS), the Survey of Consumer Finances (SCF), the Consumer Expenditure Survey (CES) and the Panel Study of Income Dynamics (PSID). We found that no existing data sets fully met the design criteria. In general, this is because a tradeoff exists between representativeness and comprehensiveness—data that are representative are rarely comprehensive, and data that are comprehensive are rarely representative.

The HMDA data include loan applications and outcomes for most mortgages with selected information about the loan, property, and borrower. The data are arguably the most representative publicly available existing data source about the mortgage market. However, it contains no information on loan performance, has little information on borrower credit-worthiness, and has up to a 21-month delay in release.

The Federal Reserve Bank of New York/Equifax Consumer Credit Panel provides a nationally representative 1-in-20 sample of individuals with credit records, observed quarterly from 1999 onward. However, little attempt has been made to clean the data of duplicates, and no additional fields have been merged to the original data. Thus, important information is missing about mortgages in the files, such as loan purpose, owner-occupancy, pricing, loan-to-value ratio, income and borrower demographics. Finally, these data have only limited accessibility to FRB staff.

The semi-annual American Housing Survey (AHS) contains comprehensive information on a nationally representative 1-in-2000 sample of mortgages of owner-occupied properties with very good property data and good borrower demographics. However, it contains no information on mortgage performance and limited information on the mortgage itself. Moreover, its public release is significantly delayed from the time the data are originally collected. The other nationally representative data sources (SCF, CES, PSID) contain no information on mortgage performance, provide only a small number of observations, and are released with significant lags.

CoreLogic and LPS McDash produce loan-level databases with performance information collected from the firms that service the mortgages. The servicing fields available from CoreLogic and LPS McDash are relatively comprehensive in both variables and size—the CoreLogic database claims about 32 million active mortgage loans, while the LPS McDash database claims about 40 million active mortgage loans. However, they offer no assurance of being representative, as they are composed of data collected from only about 25 servicers each. Moreover, mortgages cannot be tracked if servicing is transferred. Other drawbacks include limited and very costly access, minimal borrower demographics, and no information on other borrower obligations.

The credit repository data from Equifax, Experian, and Transunion are rich in credit information—by construction they incorporate data on credit card debt, installment loans, credit inquires and public records for the consumers they cover. Their marketing data add borrower characteristics including age, gender, and marital status. These data also include information on the borrowers' moves and summary measures of their addresses such as census tract. However, there are important areas that are not covered. They lack some information on borrowers (e.g., race/ethnicity and income), mortgages (e.g., loan product and contract rate), and the underlying property (e.g., location and value).

Given these diverse and incomplete existing data sources, it was clear that a new database—the NMDB—would be required to meet the design requirements. The NMDB is designed as a 1-in-20 sample of all first lien, single-family mortgages rather than a universal registry. A sample can be large enough to support many different types of analyses but small enough to manage logistically, thus dramatically reducing both dollar and administrative costs. In addition, the use of a sampling frame permits the potential creation of a public-use version of the NMDB under federal privacy guidelines.

Credit repository data offered the best source from which to draw a nationally representative sample of mortgages. The three credit repositories all actively pursue loan servicers as data providers. As a result, they obtain information on almost the entire population of non-private mortgage loans made in the United States.

DEVELOPING THE PILOT

The NMDB is unusual in its use of credit repository data as a sampling frame, which merges these data with other available sources to create a fully comprehensive data set. Given the novelty of its approach, it was critical to pilot its development prior to embarking on the creation of the complete database. Funded by Freddie Mac, the pilot enabled us to explore and resolve several critical issues. These included transforming consumer-level credit repository data to the mortgage-level NMDB and using the credit repository's archives to construct the NMDB retrospectively, as if data had been collected on newly originated mortgages since 1998.

This required extensive collaboration with credit repository staff, and involved much "learning by doing." The result of these efforts ensured that the complete version of the NMDB could successfully commence relatively shortly after being funded.

Credit repository data provides the basic terms of the sampled mortgages, monthly updates on their performance, information on any second liens on the sampled properties, and data on the other debt obligations of all the sampled mortgage borrowers and co-signers (including credit cards and car loans). The use of credit history provides information about borrowers' experiences with earlier mortgages and the continued tracking of sampled borrowers until one year after termination allows for the characterization of events following the termination of sampled mortgages. In addition, repository data allow for combining credit information on all co-borrowers to provide household measures of credit worthiness.

However, as noted earlier, the credit repository data lack key information required by the NMDB. The pilot, therefore, explored techniques for merging additionally required data to the core obtained through the repository.

The credit repository data are most effectively merged with other data using personal identifying information (PII). This presents privacy and Fair Credit Reporting Act (FCRA) "permitted purpose" challenges. Under the pilot, legally acceptable, but equally effective, procedures were developed to merge credit bureau data with data from third-party providers of property information (such as purchase price) and with HMDA data to provide borrower race, ethnicity, sex and income.

Finally, there is a survey component built into the NMDB designed to collect information on borrowers' experiences and attitudes that are not otherwise obtainable. It also provides an opportunity to collect critical information on contemporaneous issues or policy of regulatory interest.

An advisory group including participants from government agencies, non-profit organizations, consumer advocacy groups, trade and industry groups and academia provided guidance as we developed the survey instrument. Three overlapping mail surveys were developed and tested: one aimed at borrowers with newly originated mortgages; a second sent to those with active mortgages, and a third for those with terminated mortgages. The survey solicits information on financial literacy and homeownership counseling; mortgage shopping; the mortgage closing process; expectations about house price appreciation and critical household financial events; the existence of "trigger" events such as unemployment spells, large medical expenses and divorce; and detailed demographic information.

The process of administering the surveys was also examined. The FCRA restricts the NMDB survey to a mail format, which reduces costs but can substantially lower accuracy and response rates. To determine the best way encourage a high response rate, we tested several incentive strategies and cover letters.

DATA PRODUCTION

The pilot served as a proof of concept for the NMDB. Production of a complete database, however, requires permanent funding, as the database requires an extensive investment in data preparation, data cleaning, documentation and presentation. The first step, then, was securing funding. Formalizing the NMDB as a government resource was believed to be the most appropriate method likely to minimize duplicative effort while providing the best opportunity to make the resulting data publicly available. Additionally, the federal government is likely to be the major user of the NMDB. As a result, the FHFA and CFPB have taken the lead in the development of the database, with support from Freddie Mac staff.

Next, we needed to select a credit repository and other partners. The production staff issued a Request for Proposal and chose Experian as its credit repository partner. It is also working with other federal agencies, such as the Federal Housing Authority, the Department of Veterans Affairs, and the Rural Housing Service for assistance in administrative file matching, and is exploring relationships with third-party data providers.

Ultimately, the production team must build on the efforts engaged in the pilot to produce a working dataset. The primary data challenges in creating the NMDB are as follows:

- Repository data are designed to provide once-a-month snapshots; they are not designed for tracking over time.

- Repository files contain many duplicative records of a single mortgage. Duplication appears to be a particular problem for mortgages originated prior to 2007, where duplicates account for roughly 25 percent of these loans.

- The repository files contain no direct measures on the purpose of a mortgage loan (home purchase or refinance) or whether it is for an owner-occupied property, vacation home or investor property and only imperfectly classify first and second liens.

- The address of the property associated with the mortgage proves to be both important and elusive; mortgage servicers report the billing address of the mortgage borrowers, but this is not necessarily the property address, particularly for mortgages on non-owner occupied properties.

- Matching to external data sources is critical for ensuring the comprehensiveness of the NMDB. While HMDA matching has proved feasible, match procedures for other data sources are under development.

The production team must develop tools and procedures to address these issues. This includes developing and documenting mechanized data cleaning and scrubbing protocols, resolving data duplications and inconsistencies, developing tools for tracking individuals and mortgages over time, determining the "best" value of variables that are available from multiple sources, merging with external data sets, and imputing values for missing key variables. In addition, to achieve scale and consistency, the production team must develop computer algorithms and protocols for processing the data as part of regular production maintenance.

ACCESS AND AVAILABILITY OF DATA

In order to be useful, the NMDB data must be both accessible and relatively straightforward to use. These are significant challenges. The size and comprehensiveness of the database is its strength, but it also creates difficulties for users. The detailed information it contains raises privacy concerns, which poses a threat to its accessibility. The NMDB production team is exploring techniques for addressing these concerns.

Access to the NMDB likely will be provided initially only to Freddie Mac and federal government staff while privacy concerns and data complexities are resolved. The long-term vision includes the development of alternative versions of the NMDB with various levels of access depending on the type of information included. The complete dataset, including PII, will be maintained by Experian alone. PII will be used only for data matching or survey operations, which will be conducted using techniques to ensure that PII as well as other proprietary information is fully protected.

The fully "cleaned" version of the NMDB will be the primary one used for supervision, analysis and research and to create regular public reports on the condition of the mortgage market. One variant, which will be updated quarterly, may be used to track sample mortgages, with the mortgage as the unit of analysis. A second variant could be the historic database used to study the mortgage crisis, where either mortgages or borrowers can be used as the unit of analysis.

Federal employees and employees of the Federal Reserve Banks, Federal Home Loan Banks, Freddie Mac and Fannie Mae will be granted access to this full, cleaned version of the dataset, including geographic information to the census tract level.[1] These users will be held to strict security standards to ensure that potentially sensitive information is not released. NMDB project staff is also exploring ways to grant access to the full dataset to researchers outside of the federal government. One idea under consideration is the use of access processes similar to those employed by the Census Bureau.

NMDB project staff will also develop a data interface for the full dataset that facilitates a broad range of queries addressable with aggregated data. There are two goals here. First, a majority of potential users of the NMDB are expected to be interested in relatively simple questions. An interface will well serve these requests, and provide access to the NMDB for a wide variety of people and for many purposes. Second, by using only aggregated results, the interface will address privacy concerns. This expands the use and usefulness of the NMDB. A potential further version of the database could include only information on borrowers who have participated in the NMDB origination survey, and would be made available to the public once the release meets federal privacy guidelines.

Finally, if feasible, a public version of the full NMDB dataset will be made available. This requires that standards be developed to ensure that data released fully meet federal privacy and FCRA guidelines. It is not yet clear whether this database can be released at a mortgage or borrower level. Possibly, access will only be available to aggregated data, which can nevertheless be used to respond to a wide variety of queries.

LEARNING FROM DEVELOPMENT OF THE NMDB

The creation of the NMDB has not been without challenges. These can be categorized into three primary areas: accessing and merging commercially available data with less public data; providing clean rather than raw data; and granting access to the database, given restrictions from the FCRA and privacy concerns.

---

1   Because of contract restrictions, information on the lender and servicer will not be included.

The goal was to create the ideal database. All existing databases were faulty due to lack of representativeness or due to a lack of critical data fields. The tradeoff made was to sample from the most inclusive database currently available (the credit repository sampling frame) and to supplement with everything else needed. Hence, the NMDB focused on representativeness and inclusiveness. Even so, compromises were necessary, and no researcher will have everything they might like. For example, contract restrictions prevent including information on the lender and servicer and on more detailed geographic areas. Even with its limitations, the NMDB offers researchers and policymakers an invaluable resource that can contribute to better informed public policy and practice in the mortgage arena. It sets a new precedent by brokering access for public purposes to the rich information previously locked in commercial databases. Linking the credit data with critical elements from other public and private data sets can bring us closer to understanding both the complex dynamics of the mortgage market and financial implications for households.

The process of creating any database should follow the same general steps the NMDB team followed. First, start with an understanding of which questions are being raised and which answers can be sought. Second, find out whether existing databases can meet the needs. Next, assuming none exist, find the best one to start with and choose a sampling frame. Test the data collection process. Validate the data. Perfect the data to the extent possible, including processes for cleaning and removing duplication. Finally, be sure to plan for data release to allow access to the insights from the data while protecting privacy.

Our experience suggests that by following these steps, it is possible to create a database blending data from multiple sources that can be generally and widely used for a variety of purposes with substantial accuracy.

■ ■ ■

ROBERT AVERY *is the project director of the National Mortgage Database at the Federal Housing Finance Agency. He joined the FHFA after retiring as a senior economist from the Board of Governors of the Federal Reserve System. Previously, he was a professor at Cornell University and an assistant professor at Carnegie Mellon University.*

■ ■ ■

MARSHA J. COURCHANE, *vice president and practice leader, Charles River Associates, heads the Financial Economics Practice in the US/UK and is a leading expert in the areas of mortgage and consumer lending. Courchane engages in research, consulting, and litigation support with respect to mortgage markets, discrimination in lending, consumer credit, securitization, credit risk, and redlining issues.*

■ ■ ■

PETER ZORN *is vice president of housing analysis and research at Freddie Mac. He has been employed at Freddie Mac since 1994. Prior to that, he was an associate professor in the department of consumer economics and housing at Cornell University. His research interests focus on financial literacy, affordable lending, fair lending and default and prepayment modeling.*

IN BRIEF

APPLYING TECHNOLOGY ADVANCES TO IMPROVE PUBLIC ACCESS TO MORTGAGE DATA

Ren Essene and Michael Byrne
Consumer Financial Protection Bureau

"Sunlight is said to be the best of disinfectants"
—Justice Louis D. Brandeis

Recent open government initiatives view data as a "valuable national resource." Project Open Data and others are providing data sets to the general public and private-sector innovators "to promote efficiency and effectiveness in government, but also...to create economic opportunity and improve citizens' quality of life."[1]

Data can help community leaders understand how well current policies are working and advance evidence-based policymaking. The community development sector has a long history of using data and metrics alongside community members' stories to inform policymaking. Two civil rights era statutes from the 1970s, the Community Reinvestment Act (CRA) and the Home Mortgage Disclosure Act (HMDA), implicitly encourage citizen groups working to improve their communities to use data to augment the more formal regulatory and enforcement establishment.[2]

Although there continues to be a push to release more data sets, many open data advocates are also focused on the quality and value of the

---

1 Project Open Data [website]: http://project-open-data.github.io/.

2 A. Fishbein, "The Ongoing Experiment with 'Regulation from Below': Expanded Reporting Requirements for HMDA and CRA," *Housing Policy Debate*, 3 (2) (1992): 601–636.

data. The idea that public disclosure can improve market functioning, engendering both greater fairness and efficiency, depends critically on the quality and value of the public information available. As the community development sector has long understood, data need to be relevant, easily accessible, and easy to use.

In keeping with these objectives, the Consumer Financial Protection Bureau (CFPB) has developed new mortgage data tools to provide public HMDA data in more user-friendly forms to improve transparency in the mortgage market. These tools make it easier for the public to analyze market trends and emerging risks. Public officials also gain improved access to the public data to conduct analyses that may inform future policymaking and research.

HMDA BACKGROUND

In response to community development issues in the 1960s and 1970s, including urban blight caused by mortgage redlining by thrift institutions and banks, Congress passed a series of federal laws to prevent discrimination, discourage redlining, and encourage reinvestment in the nation's cities.[3] Enacted in 1975, HMDA provides communities with greater transparency about local lending activities as a way to encourage a fair and functioning mortgage market, particularly for low-income and minority neighborhoods. At its core, HMDA is a simple statute: it ensures transparency by requiring many mortgage lenders to collect, report, and publicly disclose data about their home lending activities. HMDA data currently capture the majority of mortgage loans made, loans sold, and applications received for home purchase, refinance, and home improvement in metropolitan areas.[4]

Initially, Congress was focused on discrimination at the neighborhood (census tract) level. The two original purposes of HMDA include: 1) to help determine whether financial institutions were serving the housing needs of

---

3 P. McCoy, "The Home Mortgage Disclosure Act: A Synopsis and Recent Legislative History," *Journal of Real Estate Research* 29 (2007): 381–397. These laws include Title VIII of the Civil Rights Act (1968), the Equal Credit Opportunity Act (1974), the CRA (1977), and HMDA (1975).

4 Financial institutions that meet the metropolitan statistical area (MSA) asset and loan threshold tests report their lending activities in non-MSA areas, while financial institutions that do not have a home or branch office in an MSA generally do not report their lending activity. See FFIEC, "A Guide to HMDA Reporting: Getting it Right!" (Washington, DC: FFIEC, December 30, 2013), available at www.ffiec.gov/hmda/guide.htm.

their communities; and 2) to help public officials distribute public-sector investment to attract private investment to needed areas. In the late 1980s, studies highlighted potential race-based lending discrimination, and Congress responded with broad changes to HMDA. In particular, Congress amended HMDA to require itemization by "racial characteristics," which assists in identifying possible discriminatory lending patterns and enforcing antidiscrimination statutes.

HMDA's statutory text and legislative history show that the law was designed to put data in the hands of the public as well as government officials. Spurred by community advocates and in response to changing market products and practices during the past 39 years, Congress and the Federal Reserve Board have updated, respectively, HMDA and its implementing Regulation C significantly to improve the volume and types of information publicly available. For example, in 1980, the Federal Financial Institutions Examination Council (FFIEC) was directed to compile data for metropolitan areas and produce aggregate tables for institutions by categories such as census tracts, age of housing, income, and race.[5] Following additional statutory changes in 1989, Regulation C was revised to require financial institutions to record loan-level information on the "Loan/Application Register" (LAR), including information about race, ethnicity, sex, income, and application disposition.

Today, HMDA is the preeminent source of data about the US mortgage market and is used by community advocates, economists, social scientists, the news media, government agencies, and financial institutions. HMDA data have been used to understand community lending patterns across different characteristics, such as income, race, and ethnicity. This understanding has driven policy related to community investment strategies, helped bank regulators and other agencies supervise financial institutions, ensured greater compliance with the CRA, and aided in the enforcement of fair lending laws. In response to the Great Recession, Congress passed

---

5   The FFIEC is a formal interagency body empowered to prescribe uniform principles, standards, and report forms for the federal examination of financial institutions by the Board of Governors of the Federal Reserve System (FRB), the Federal Deposit Insurance Corporation (FDIC), the National Credit Union Administration (NCUA), the Office of the Comptroller of the Currency (OCC), and the CFPB, and to make recommendations to promote uniformity in the supervision of financial institutions. In 2006, the State Liaison Committee (SLC) was added to the Council as a voting member. The SLC includes representatives from the Conference of State Bank Supervisors (CSBS), the American Council of State Savings Supervisors (ACSSS), and the National Association of State Credit Union Supervisors (NASCUS). See http://www.ffiec.gov/.

the Dodd-Frank Act, which transferred HMDA rulemaking authority to the newly established CFPB and added new reporting requirements.

MODERNIZING HMDA

The CFPB's modernization efforts address the three stages of HMDA data: collection, reporting and processing, and publication. In implementing the Dodd-Frank Act changes to HMDA, the CFPB has proposed to reform the HMDA data collection.[6] Alongside this rulemaking, the CFPB is working to modernize and improve the reporting and processing of the future HMDA data set to mitigate burden and increase efficiency for industry. The CFPB has also worked to improve data publication, as robust public access allows for greater public transparency and utility, ultimately better serving the purposes of HMDA.

HMDA has an established history as a high-quality public data source for technically sophisticated users analyzing mortgage market applications, originations, and loan purchase activity. These users are generally academic, industry, or government researchers with statistical analysis and statistical software skills. Although full data files are available to the public on the interagency FFIEC website, the size and complexity of the data can be hard for the public to digest and understand. Beyond the data files, the FFIEC also releases aggregate and disclosure reports that aggregate and display the data by different geographies and financial institutions.[7] However, some of the primary audiences have found the information difficult to use. Although the data have become more accessible as technology has advanced, community advocates continue to call for the information to be more user-friendly.[8]

The CFPB employs a user-centric design approach to technology development. Therefore, to understand better the challenges that HMDA data

---

6 On July 24, 2014, the CFPB issued on its website a proposed rule to implement the Dodd-Frank Act changes to HMDA and make other improvements in Regulation C. See: http://www.consumerfinance. gov/newsroom/cfpb-proposes-rule-to-improve-information-about-access-to-credit-in-the-mortgage-market/. The proposed rule was published in the Federal Register on August 29, 2014. *See* 79 Fed. Reg. 51732 (August 29, 2014).

7 For a listing of reports see FFIEC, "HMDA Aggregate and Disclosure Reports" [website] (Washington, DC: FFIEC), available at https://www.ffiec.gov/hmdaadwebreport/abouthmda.htm.

8 The Federal Reserve Board conducted hearings on HMDA reform in 2010 to gather suggestions for improvements. Many panelists called for improved public access to the data. For more detail on the hearings, see www.federalreserve.gov/communitydev/hmda_hearings.htm.

users face, the CFPB reached out to community groups, think tanks, academia, and other regulatory agencies asking how they currently use HMDA data and what barriers exist to greater use. These initial user interviews suggested that local government, community groups, and students, in particular, would benefit from more accessible HMDA data. Users expressed interest in a web layout, default data, download options, custom geographies, save search function, user forums, mapping capabilities, and panel data that are more intuitive and easier to use. Users also wanted improved data documentation.

Once the problem was clear, the initial solution prioritized broadening the user base and helping less technically sophisticated users to download smaller slices of HMDA data. The CFPB then put its technology experts to the task of designing a web-based solution. The initial result is a new public data platform that enables queries to the data to be processed almost instantly, providing data users with both a simple summary statistic and the complete underlying data used to develop that summary. This technology approach is a great step forward for large data delivery to less sophisticated users.

NEW MORTGAGE DATA TOOLS

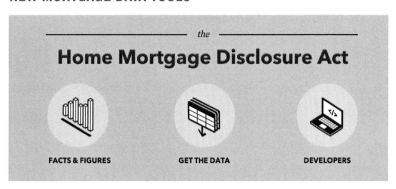

The CFPB's open source HMDA public data platform (available at www. consumerfinance.gov/hmda) provides information for a variety of users. Basic *facts and figures* provide a snapshot of annual mortgage data; *get the data* allows users to filter and download just the data they need; and *developers* offers access to the underlying application programming interface (API) to allow developers to build their own tools and contribute to the open source tools.

Facts & Figures

Homepage: The homepage shows some basic trends and infographics to orient the user, along with linking to a video that describes what is in the data.

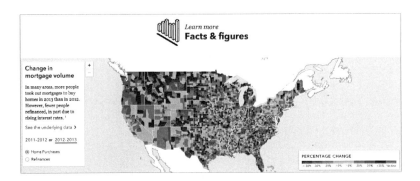

Get the Data

Users can either extract a bulk download or download filtered data since 2007, allowing users to better understand the mortgage market trends in their communities. For less sophisticated users, the tools allow users to construct custom filters and queries and download the data in multiple formats, depending on the users' software options. Users can also share filtered data through the new platform's "share" function to encourage a robust civic debate.

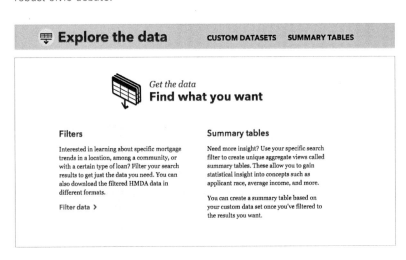

Custom Filters: Through links from the homepage, users can choose to see only the data that interest them. The data can be filtered by geography (state, metropolitan area, county, and census tract), loan characteristics, property type, and more. The website provides some suggested filters to help users get started.

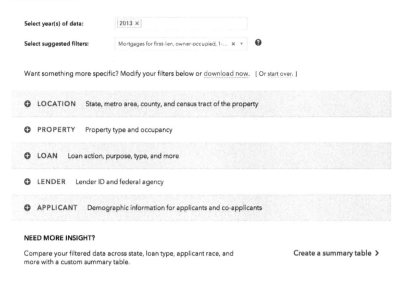

Filter the data

Select year(s) of data: `2013 ×`

Select suggested filters: `Mortgages for first-lien, owner-occupied, 1-... × ▾` ❓

Want something more specific? Modify your filters below or download now. [Or start over.]

⊕ LOCATION   State, metro area, county, and census tract of the property

⊕ PROPERTY   Property type and occupancy

⊕ LOAN   Loan action, purpose, type, and more

⊕ LENDER   Lender ID and federal agency

⊕ APPLICANT   Demographic information for applicants and co-applicants

NEED MORE INSIGHT?

Compare your filtered data across state, loan type, applicant race, and more with a custom summary table.

Create a summary table ❯

Custom Summary Tables: Similarly, users can create summary tables of information. For example, users can compare refinances and home purchases over the past few years, or see county-level trends in federally related mortgages.

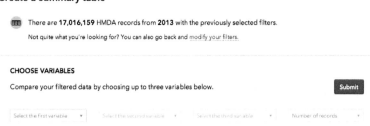

Create a summary table

▦ There are **17,016,159** HMDA records from **2013** with the previously selected filters.

Not quite what you're looking for? You can also go back and modify your filters.

CHOOSE VARIABLES

Compare your filtered data by choosing up to three variables below.   **Submit**

| Select the first variable ▾ | Select the second variable ▾ | Select the third variable ▾ | Number of records ▾ |

Data Downloads: Once users select the data they want, they can download that data in a variety of formats, including CSV, which is compatible with most spreadsheet programs, and JSON, JSONP, and XML, which are standards commonly used by software developers. Users can also preview the first 100 records returned before downloading the data.

Save and Share Results: With a click on the "share" button, the user is provided a link to a unique web address for the query to share. This link can be pasted into a document, an email, or into social media, such as a Facebook post.

TOOLS FOR DEVELOPERS

Software developers can use and contribute to the API. Developers who want to build their own tools using the API can browse the documentation, and if there are technical questions, they can engage with CFPB developers using GitHub issue tracking.[9]

The new HMDA platform was built entirely on GitHub, an open source collaborative tool for developing software. Software engineers and developers interested in improving the underlying public data platform can also get involved on GitHub.[10]

POTENTIAL ENHANCEMENTS

Launching a new platform for data publication is only the first step. The work to date addresses today's primary consumers of public HMDA data: community-based researchers. Although this is an important constituency, the same public data could be used by a broader audience, such as financial institutions, vendors, software developers, and industry researchers. For example, some data users may want to generate interactive data products, such as community-level maps and dynamic data visualizations. To support these applications, the CFPB could invest in the development of APIs to deliver data more efficiently and effectively than a point-and-click user interface.

---

9   The API is available at: https://api.consumerfinance.gov/data. The HMDA API Documentation is available on GitHub at: http://cfpb.github.io/api/hmda/. GitHub issue tracking for HMDA or "project qu" is available at: https://github.com/cfpb/qu/issues?q=is%3Aopen.

10 Project qu, or HMDA, can be found on the collaborative GitHub tool, available at: https://github.com/CFPB/qu.

Moving forward, the CFPB aspires to continue to implement best-in-breed technology that serves the public good and furthers the goals of HMDA and Regulation C. The CFPB remains committed to open source platforms and to designing technology with smaller, decoupled components as discussed above. Open source platforms enable collaboration and transparency between the CFPB and regulated institutions, helping to reduce regulatory burden by providing opportunities for program enhancements and efficiencies. These strategies also hold the potential to reduce the long-term cost of maintaining out-of-date disparate technology and reduce the large, ongoing costs of proprietary software contracts, allowing for more efficient use of government resources. Although technology gains have improved access to data, these gains may also help to ensure greater consumer protections as well. Meanwhile, future data publications will need to balance concerns for consumers' privacy with the benefits of broad public access.

CONCLUSION

Ultimately, public data and the related open-source software are a public good. With the continuing drive toward data-driven policymaking, public data may become a vital part of the next generation of civic infrastructure.[11] Government has an important role to play in ensuring that the data are relevant, accessible, and easy to use by a broad set of stakeholders, including the public, community groups, government agencies, regulated entities, and researchers more generally. This continued modernization is responsive to user needs and provides for greater use and transparency, allowing for greater democratic participation in housing and mortgage policies.

Specifically, technology advances help to improve the methods of data publication. Data consumers, whether they are community leaders, researchers, financial institutions, or the general public, typically have at least a basic ability to manipulate digital data and an expectation that data will be delivered via interactive web-based tools. The CFPB has released new HMDA data tools as a first step to meeting these open data and new technology demands. Ultimately, increased access to public data can help community leaders foster a healthy conversation about community issues and further the purposes of HMDA.

---

11 A. Howard, "The Art and Science of Data-driven Journalism." (New York: Tow Center for Digital Journalism, Columbia Journalism School, May 2014), p. 15.

■ ■ ■

REN ESSENE *currently serves as the program manager of mortgage data assets in the Division of Research, Markets and Regulations at the Consumer Financial Protection Bureau (CFPB) and is the HMDA team lead. Previously she served as a supervisory policy analyst for the Board of Governors of the Federal Reserve System and co-authored a book chapter with Allen Fishbein entitled "The Home Mortgage Disclosure Act at Thirty-Five: Past History, Current Issues" in Moving Forward: The Future of Consumer Credit and Mortgage Finance (Brookings Press). Prior, Ren conducted research and engaged in policy efforts at the Federal Reserve Bank of Boston and the Joint Center for Housing Studies at Harvard.*

■ ■ ■

MICHAEL BYRNE *is currently a project director in the Technology and Innovation Division at the Consumer Financial Protection Bureau. He is the lead for implementing the technology supporting Home Mortgage Disclosure Act activities for CFPB. Prior to joining CFPB, he was the geographic information officer at the Federal Communications Commission. Prior to that, he was the geographic information officer for the State of California.*

The views expressed are those of the authors and do not necessarily reflect those of the Consumer Financial Protection Bureau or the United States.

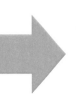

This essay lays out three policy trends related to data: open data, My Data, and smart disclosure. It highlights opportunities for practitioners to tap into each trend to further their missions, from augmenting traditional activities to creating activities that may be less familiar, such as holding hackathons for software developers to build apps that help residents access community services. The essay provides real-world examples of how community groups are taking advantage of these trends and includes practical steps groups can take to start harnessing open data, My Data, and smart disclosure to support families and strengthen communities.

THREE DATA ACCESS TRENDS SHAPING THE FUTURE OF COMMUNITY DEVELOPMENT: OPEN DATA, MY DATA, AND SMART DISCLOSURE

Amias Gerety
U.S. Treasury Department Office of Financial Institutions

Sophie Raseman
U.S. Treasury Department Office of Consumer Policy

The rise of data has emerged as a major force shaping our lives and communities. There is a growing recognition that expanding access to data can further social and policy goals, including those in community development. The community development field has increasingly turned its attention to how to use data effectively to drive decision making within organizations and to inform policy—an issue covered in depth by this book. Our essay lays out three key policy trends related to data that have received somewhat less attention in the field: open data, My Data, and smart disclosure. We highlight opportunities for community development practitioners to tap into each trend to further their missions in various ways, from augmenting traditional activities such as planning, to creating activities that may be less familiar, such as holding hackathons for software developers to build apps that help residents access community services. Along the way, we provide real-world examples of how community groups are taking advantage of these trends. We conclude by sharing a few practical steps community groups can take to start harnessing open data, My Data, and smart disclosure to support families and strengthen our nation's communities.

TREND #1: OPEN DATA

The first trend is open data—the release of data that the public can easily access and use. Government agencies are often thought of as the primary publishers of open data; however, business, nonprofit organizations, researchers, and other private entities are increasingly adopting open data policies as a core practice.

What makes data open?[1] Open data should be as easy to use as possible. This means data formats should be "machine readable"—that is, able to be processed by readily available software.[2] Open data should involve nonproprietary data formats (e.g., CSV) so that users are not obliged to license particular software to use the data. Finally, open data should be easy to access. For example, an open data publisher may allow the public to download the data in bulk or access the data through an application programming interface (API) that allows developers to write software that can automatically request data. The public should also have legal rights to reuse data—the broader the public's rights to reuse, the more open the data.[3]

Open data have taken root at the federal, state, and local levels. The Obama administration has created Data.gov, a platform that allows the public to search tens of thousands of federal open data sets. In May 2013, President Obama directed steps to increase the amount of open

---

1   The federal Open Data Policy defines open data as "publicly available data structured in a way that enables the data to be fully discoverable and usable by end users." Office of Management and Budget, "Managing Information as an Asset." OMB Memorandum M-13-13 (Washington, DC: OMB, May 9, 2013) [hereinafter the federal Open Data Policy], http://www.whitehouse.gov/sites/default/files/omb/memoranda/2013/m-13-13.pdf. For an in-depth discussion of the definition of open data from one nongovernment organization's perspective, see Open Knowledge Foundation, *Open Data Handbook* (Cambridge, UK: Open Knowledge Foundation, 2012), http://opendatahandbook.org/en/index.html. Tim Berners-Lee, Director of the World Wide Web Consortium (W3C) and member of the UK government's Transparency Board, has proposed a five-star continuum of linked open data. See post, "Linked Data" (July 27, 2006), http://www.w3.org/DesignIssues/LinkedData.html. The Sunlight Foundation, a nonprofit organization advocating for government transparency and accountability, has developed 10 principles for open data, available here: http://sunlightfoundation.com/policy/documents/ten-open-data-principles/.

2   For a more comprehensive introduction to some of the key technical concepts involved in open data, such as machine readability and application programming interfaces, see Data.gov, "A Primer on Machine Readability for Online Documents and Data" (Washington, DC: Data.gov), www.data.gov/developers/blog/primer-machine-readability-online-documents-and-data.

3   In some cases, governments or private entities may use alternative or hybrid types of open licenses, such as licenses that allow for the free reuse of data for noncommercial purposes. See, e.g., the Open Knowledge Foundation's Open Data Commons, http://opendatacommons.org/ (free legal tools to help the public provide and use open data, including model licenses).

OPEN DATA ARE AFFECTING COMMUNITIES ACROSS THE COUNTRY IN A NUMBER OF WAYS. FOR EXAMPLE:

Thirty-five communities participating in the National Neighborhood Indicators Partnership (NNIP) coordinated by the Urban Institute have created neighborhood-level information systems to support community building and local decision making.[1] Although some of these groups have been collecting government data for more than 20 years, open data efforts by government agencies have expanded the data available for these systems. For example, Urban Strategies Council, the NNIP partner in Oakland, California, launched InfoAlamedaCounty. Using Home Mortgage Disclosure Act (HMDA), foreclosure, and other data to create maps that illuminate trends affecting community residents, InfoAlamedaCounty draws on data sources from federal and local agencies to help support data-driven decision making in Alameda County.[2] Long before the term *open data* was common, community development groups used published data, at no cost, from government sources to understand the needs and opportunities in their communities, identify community assets, and measure changes to shed light on program effectiveness. Advances in open data have fueled growth in the scale and scope of these efforts.

The US government provides the Global Positioning Service (GPS) for civilian use, free of direct user fees. GPS has unleashed innovations that contribute an estimated $90 billion to the U.S. economy each year. GPS also powers mobile apps such as iTriage, which helps consumers find nearby federally subsidized community health centers.[3]

The nonprofit organization OpenPlans has created easy-to-use tools that community groups can employ to collect data to contribute to shaping the future of their neighborhoods and cities. One of its tools, called Shareabouts, allows community groups to collect their own data, visualize the data with mapping software (powered by open map data), facilitate community dialog, and survey residents—and then use that data to influence local planning.[4]

---

1   National Neighborhood Indicators Partnership, http://www.neighborhoodindicators.org/. See T. Kingsley, K. Pettit, and L. Hendey, "Strengthening Local Capacity for Data-Driven Decisionmaking" (Washington, DC: National Neighborhood Indicators Partnership, June 2013), http://www.urban.org/UploadedPDF/412883-Strengthening-Local-Capacity-For-Data-Driven-Decisionmaking.pdf.

2   InfoAlamedaCounty Map Room, http://www.viewer.infoalamedacounty.org/. InfoAlamedaCounty's data sources are listed at http://www.infoalamedacounty.org/index.php/Data/Metadata-Sources.html.

3   For more background on iTriage, see Health Resources and Services Administration, US Department of Health and Human Services, "Health Centers and Look-alike Sites Data Download," http://catalog.data.gov/dataset/health-centers-and-look-alike-sites-data-download. The clinic locations themselves are also available as open data from Health and Human Services.

4   OpenPlans, Shareabouts, http://openplans.org/work/shareabouts/.

data available to the public.[4] Under the new policy, all newly generated government data must be made available in open, machine-readable formats that are designed to ensure privacy and security.

States and local governments have also embraced open data. Cities including Chicago, New York, and San Francisco, for example, have released a wide variety of data sets on local issues, ranging from crime data, to real-time bus routes, to the locations of grocery stores.

Standards are particularly important to make local data usable at national scale. A growing number of local officials and advocates are working to standardize local data formats for data on topics that are common across geographic areas. For example, communities have worked together to promote Open311, a standard, open protocol for nonemergency municipal service requests.[5]

Open data have created new opportunities for innovation throughout the community development field, including in housing, health, education, transportation, workforce development, and financial empowerment. One of the most substantial opportunities for community development organizations is to use open data to enhance data-driven decision making, such as using open data to enhance the mapping of community needs and assets, program evaluations, and planning and participation efforts. Open data can help create tools to map, visualize, and analyze community assets and needs. Data can be used to develop insights on the nature and causes of issues, and to evaluate solutions. Organizations can also take advantage of various free and low-cost software tools to enable residents to interact with—and even help create— open data to learn about issues and to engage in dialog and action.

Data Driven Detroit, an NNIP member, and technology firm Loveland Technologies have used open data to help drive evidence-based planning in their community. The organizations have joined forces to conduct the Motor City Mapping project, in which more than 100 residents helped

---

4 On May 9, 2013, President Obama signed Executive Order No. 13642, "Making Open and Machine Readable the New Default for Government Information." See www.whitehouse.gov/the-press-office/2013/05/09/executive-order-making-open-and-machine-readable-new-default-government-. The Executive Order directs agencies to follow the federal Open Data Policy.

5 See www.Open311.org for more background on the Open311 standardization effort.

to collect and map data about every parcel in Detroit.[6] The project will enable city government, community groups, philanthropists, and the private sector to have a common understanding of the size and spatial pattern of problem properties, and it will help in formulating informed approaches to tackle blight in the city.[7]

Another major opportunity for community organizations is using open data to help connect residents to community services and resources. Community groups can use open data on social services and benefits that already exist in some communities to create tools that help residents access local services. In addition, community groups can use resident feedback and other service quality data to help residents access the highest-quality services available and to inform campaigns to improve services.

Community groups can engage with efforts underway to release and standardize open data on public benefits and social services.[8] For example, the Open Referral Initiative is an effort to develop common standards and open platforms for sharing community resource directory data (e.g., local 2-1-1 systems).[9] It will be important for the community development field to have a voice in these standards development processes so that the standards reflect the unique expertise of the field and the specific needs that community development organizations will have when they use the data.

Finally, privacy must be a cornerstone of any open data effort. In some cases, open data are released in anonymized form (i.e., after being stripped of details, such as names and addresses, that could identify

---

6 For a description of the project, see Skillman Foundation, "Video: See How the Biggest Data Set of Detroit Blight is Being Built" (Detroit, Skillman Foundation, February 7, 2014), available at www. skillman.org/Knowledge-Center/A-Rose-for-Detroit-Blog/Motor-City-Mapping-Detroit-blight-Skillman-Foundation#sthash.x9ugymHl.dpuf.

7 A detailed description of the Motor City Mapping Project and the full report of the Detroit Blight Removal Task Force can be found at the Detroit Blight Removal Task Force site at www.time-toendblight.com.

8 For background on efforts to standardize social service data, see Greg Bloom, "Towards a Community Data Commons." In *Beyond Transparency: Open Data and the Future of Civic Innovation,* edited by Brett Goldstein with Lauren Dyson (San Francisco, CA: Code for America Press, 2013). http://beyondtransparency.org/chapters/part-5/towards-a-community-data-commons/.

9 Open Referral, http://openreferral.org/.

individuals), or in the form of aggregated data derived from data sets that contain personal information. Data must be carefully reviewed so that personal information, particularly sensitive personal information, is not released in a manner inconsistent with the standards or requirements applicable to the entity that maintains the data. Such reviews must consider the mosaic effect, which occurs when the information in an individual data set, in isolation, may not pose a risk of identifying an individual, but when combined with other available information, could pose such risk.

TREND #2: MY DATA

Another key data trend that will help reshape the community development field is "My Data," which involves making data on a particular individual available to that individual in a usable format. The data are provided in a manner designed to ensure privacy and security. My Data efforts aim to help individuals unlock the value of the large amounts of personal data they generate in their daily lives.

Governments, nonprofit organizations, and businesses are embracing My Data in areas including health, education, energy, and personal finance. Patients, for example, are downloading their electronic medical records to share vital information with their doctors. Homeowners are analyzing their energy use data to save money on their bills. Commercial building operators are using data on their electricity use to improve energy efficiency. Students are using their personal data to determine eligibility for college grants and loans.

The technical implementation of My Data has many parallels to open data. The goal of My Data is to make it as easy as possible for an individual to access and use his or her personal data or share the information with trusted third parties. Ideally, individuals can thus access their My Data in open, machine-readable formats on the internet. In addition, as in the case of open data, data providers make My Data available to the individual for download and through APIs.

Privacy and security are paramount for My Data. Data providers must take steps to verify the identity of the individual requesting the data (a step known as "authenticating" the individual) and that the data are delivered securely. My Data providers often use customized systems to authenticate the individual (such as asking the individual to provide information that can be checked against the provider's own internal records), widely used commercial authentication solutions offered by credit bureaus or others, or a combination of the two.[10]

Using personal data for income and asset verification illustrates how My Data can positively affect community development, social services, and beyond. Today, many agencies, companies, and organizations in the housing ecosystem must collect personal financial information from individuals. Lenders use this information to establish eligibility and to price loans. Servicers require this information before providing foreclosure assistance. Low-Income Housing Tax Credit property managers verify tenant income. Public housing authorities verify eligibility for affordable housing programs such as the Section 8 Housing Choice Voucher Program.[11]

These paper-based data collection and verification processes exact a toll on the housing ecosystem (as they do throughout the social service ecosystem). They create friction that impedes enrollment in programs. They increase administrative costs for housing providers, including costs for cash-strapped nonprofit organizations and public agencies. Furthermore, they add to the stress and burden of residents who are already under pressure—at worst leading families in need to give up on accessing benefits or services owing to frustration or confusion. In the course of a year, a low-income resident may have to satisfy multiple *verifiers*—a term for the organization that is verifying the resident's financial information—whether for housing or for other program administrators (e.g., nutrition assistance). Each verifier may require different documents, such as tax returns; W2s; pay stubs; letters from employers to confirm employment and salary; bank account statements;

---

10 The ubiquity of e-commerce and other transactions involving sensitive personal data exchange via the internet has increased a wide range of readily available technical solutions for entities considering implementing My Data initiatives.

11 Public housing authorities are also required to use the Department of Housing and Urban Development's Enterprise Income Verification system (EIV) to verify income reported by program participants. For more background on this system, see U.S. Department of Housing and Urban Development, "Enterprise Income Verification (EIV) System" (Washington, DC: HUD, 2013), available at http://portal.hud.gov/hudportal/HUD?src=/program_offices/public_indian_housing/programs/ph/rhiip/uivsystem.

documentation related to assets such as vehicles; letters to certify benefits received (e.g., disability benefits); and evidence of expenses (e.g., child care). Residents often need to produce documents in person, by mail, or by fax.

Access to personal financial data via My Data can free residents, lenders, housing providers, and program administrators from burdensome paperwork. Government has a major role to play, as state and federal agencies must already collect certain financial records electronically, such as income tax returns, benefits records, and wage reports.

The federal government has made progress in making it simpler for individuals to access and share critical financial records electronically. For example, in 2013, the IRS made it easier for taxpayers to share tax returns with lenders and other third parties through the IRS's Income Verification Express Service (IVES) by making it possible for taxpayers to electronically sign the request to share their returns.[12]

In addition, the Social Security Administration (SSA) has made it easier to access the letters it has historically provided as proof of benefits information.[13] Community residents may need to provide these letters to prove their income when applying for a mortgage, housing, or other benefits.[14] The SSA now allows beneficiaries to download an electronic copy of this letter via the online mySocialSecurity account, increasing convenience for both beneficiaries and verifiers.

Community development practitioners should consider helping residents take advantage of new My Data systems, such as the new My Data resources accessible from the IRS and SSA. Such systems can help streamline and reduce administrative costs, reduce burdens, and ultimately ensure that more families have access to affordable housing, homeownership, and critical social services.

---

12 Income Verification Express homepage, http://www.irs.gov/Individuals/Income-Verification-Express-Service.

13 These letters are known as "budget letters," "benefits letters," "proof of income letters," or "proof of award letters."

14 The letter can also be used to establish current Medicare health insurance coverage, retirement status, and disability status.

TREND #3: SMART DISCLOSURE

The last data trend is smart disclosure, which is the release of data that helps consumers make more informed decisions and adopt positive behaviors—all by enabling innovators to build data-driven tools for consumers called choice engines, such as comparison shopping apps or personal dashboards.

Why should community development practitioners care about consumer issues, including smart disclosure? Every day, residents make decisions in consumer markets that can have significant and long-lasting effects on their lives, as well as the lives of their neighbors—whether they are deciding where to buy a home, where to go to college, or what kind of car to drive. Consumer decisions can ultimately affect the entire nation, as the mortgage crisis showed.

The promise of empowering consumers is why the Obama administration has promoted smart disclosure throughout the U.S. government, including creating the Task Force on Smart Disclosure and creating Consumer.Data.gov, a centralized platform for federal smart disclosure data sets and resources that community development organizations can start taking advantage of today.[15]

Two types of smart disclosure exist: The first is composed of open data relevant to consumer decisions, such as data on product recalls or college graduation rates. The second is composed of My Data relevant to consumer decisions, such as a consumer's own electricity use data, which consumers can use to evaluate which services may best meet their needs. Figure 1 shows the relationship between smart disclosure, open data, and My Data, which illustrates that a smart disclosure initiative can involve the release of open data, My Data, or a combination of both.

Some tech-savvy consumers may analyze smart disclosure data directly. However, for the vast majority of consumers, smart disclosure will have

---

15 A comprehensive overview of smart disclosure, including examples of smart disclosure initiatives at the federal level, can be found in the White House Task Force on Smart Disclosure Final Report, "Smart Disclosure and Consumer Decision Making: Report of the Task Force on Smart Disclosure." (Washington, DC: White House Task Force on Smart Disclosure, May 2013), available at www. whitehouse.gov/sites/default/files/microsites/ostp/report_of_the_task_force_on_smart_disclosure.pdf.

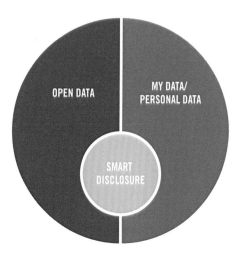

Figure 1. The large circle represents government policies to expand access to data. Smart Disclosure can involve open data, My Data, or both.

an effect by enabling third parties to create choice engines—software-based tools that help consumers make more informed decisions. Today, many consumers use popular data-driven choice engines to compare airline flights, for example. Nonprofit organizations are also creating choice engines, such as GreatSchools, which helps parents choose a local school using government data.

Smart disclosure also helps create market pressure on suppliers of goods and services to improve. For example, the nonprofit organization Code for America, the City of San Francisco, and Yelp have worked together to make restaurant health inspection data available as standardized open data.[16] Yelp now prominently displays health scores on restaurant search pages. In the short term, consumers can choose to eat at restaurants with higher ratings. In the long term, restaurants may come under pressure to improve their food safety practices to stay competitive.

Several services are appearing that use smart disclosure data to help residents choose healthier options. The Healthy Shoppers Reward

---

16 Code for America and Yelp are working to expand the number of localities that adopt the restaurant inspection open data standard used in San Francisco, known as LIVES. See "Foodies and Open Data Enthusiasts Rejoice," Code for America Blog (January 17, 2013), http://www.codeforamerica.org/2013/01/17/foodies-and-open-data-enthusiasts-rejoice/.

Program, led by the Lerner Center for Public Health Promotion at Syracuse University, illustrates the potential for smart disclosure to improve community health by enabling residents to make healthier food shopping choices.[17] Residents see a simplified nutrition score for food items at a local grocery store partner, so they can easily compare the health effects of foods. They can also choose to share the data on the scores and food items they purchase with physicians at a nearby health center, who can then provide personalized care informed by the patients' diets—and even write prescriptions for vegetables. Some simpler apps aim to tackle a narrower—but nonetheless important—problem: helping consumers locate healthier food options. For example, several apps help residents find farmers' markets and other fresh food in their neighborhoods using public data. In addition, many apps use open nutrition data from the U.S. Department of Agriculture to help individuals make healthier eating choices.

Housing is an example of an area ripe for innovation using smart disclosure data. Commercial real estate and rental sites are already actively embracing smart disclosure to make it easier for families to decide where to live using open data, often from federal, state, and local governments. Trulia and Zillow, two popular real estate and rental search sites, for example, leverage data from government agencies to help individuals make informed decisions on where to live. Community groups and coalitions have an opportunity to build on these mainstream housing search innovations by developing the next generation of choice engines tailored to the unique needs of individuals looking for affordable housing options, including filters such as income eligibility, acceptance of Section 8 vouchers, and proximity to social services a family may need.

HOW TO START TAKING ADVANTAGE OF OPEN DATA, MY DATA, AND SMART DISCLOSURE TO BUILD STRONGER COMMUNITIES

For those who have not begun to incorporate open data, My Data, and smart disclosure into their toolkits, there are simple ways to

---

17 Lerner Center for Public Health Promotion, "New Program Rewards Healthy Shopping" (Syracuse, NY: Lerner Center, 2014), available at http://lernercenter.syr.edu/projects/Healthy-Shopper-Rewards.html.

begin putting valuable data to work immediately in communities. The approaches described below are designed to be accessible to a range of organizations. Some community organizations may choose to use these approaches as part of a comprehensive data strategy. Organizations facing significant capacity constraints can use the list to select small-scale, manageable ways to begin leveraging data as a part of their missions. In addition, community groups can work through coalitions to engage in efforts that require more resources than are available at the local level.

Become a more data-driven organization by leveraging open data, My Data, and smart disclosure

Not only is government opening its data, but increasingly government- and foundation-sponsored community development programs are requiring grant recipients to offer data-driven diagnoses of their local needs, or data-driven assessments of local assets to demonstrate that a plan is workable. Furthermore, federal programs increasingly want recipients to rigorously measure results. Organizations may consider how open data can help them streamline the work of diagnosing need or measuring results. There are a variety of methods to find the most relevant data resources. For example, you can use government open-data search platforms to regularly discover new data sets relevant to your work. Platforms such as the federal government's Data.gov can help you search for data relevant to your existing programs. Depending on your topic or complexity of the data, you may need to enlist the assistance of your expert allies to locate and process needed data.

Become a data provider yourself—that is, create and/or publish open data, My Data, or smart disclosure data that others can use

Does your organization have data sets that could be valuable if released as open data, made available to individuals as My Data, or used to support smart disclosure? The San Francisco–based nonprofit social service referral system One Degree, for example, has announced that it will publish the database of social service nonprofit organizations and agencies it has built, including customer reviews and feedback.[18] A first step could be taking an inventory of the data assets your organization possesses and prioritizing the release of data sets based on your mission

---

18 One Degree, "One Degree Resource Server" (beta). See https://data.1deg.org.

objectives. Outside individuals and groups may have useful insights into which data sets would be valuable. For example, you can write a blog post listing the data sets you maintain and ask stakeholders to comment on which should be released.

Releasing open data does not have to be difficult given the tools and best practices that have become available in recent years. Becoming a publisher can be as simple as adding several links to your website to download a few valuable data files. For organizations with very large data inventories, off-the-shelf solutions are available for publishing open data catalogs. A number of nongovernmental organizations have used the open source open data platform CKAN, for example, including the community-driven OpenOakland data catalog.[19] Community groups interested in publishing anonymized open data on individuals, or information derived from data about individuals (such as statistical data), should consult with experts—such as nonprofit organizations specialized in open data or privacy—about best practices and legal compliance.

Successful data providers embrace open data or My Data as a core part of organizational culture. Consider developing challenge goals for your organization, such as releasing the underlying data for every report your organization publishes. Or consider adopting an "open-by-default" presumption that all your organization's data should be made accessible while protecting privacy and security—similar to the new federal Open Data Policy that makes newly generated data sets open by default.

Identify and fill data gaps

You may need new data initiatives to further your organization's mission. In this case, your organization can identify data gaps and work to fill them. Sometimes an organization can fill these gaps directly, either by collecting and releasing new data sets or funding such collection and release.

Often the needed data sets are already in the government vaults. At the national level, under the terms of the new federal Open Data Policy, any

---

19 OpenOakland, Open Oakland Data Catalog, data.openoakland.org. CKAN was developed by the nonprofit organization Open Knowledge Foundation and is overseen by the CKAN association. For more examples of organizations using CKAN, see "CKAN Instances Around the World," www.ckan.org/instances and CKAN case studies, www.ckan.org/case-studies.

data sets in the agency's data inventory that can be made publicly available must be listed on the agency's website to the extent practicable.[20] This includes data sets that can be made publicly available but have not yet been released. Community groups are now able to review data sets that could be released in an easy-to-use catalog on Data.gov and provide feedback to agencies.

In addition, various public disclosures and notice laws, as well as freedom of information laws, provide a view of what information government bodies already collect. For example, at the federal level, the Privacy Act of 1974 requires that agencies publish certain notices in connection with information systems that contain personally identifiable data. These notices can be used to identify many potentially valuable personal databases maintained by federal agencies.[21] The Paperwork Reduction Act requires that detailed descriptions of many forms, known as *information collections*, be made available to the public.[22] Paperwork Reduction Act notices can also be used to discover potentially valuable databases housed at federal agencies that could be made available to the public.

If you have an agency data set identified, government bodies often have channels for the public to provide feedback on data. Under the federal Open Data Policy, for example, all federal agencies must establish a process to solicit feedback on open data, which should be disclosed on their agency websites. Public officials rely on domain experts to generate

---

20 Agency open data pages are typically available by typing the agency's main URL and then adding "/data" at the end, so that the ultimate URL looks like www.[agency].gov/data (e.g., www. treasury.gov/data).

21 A directory of federal agency System of Records Notice (SORN) homepages can be found at https:// cio.gov/about/groups/privacy-cop/privacy/. For an example of SORN, see the Consumer Financial Protection Bureau's SORN providing notice of its Consumer Response System, https://www. federalregister.gov/articles/2012/10/19/2012-25487/privacy-act-of-1974-system-of-records#h-11. The CFPB publishes anonymous complaints from the Consumer Response System as open data at http:// www.consumerfinance.gov/complaintdatabase/.

22 The Office of Information and Regulatory Affairs makes information about federal information collections available for search and for download in machine readable formats at Reginfo.gov. See http://www.reginfo.gov/public/do/PRASearch (to search all information collections from federal agencies) and http://www.reginfo.gov/public/do/PRAXML (to download a listing and description of all federal information collections in XML format). For an example of the information available on Reginfo.gov associated with each information collection, see the record for the Consumer Financial Protection Bureau's (CFPB) "Consumer Response Intake Form" at http://www.reginfo.gov/public/do/ PRAViewICR?ref_nbr=201311-3170-001. The record allows members of the public to view the form that the CFPB is using, including all the individual questions asked.

ideas for how data sets could be used. In addition, community groups have also participated in passing data laws, such as local open data laws that have been enacted New York City, Oakland, and other localities.

Community organizations can also work with private sector data custodians. Many businesses have an interest in adopting open data, My Data, or smart disclosure initiatives. Corporate data access initiatives may be motivated by commercial imperatives and corporate values; in addition, laws or regulations sometimes require entities to provide individuals with access to their personal records or open data (e.g., personal information in the health, education, and finance sectors). Many companies release free open data through APIs for commercial purposes.

Community organizations can facilitate access to data held by companies by making the case that investing in data initiatives will benefit the company and advance values aligned with the company's mission. There are several examples of successful public sector- and nonprofit-led initiatives to encourage companies to voluntarily adopt open data, My Data, and smart disclosure. For example, utilities throughout the country have voluntarily given customers access to their own energy use data.[23] Hospitals, doctors, and others have also voluntarily given patients access to electronic health records.[24] The nonprofit organization Health Data Consortium fosters collaboration among government, nonprofit, and private-sector organizations working to increase the availability and use of data to improve health, including data from private-sector providers.

Foster the development of a vibrant ecosystem of companies, nonprofit organizations, and others working to solve problems in your field.

One effective tactic is to raise awareness of data to help address the "last mile" challenge common to many open data, My Data, and smart disclosure efforts—that is, the problem that data cannot simply be published; rather, data must be put to work by companies and nonprofit organizations to be genuinely effective. You can help increase awareness

---

23 See John P. Holdren and Nancy Sutley, "Green Button Giving Millions of Americans Better Handle on Energy Costs," White House Blog (March 22, 2012), http://www.whitehouse.gov/blog/2012/03/22/green-button-giving-millions-americans-better-handle-energy-costs.

24 HealthIT.gov, "Your Health Records: About Blue Button" (Washington, DC: HealthIT.gov, September 15, 2013), available at www.healthit.gov/patients-families/blue-button/about-blue-button.

of data resources to ensure a positive impact in your community. Actively publicizing data resources is a critical part of ensuring that nonprofit organizations, businesses, and others ultimately discover and use the data in ways that benefit the public.

A basic way to begin this process is becoming a data curator: developing and maintaining public listings of data resources in one area or that are relevant to a particular challenge. The NNIP community-based curated open data portals exemplify this type of approach. Although many government platforms such as Data.gov make it easy to search within a particular government body's data, solutions are needed for searching for data across multiple sources by topic. You can easily create and maintain a simple webpage with a directory of data sets from various sources that are relevant for your mission.

Another potentially powerful outreach tactic is using challenges, such as offering a prize for the top solution to a problem. Difficult and meaningful problems are the most likely to attract participants. Free resources are available to help learn more about how to structure a prize for maximum effect, as well as entities that specialize in helping others administer prizes.[25]

Organizations can also sponsor short, focused events where individuals come together to build applications or analyze data with or without the structure of a prize. Such events, including hackathons, hack nights, and code sprints, are common throughout the technology world. They are often most useful for building community and generating simple prototypes and ideas, rather than creating full-fledged software applications. For example, a community-based hackathon held in Minneapolis yielded projects to assess the use of bus stops; facilitate dialogue between parents and schools; promote a local child care center; and visualize local crime data.[26] The field is building a set of best practices

---

25 See, e.g., McKinsey & Company, "And the Winner Is... Capturing the Promise of Philanthropic Prizes" (New York, NY: McKinsey & Company, 2012), http://mckinseyonsociety.com/downloads/reports/Social-Innovation/And_the_winner_is.pdf.

26 The Federal Reserve Bank of Minneapolis, "Techies and Neighborhood Groups Hack Their Way to Community Solutions" (Minneapolis: FRB, October 1, 2013). www.minneapolisfed.org/publications_papers/pub_display.cfm?id=5170&.

for making these days the most productive with closer connection to community needs.[27]

Depending on the context, the last mile problem may be solved by engaging or creating an ecosystem of data innovators. Community members may help you achieve your mission using a range of ways, whether by creating new products and companies, conducting new analyses, generating new ideas and feedback, or even serving as a recruitment pipeline for your organization.

It is important to identify goals that are broad enough to sustain an ongoing community. Particularly in smaller communities, you may need to extend your geographic reach to locate enough potential community members, such as by partnering with national organizations or other local groups. If your issue or problem is too narrow or time-limited to attract a dedicated, ongoing community of data users, you can also join existing communities, such as mission-driven civic hackers, that are often looking for interesting projects or challenges.

Build Capacity

To implement any of these strategies, you may need to build capacity in your organization to work with data. This may entail securing resources to hire additional staff with expertise in data, such as software engineers and data analysts. Consider expanding your capacity in this area by taking advantage of free resources and partnering with data and technology-savvy partners. Many organizations and companies provide technical assistance, tools, and learning opportunities for those who want to learn to use open data.[28] In addition, an increasing number of

---

27 See, e.g., Open Data Society, "Open Data Hackathon How-To Guide" (British Columbia, Canada: Open Data Society, October 2012), available at https://docs.google.com/document/d/1fBuisDTliBAz9u2tr7sgv6GdDLOV_aHbafjqHXSkNB0/. For an example of a hackathon, see Center for Urban and Regional Affairs, "Visualizing Neighborhoods: A Hackathon for Good" (Minneapolis: University of Minnesota, CURA, May 25, 2013), available at www.cura.umn.edu/visualizingneighborhoods.

28 See, e.g., The Open Knowledge Foundation, *Open Data Handbook*; and Open Data Commons (legal tools for open data), http://opendatacommons.org/guide/; see also the European Journalism Centre and Open Knowledge Foundation, *The Data Journalism Handbook* (New York: O'Reilly Media, July 2012), available at http://datajournalismhandbook.org/; and Brett Goldstein with Laura Dyson (eds.), *Beyond Transparency: Open Data and the Future of Civic Innovation* (San Francisco, CA: Code for America Press, 2013), http://beyondtransparency.org/.

free tools are available to teach the basics of software programming and data analysis.

An increasing number of nonprofit organizations, foundations, independent citizens, and others have extensive expertise in open data, My Data, and smart disclosure. They frequently partner with community-based organizations and can help supplement organizations' capacity to engage in data and technology projects. For example, through the Code for America Brigade program, citizens, technologists, community groups, and others come together to tackle problems in their cities using open data and other technology-based approaches. Data Science for Social Good is a fellowship program that places highly skilled data analysts in nonprofit organizations to tackle problems with a social impact. They have partnered with the Cook County Land Bank and Institute for Housing Studies at DePaul University to build an open source analytics tool to help the land bank make data-driven decisions on which properties to acquire and redevelop.[29]

Some important movements and groups for community organizations to connect with include civic hackers[30] (focused on using technology to improve government and civic life, often at the local level); civic startups (often focused on building commercially viable products that benefit communities or citizens); open government and transparency advocates; community data organizations; data journalists; privacy and personal data access advocates; urban planners; and participatory budgeting groups. Often, these groups are actively seeking partners with specific domain expertise.

THE ROAD AHEAD FOR COMMUNITY DEVELOPMENT, OPEN DATA, MY DATA, AND SMART DISCLOSURE

Community development practitioners now enjoy a tremendous variety of opportunities to innovate by building on the growing tide of data access initiatives at the federal, state, and local levels. For many organizations, taking advantage of these opportunities will require significant

---

29 Data Science for Social Good, "2013 Projects." www.dssg.io/projects.

30 *Hacker* is used in a positive way to refer to a programmer throughout the software community. Sometimes the term refers specifically to someone who embodies the principles of such a programmer while making a difference in other domains.

investments. Organizations will need to augment their technical capacity and, in some cases, hire staff with new types of expertise. Organizations will need to engage in new ways of doing business, such as working with private-sector software developers or holding contests open to the public. The examples in this chapter illustrate that many organizations have already started this transition, with powerful dividends for their local communities. Going forward, the community development field should continue to push the boundaries of how data can be used to lift people out of poverty, promote well-being, strengthen neighborhoods, and contribute to a more vibrant economy. In addition, the field should continue to explore broader ways to raise capacity of the sector to ensure that the benefits of open data, My Data, and smart disclosure reach all communities.

■ ■ ■

AMIAS GERETY *serves as the Acting Assistant Secretary for Financial Institutions. In this role, Mr. Gerety is responsible for developing and coordinating Treasury's policies on issues affecting financial institutions, and for overseeing Treasury programs including the Community Development Financial Institutions (CDFI) Fund, the State Small Business Credit Initiative, and the Small Business Lending Fund. He previously served as Deputy Assistant Secretary for the Financial Stability Oversight Council, and as Senior Advisor to the Assistant Secretary to Financial Institutions.*

■ ■ ■

SOPHIE RASEMAN *is the Director for Smart Disclosure in the U.S. Treasury Department Office of Consumer Policy. In that capacity, she works to promote open data, my data, and smart disclosure policies that fuel innovations benefiting financial consumers. She has served as the Co-Chair of the White House's Task Force on Smart Disclosure and leads the federal Smart Disclosure Network.*

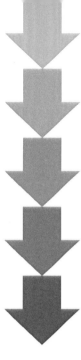

IN BRIEF

CAN DATA FROM NONPROFIT HOSPITAL TAX RETURNS IMPROVE COMMUNITY HEALTH?

Erik Bakken and David Kindig
University of Wisconsin, Madison

Nonprofit hospitals play a key role in improving the overall health of their communities. New opportunities, though, are arising through Affordable Care Act's (ACA) emphasis on community-level data for community health planning. The ACA requires nonprofit hospitals to draft a Community Health Needs Assessment (CHNA) triennially as part of their IRS tax-exempt status. The assessment researches and identifies the health needs of their communities and details plans to address these needs. The CHNAs could also improve efficiency, eliminate overlapping programs, and better coordinate community-wide health resources if they were jointly carried out with other hospitals or stakeholders. If aligned with other community-level data projects, CHNAs could coordinate investments from other key sources of community improvement, such as funds from Community Reinvestment Act–motivated banks, community foundations, socially motivated investors, and local governments. CHNAs could also ensure that community benefit dollars are better aligned with community health improvements. This essay summarizes the current status of such community benefit allocations recently made available through new IRS reporting.

IRS COMMUNITY BENEFIT POLICY

For nonprofit hospitals to qualify for tax exemption, they must provide charitable health-promoting activities (community benefit) to their communities. In 2007, the IRS announced new rules defining how hospitals must report their community benefit allocations as part of their tax filing to qualify for exemption. Schedule H, a new section of the 990 tax-exemption form (Form 990) that was added for hospitals, codified and strictly defined what hospitals could count as community benefit.[1] Hospitals now were required to report their annual community benefit provisions in total and by qualifying categories. In addition, certain qualitative information regarding internal hospital policies, organization, and mission was made mandatory. The definitions of community benefit categories have remained unchanged since their introduction in 2008 and can be defined as follows:

- **Financial assistance at cost,** commonly referred to as "charity care." This is free or reduced-price care provided to those financially unable to afford treatment, such as the underinsured or those eligible but not enrolled in Medicaid.

- **Unreimbursed Medicaid,** which is the "net cost" to the organization for providing these programs. It is the disparity between cost of treatment for Medicaid patients and the government reimbursement rate.

- **Other unreimbursed means-tested government programs,** which is the net cost to the organization for providing these programs. It is the disparity between cost of treatment for these patients and the government reimbursement rate.

- **Subsidized health services** are clinical inpatient and outpatient services that are provided by the hospital despite a financial loss or that would be otherwise undersupplied to the community. Typically, these are services with thin or negative profit margins for the hospital, such as burn units, and they are meant to insulate the hospital financially for providing these services.

- **Community health improvement services** include activities or programs subsidized by the organization for the express purpose of community health improvement, documented by a Community Health Needs Assessment. Examples include immunization programs for low-income children or diabetes health education courses.

---

1   L. Wright, T. Clancey, and P. Smith, "Unraveling the New Form 990: Implications for Hospitals," *Journal of Healthcare Finance* 35 (4) (2009): 83–92.

- **Health professional education** includes the net cost associated with educating certified health professionals.

- **Research** includes the cost of internally funded research and the cost of research funded by a tax-exempt or government entity.

- **Cash and in-kind contributions** include contributions, monetary or otherwise, to community benefit activities that the organization makes to community groups. [2]

The IRS also requires reporting in three supplemental, optional categories in the community benefit section of Form 990. These are not counted as community benefit because of IRS rulings, but must be reported if allocations exist. These supplemental categories are:

- **Bad debt,** which includes the portion of hospital billings that is unpaid and the organization believes could be of community benefit.

- **Unreimbursed Medicare,** which includes the surplus or shortfall from the organization's Medicare Cost Report.

- **Community-building expenses,** which protect or improve community health and safety, including housing, economic development, environmental improvement, leadership development, and coalition building. [3]

HOW IS COMMUNITY BENEFIT ALLOCATED?

Even with the new standardized reporting, findings on how hospitals were allocating community benefit dollars were slow to emerge. Data is not directly available from the IRS, but individual hospital Schedule H filings can be viewed on the GuideStar website. [4] There is however a several-year delay in data availability. In 2012, we published the first peer-reviewed results from the new Schedule H, examining community benefit levels in Wisconsin for 2009 (Figure1). In a modestly sized state such as Wisconsin, reported community benefit totaled more than $1 billon for the 2009 financial year. Hospitals varied in their levels of community benefit spending, but on average community benefit amounted to 7.5

---

2   Internal Revenue Service, Instructions for Schedule H (Form 990) (Washington, DC: IRS, 2012).

3   Ibid.

4   GuideStar. http://www.guidestar.org/. Accessed January 17, 2012.

COMMUNITY BENEFIT CATEGORIES	TOTAL (DOLLARS)	AVERAGE % OF COMMUNITY BENEFIT EXPENDITURES	AVERAGE % OF TOTAL HOSPITAL EXPENDITURES
Charity Care	$96,629,458	9.1%	1.3%
Unreimbursed Medicaid	$536,292,658	50.4%	4.0%
Other Means Tested Government Programs	$12,908,862	1.2%	0.1%
Community Health Improvement Services	$47,137,597	4.4%	0.4%
Health Professionals Education	$136,358,971	12.8%	0.4%
Subsidized Health Services	$121,300,534	11.4%	1.3%
Research	$15,951,185	1.5%	0.0%
Cash and In-kind Contributions	$18,194,501	1.7%	0.2%
Community Benefit Total	$1,064,802,784	100%	7.5%

Figure 1. Wisconsin Community Benefit Reported by Category in Wisconsin, 2009

percent of total hospital expenditure (Figure 2). Interestingly, although hospital tax exemption stems historically from the provision of free care to the uninsured, traditional charity care amounted to only 9 percent of overall community benefit. More than one-half of the total came from the unreimbursed costs of Medicaid. Subsidized services were also a significant category, totaling 11 percent of the community benefit share. The community health improvement category amounted to only 4.4 percent of total community benefit dollars in the state. In addition, these dollars were asymmetrically distributed, with many hospitals allocating nothing to community health improvement, whereas others put considerable funds into this category.[5]

In 2013, the first national study of Schedule H was published in the *New England Journal of Medicine* from the same 2009 GuideStar data set,

---

5 E. Bakken and D. A. Kindig, "Is Hospital 'Community Benefit' Charity Care?" *Wisconsin Medical Journal*,111 (5) (2012): 215–219.

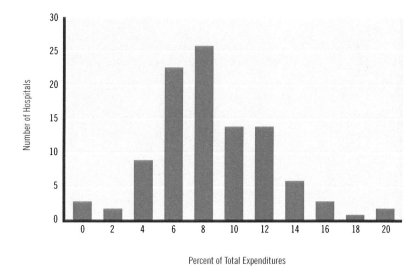

Figure 2. Distribution of Community Benefit as Percent of Total Expenditures in Wisconsin in 2009. Hospitals vary in their community benefit spending; on average, community benefit spending equaled 7.5% of total hospital expenditures.

with generally similar results for the entire country (data not shown).[6] Total community benefit was 7.5 percent of expenditures. Twenty-five percent was reported for charity care, while only 5 percent was reported for community health improvement. Forty-five percent was reported for unreimbursed Medicaid, and 15 percent was reported for subsidized clinical services.[7]

USING SCHEDULE H INFORMATION FOR POLICY

As this data becomes more widely available, it may be more actively used for hospital and local public health decisions. Specifically, it would allow hospitals to better link dollars toward the triennial CHNA required by the Affordable Care Act (ACA). The CHNA defines the community that the hospital is serving, identifies the particular needs of that community, and must contain a plan to address these established needs.[8] A fine-based compliance mechanism will be imposed for those failing to meet CHNA requirements.

---

6 G. J. Young et al., "Provision of Community Benefits by Tax-Exempt U.S. Hospitals," *New England Journal of Medicine*, 368 (16) (2013): 1519–1527.

7 Ibid.

8 E. Bakken and D. A. Kindig, "Is Hospital 'Community Benefit' Charity Care?"

The IRS community benefit requirements represents a potentially unique, dedicated funding stream for activities that meet the needs identified in a CHNA and yield real public health improvement. More transparent access to data about community health needs and improvement activities would allow hospitals to better coordinate community benefit dollars to tackle large projects or improve efficiency by eliminating redundant programs. In some markets, community health needs are likely to be similar among facilities. With better access to information, hospitals in multi-facility markets would be able to coordinate their public health pursuits to jointly address a single issue, or agree to address different programs in overlap areas. Recent policy changes indicate policymakers' growing awareness of the need for community benefit to extend beyond the traditional boundaries of health care to support community development activities. Although the supplemental community-building category remains uncounted as a community benefit broadly, hospitals can now count some community-building activities in certain circumstances. An activity is now eligible for the community health improvement category if the activity addresses an identified CHNA issue and directly improves health outcomes.

As we have indicated, however, retrieving information about how hospitals are allocating community benefit dollars from the GuideStar website is burdensome. To help communities obtain and use this data more easily, the Department of Health Policy at George Washington University, with support from the Robert Wood Johnson Foundation, will be working to develop a web-based database for Form 990.[9] This database is intended for public health practitioners, researchers, community stakeholders, policymakers, and others to have ready access to community health investment by hospitals. The project will allow users to search by hospital, geographic area, size of facility, and other factors. A major hindrance to linking community benefit dollars to community health improvement is lack of information.[10] With this database tool, the Department of Health Policy at George Washington University intends to improve information access so that community benefit dollars may be better spent in each community. Better tools and more transparent information may also push hospitals to allocate more funds away from covering Medicaid shortfalls or subsidizing unprofitable services to community health improvement activities.

---

9   Personal communication with Sara Rosenbaum, principal investigator.

10 Ibid.

Whereas the authors of the recent national study commented that "the availability of new sources of data and research… will at least make the debate an informed one," we conclude that community benefit policy is too important, and the needs for population health improvement resources are too great for there not to be more explicit allocation standards.[11] The need for additional resources for tackling upstream health determinants has been recently underscored by the documentation of our shockingly poor health outcome performance compared with other high-income countries.[12] Although other financing mechanisms, such as increased state and federal categorical funding, shared savings from Accountable Care Organizations, and global budgeting approaches need to be fully examined as well, community benefit policy seems like an unusually appropriate opportunity. The information now being made available by Schedule H should assist in aligning these needs with much-needed resources.

■ ■ ■

ERIK BAKKEN *is a project assistant at the Department of Population Health Sciences at the University of Wisconsin. Erik's previous work has focused on public health policy, non-profit hospital policy, and alternative funding mechanisms for public health programs. He received his Master of Public Affairs at the La Follette School of Public Affairs at the University of Wisconsin-Madison and his BA in Political Science from the University of Wisconsin-Madison.*

■ ■ ■

DAVID KINDIG, *MD, PhD, is emeritus professor of Population Health Sciences at the University of Wisconsin-Madison School of Medicine and Public Health. He is co-chair of the Institute of Medicine Roundtable on Population Health Improvement. He co-directs the Wisconsin site of the Health and Society Scholars program, and was founder of the University of Wisconsin Population Health Institute which produces the County Health Rankings and the Culture of Health Prize for the Robert Wood Johnson Foundation.*

---

11 Wright, Clancey, and Smith, "Unraveling the New Form 990: Implications for Hospitals."

12 D. A. Kindig, "What is Population Health?" Blog post. "Improving Population Health," a blog of the Population Health Sciences at the University of Wisconsin, n.d., www.improvingpopulationhealth. org/blog/what-is-population-health.html; D. A. Kindig, "Population Health Financing: Beyond Grants." Blog post. "Improving Population Health," a blog of the Population Health Sciences at the University of Wisconsin, January 31, 2013, www.improvingpopulationhealth.org/blog/2012/01/ population_health_financing_beyond_grants.html.

A youth sector is comprised of a broad array of actors and agencies that affect youth learning and development. The success of a youth sector collaborative—a formal effort among these organizations to work together in a coordinated way—depends in large part on the availability of cross-institutional integrated data. In this essay, we use the experience of the Youth Data Archive to illustrate how an integrated database linking administrative and program data from several agencies allows community partners to define issues affecting youth that transcend specific institutional responsibilities, as well as to conduct research and identify opportunities for joint action.

THE YOUTH SECTOR: SUPPORTING CROSS-INSTITUTIONAL COMMUNITY COLLABORATION THROUGH SHARED DATA

Rebecca A. London
University of California, Santa Cruz

Milbrey McLaughlin
Stanford University

Young people engage with multiple institutions and organizations as they grow up. Most youth attend school and interact with public and private health and recreational organizations; many youth connect with social service institutions of various stripes; some youth find themselves involved with the criminal justice system. However, these diverse institutions rarely coordinate their service strategies or goals with one another to better serve youth, and because of institutional silos, they often fail to capitalize on the close interrelationships among youth's social, emotional, cognitive, and physical development. As a result, they fail to provide the "web of support" policymakers and practitioners intend. This institutional isolation can also lead to misallocated funding and disappointing outcomes because services do not cover all youth needs or are unnecessarily duplicated. Ultimately, this can result in a failure to provide the necessary investments to support positive development for all young people.

A better alternative is to foster the establishment of holistic "youth sector" collaboratives, where myriad agencies can find opportunities to work collectively toward shared goals. A shared data framework can hold these collaboratives accountable to reaching those goals. This essay examines possibilities for using shared data systems to support and sustain youth sector collaboratives through the experience of the Youth Data Archive (YDA), an initiative of the John W. Gardner Center for Youth and Their Communities at Stanford University. The YDA links data from schools, public agencies, and community-based organizations to help ask and answer key questions about the youth the partnering organizations serve. Participating agencies collectively identify shared questions that no single agency can answer alone. Ultimately, the YDA supports partners in understanding the resulting analyses and in making data-driven policy and program decisions to improve outcomes for youth.

WHAT IS A YOUTH SECTOR?

A youth sector includes all the public and private organizations addressing a complex youth-related issue, such as child and infant health, social and emotional development, or college access. Some communities recognize how the missions of these agencies overlap and look beyond single institutions or existing policy systems to identify resources and relationships that will promote common goals for youth across sectors (e.g., health and education). In most communities, however, much of the work often happens in silos, with each agency independently pursuing its own goals with little knowledge of the work of other agencies serving some of the same children and youth. For instance, schools and district personnel are charged with the difficult task of educating all students and meeting federal and state standards to show their progress. They operate under shrinking budgets and unfunded mandates, leaving little room to focus on anything other than educational outcomes. Yet, research shows—and most educators know—that healthy students are more successful students. By participating in a youth sector collaborative, a school district could access information, and possibly resources, from partners to achieve both health and education goals. A collaborative approach reframes the policy space from a set of disconnected institutional policies and programs, each focused on a specific aspect of youth policy, to an approach in which youth initiatives are collectively developed, implemented, and evaluated. By considering how various service strategies are mutually reinforcing, youth sector initiatives can invest in youth development more effectively and efficiently. In addition, a youth-sector frame supports communities in tackling complex and entrenched social issues that no institution can address alone.

At their core, youth sector initiatives require sustained cross-sector collaboration undergirded by data sharing and strategic alignment, but can look different depending on a collaborative's particular goals. The Promise Neighborhoods initiative, for instance, funded by the U.S. Department of Education and based on the Harlem Children's Zone project, promotes coordination among youth-serving organizations from many sectors. The initiative has a strong commitment to using real-time data to measure progress and hold partners accountable to the program goals of improving educational and developmental outcomes of children and youth in distressed communities, and in the process transforming those communities.[1] Locally, many communities are forming their own youth sector collaboratives. For instance, Redwood City 2020 is a collaboration among multiple city and county agencies, school districts, nonprofit organizations, and business partners focused on improving youth outcomes through data-sharing, collaborative planning, and joint funding.[2] One scaffolding for these types of collaboratives is "collective impact," which emphasizes shared measurement as a way to move partners toward common goals.[3]

CREATING AN EFFECTIVE YOUTH SECTOR COLLABORATIVE

Although collaboration and collective action among youth-serving institutions makes intuitive sense in terms of maximizing a very limited set of resources available to serve youth, in practice, this is not an easy undertaking. Collaboration among institutions within a single sector (such as health or education), let alone *among* sectors, has been notoriously difficult to achieve or sustain. Competition for scarce resources, different models for addressing problems, and incompatible policy

---

1 U.S. Department of Education, "Promise Neighborhoods and the Urban Institute: Measuring Performance—A Guidance Document for Promise Neighborhoods on Collecting Data and Reporting Results" (Washington, DC: US Department of Education, 2014), www2.ed.gov/programs/promise-neighborhoods/index.html.

2 Redwood City 2020. www.rwc2020.org/.

3 J. Kania and M. Kramer, "Collective Impact," *Stanford Social Innovation Review* (Winter 2011). www.ssireview.org/articles/entry/collective_impact.

frames and accountability requirements can often interfere.[4] Similarly, differing financial resources, personnel or time constraints, or lack of political or community support can frustrate collaboration and threaten the trust-building that is essential to a cohesive youth sector.

Experience suggests that meaningful and sustained collaboration depends on at least four factors. The first factor is time. It takes time for partners to establish the relationships, trust, and new routines fundamental to this approach. A second factor is a shared sense of urgency to address a specific problem, to think beyond business-as-usual responses. Successful collaborations are forged when a critical concern—such as poor educational outcomes or increased youth violence—motivates joint action.

A third factor is the presence of an independent, neutral convener. This entity provides stability in the face of institutional churn and other challenges, and offers a neutral stance on data and findings. Such conveners also function as collective capacity builders. They manage the opportunities and issues that emerge in a collaborative setting and integrate knowledge and resources among participants.

The final requirement essential to success is integrated data; that is, data collected by each participating organization and linked across agencies. An integrated database can foster a shared mission and collective responsibility while providing a reason to continue collaborating. By themselves, good will and a shared goal of improving youth outcomes are insufficient to create the new relationships required to engage in joint action to tackle complex issues. Also needed are an agreed-upon set of outcomes and cross-institutional data to inform both the urgency and the outcomes of the collaboration. Promise Neighborhoods initiatives, for example, are required to implement a shared service-provider data system to allow providers to see the services used by participating families across service providers. Likewise, the Next Generation Afterschool System Building Initiative supports the creation of citywide data systems to track program participation and improve

---

4 R. Friedland and R. Alford, "Bringing Society Back In: Symbols, Practices and Institutional Contradictions." In *The New Institutionalism in Organizational Analysis*, edited by W. Powell and P. Dimaggio (Chicago: University of Chicago Press, 1991); E. Weber and A. Khademian, "Wicked Problems, Knowledge Challenges, and Collaborative Capacity Builders in Network Settings," *Public Administration Review* 68 (2) (2008): 334–49.

quality.[5] Linking data across institutions allows actors and agencies from different sectors to consider youth outcomes in broad terms, align investments, and identify shortfalls. Shared data become the glue that binds and deepens the relationships among partner organizations.

THE YOUTH DATA ARCHIVE: USING SHARED DATA TO SUPPORT COMMON GOALS

The Youth Data Archive (YDA) houses longitudinal data collected by public and nonprofit youth-serving agencies and organizations in a community, harnessed by partners to ask and answer questions that no one agency could answer alone.[6] At its core, the archive creates actionable knowledge that communities can use to support improved policies and practices for all children and youth. The YDA contains data from a wide range of agencies, including data such as student attendance and test scores, afterschool program participation, child welfare involvement, health indicators, and surveys on youth attitudes. It currently covers three California counties (San Mateo, Orange, and San Francisco) and is in development in Santa Clara and Alameda counties.

Researchers at the Gardner Center work with community partners to obtain and link data, which are maintained on a secure server at Stanford University. Partners retain ownership of their data and give consent for their data to be used for analysis. They must also approve any resulting reports or publications before they are disseminated. The YDA supports only research; partners do not have access to other organizations' data for case management or service provision.

Collaboratives that have used the YDA vary considerably, and many of the efforts have included broad partnerships among county health and human services agencies, county First 5 Commissions,[7] school districts, community college districts, city police and parks and recreation

---

5   Next Generation initiative is a Wallace Foundation effort to strengthen systems for coordinating local afterschool opportunities in grantee cities. See National League of Cities, "Communities Learning in Partnership": http://www.nlc.org/find-city-solutions/institute-for-youth-education-and-families/education/higher-education/communities-learning-in-partnership.

6   M. McLaughlin and R. London, eds., *From Data to Action: A Community Approach to Improving Youth Outcomes* (Cambridge, MA: Harvard Education Press, 2013).

7   First 5 California distributes funds through county First 5 County Commissions to support education, health services, childcare, and other programs for children ages 0 to 5 and their parents and caregivers. See http://www.ccfc.ca.gov/.

departments, city mayor's offices, afterschool providers, providers of counseling services, and others.[8] In one project, multiple school districts and the county human services agency engaged the YDA to examine the causes, consequences, and correlates of truancy and chronic absenteeism in an effort to help affected students. In another project, the County Office of Education, First 5 Commission, and a local school district partnered to understand how student participation in Preschool for All programs supported their transition to elementary school, with particular attention to the needs of low-income and minority students. County and district personnel use the research to support subsidized high-quality preschool and the alignment of preschool and elementary school standards and goals.

At the heart of the YDA is a university-community partnership, but this arrangement is not essential to its success. What is essential is identifying a host agency with the capacity and infrastructure to support the storage and analysis of shared data. In the YDA case, the data analysts have a place at the table when partners are building their capacity to understand and interpret the data. The researchers are neutral supporters of the collaborative, which can be particularly helpful in contexts where partner organizations are more accustomed to blaming one another than working together.

CREATING A DATA-SUPPORTED YOUTH SECTOR COLLABORATIVE

Developing an archive of shared data that can inform cross-institutional action is not necessarily a linear process, but conditions build on each other in mutually reinforcing, or inhibiting, ways. Six factors help ensure success.

Establishing Trust

Establishing trust among partners is critical.[9] Previous competition among partners for scarce community resources, lack of experience with cross-sector interactions, and concerns that someone outside the

---

8   See John W. Gardner Center, "The Youth Data Archive," http://gardnercenter.stanford.edu/our_work/yda.html.

9   I. Nelson, R. London, and K. Strobel, "Reinventing the Role of the University Researcher" (Stanford, CA: John W. Gardner Center for Youth and Their Communities, 2013).

organization could misuse or misreport data can derail any data-sharing efforts. The YDA addresses some of these concerns by using written agreements that data will not be shared with any other parties and that findings will be released only with permission from all who have contributed data. These assurances make partners more comfortable with sharing data and less concerned that they will be taken by surprise in seeing findings from their own data presented in a public forum.

Strong Leadership

Strong, committed leadership is also key to success. Agency heads unaccustomed to thinking of their work in the context of the broader youth sector will need to become comfortable with new norms of practice and organizational relationships. Although members of a youth sector collaborative will have committed to a joint agenda for supporting children and youth, they are still individually accountable for specific outcomes to funders and governing agencies. Negotiating this dual responsibility requires the agency leader to understand the importance of placing his or her work in community context and extending this understanding to operations of the organization.

Establishing a Shared Research Agenda

In coming to agreement on a research agenda, a key step involves selecting shared outcomes to track. When community organizations come together for common purpose, it is often to achieve a lofty goal, such as reducing childhood obesity or improving graduation rates. The factors underlying such problems are highly complex and not rooted in the system charged with addressing the problem (e.g., a health department or school district), and thus are ripe for a cross-sector approach. However, rates of obesity or high school graduation change slowly, and even if the community is making some progress in addressing the problem, it may take a decade or longer before success is evident. It is important, then, to consider progress on interim outcomes. These can include tracking whether communities are providing opportunities for youth to engage in physical activities and access healthy foods, or creating culturally responsive school environments that enable and encourage youth to stay in school.

Even with shared outcomes in mind, agreeing on research questions can be challenging for agency heads who are accustomed to asking questions about their own programs or populations but not about how those programs or populations intersect with others or about opportunities for joint approaches to complex problems. A good research agenda should have three characteristics:[10]

- Aligned: Does the question represent or support a core goal of the collaborative?

- Answerable: Can the question be answered with data that partners collect?

- Actionable: Will partners be able to take action when they have results?

Questions should first be *aligned* with the mission of the collaborative. If the mission is to improve college attendance rates for inner-city high school students, the collaborative should specifically consider the process leading to high school completion and college enrollment, as well as students' early college experiences. This may require educational leaders focused on K-12 to extend their traditional commitment to students beyond graduation and postsecondary leaders to consider factors that influence student success even before they enter college. Data could be combined from various agencies to understand students' supports and experiences during high school, although it is not essential that data from every collaborative member be used in each analysis.

The questions asked must also be *answerable* with data collected by contributing organizations. Administrative data—data collected by agencies or service providers as part of their daily operations —help agencies track the number of youth they serve, the types of services received, or selected outcomes. Organizations may collect information on young people's experiences to comply with state and federal government regulations or to satisfy foundation requirements. However, administrative data may not capture the measures most appropriate for

---

10 John W. Gardner Center for Youth and Their Communities, "From Data Collection to Data Utilization: Presentation to St. Paul Next Generation Afterschool Initiative" (Stanford, CA: John W. Gardner Center, 2013).

a particular analysis. For instance, many agencies are focused on social and emotional development. However, no single method for measuring social and emotional development exists, and partners are most likely not collecting this information routinely. If the collaborative determines that providing positive developmental experiences is a shared goal, agency partners will need to find or develop new metrics or use different types of data to measure current conditions and progress.

Answers to partners' questions may require other types of data collection, such as student or parent surveys, interviews, or focus groups. Parent or survey data that include identifiers can be linked to other administrative records. In contrast, interview or focus group data, which may involve few respondents or group-level data (in the case of focus groups) would not be integrated into the overall database but can still be important to understanding questions about program implementation or respondents' perceptions.

The most challenging of these three criteria is whether the research is *actionable*. How will partners know in advance whether the findings will lead them to act? There is no way to know in advance whether the findings will help leaders to act, but if the analysis is relevant to the decision-making process, even a decision for the status quo may be 'action.' The YDA research team has adopted a definition of *action* that takes many forms along a continuum, including any change in policy, practice, or programming; continuing with existing efforts; or the intention to use research to discuss making changes or continuing with the status quo.[11] Partners may take action on a given set of findings immediately or in the future. Several YDA analyses have gained the attention of state and local policymakers, which broadens the potential for action beyond the contributing partners' use of the findings.

Building Capacity
The process of establishing a youth sector collaborative and sharing data to support a shared mission creates opportunities to build capacity for the partners to use cross-sector data for their shared endeavor. It also allows partners to identify gaps in their own data collection or

---

11 K. Dukakis and R. London, "What Makes the Youth Data Archive Actionable?" In From *Data to Action: A Community Approach to Improving Youth Outcomes,* edited by M. McLaughlin and R. London (Cambridge, MA: Harvard Education Press, 2013).

in the entire collaborative's data collection process. Collaborators can build on the strengths of existing data to collect more robust and helpful information about the youth they jointly serve.

Asking cross-sector questions across agencies in support of positive youth outcomes is new for many agencies. Agreeing on a shared research agenda with common research questions, using data to respond to these questions, and coming together to make decisions in support of youth based on the findings can be, at first, challenging for partner organizations and may require a research partner. As agency partners become more familiar with these processes, they will be able to ask and answer increasingly more relevant and complex questions.

Sharing Data

Establishing a shared data archive also requires collaborating partners to: (1) reliably collect the necessary data in a useable format; (2) agree to share information among agencies and sectors for common purposes; (3) have a technological platform for sharing information either with one another or an external partner; (4) understand and abide by federal and state regulations that govern the sharing of confidential data; and (5) agree on a common agenda for accessing and using the data to make changes to policy and practice.[12]

However, many community organizations do not have sufficient financial resources or time to accomplish these steps. It is a leap of faith to believe that with shared goals and actions come pooled resources and support, yet organizations need to make this leap. In some cases, external funders can help (e.g., Promise Neighborhoods). In other cases, collaboratives may be able to harness seed funding for their work by offering a voice at the table to local businesses, community foundations, health care foundations, and others. They can write joint funding proposals or find funds within each organization to support ongoing work. These are not simple solutions, and funding for this type of work is not easily won. In the case of the YDA, funding comes from various sources, including partners' own contributions and grants from external funders, and resources from the Gardner Center itself.

---

12 McLaughlin and London, *From Data to Action.*

Another common impediment to success is that many community agencies have not invested in collecting high-quality, consistent, and wide-ranging data on the youth they serve. With missing or inaccurate data on student names, birth dates, and addresses, it is difficult to link individual records from disparate databases. Additionally, if agencies have not populated their database with the kinds of information needed to answer the questions generated, the analysis will stall out. For instance, if collaborative partners want to understand the effects of regular afterschool program participation on students' academic achievement, the participating afterschool provider would need to keep ongoing records on students' attendance in its program. Yet many providers do not keep these types of records. Participation in a collaborative provides an opportunity for organizations to learn about others' data collection and improve and expand their own data in the process.

Agreements for how to share and store data, all the while ensuring compliance with regulations on data security and privacy, are critical to a cross-institutional data-sharing initiative. Agreements to share data require consideration of who may access the data and how permissions to use and report the data will be managed. As mentioned earlier, the YDA operates on the principle that contributing agencies retain full ownership of their data. Partners report that this aspect of the YDA is critical for them to feel comfortable contributing their confidential data. Data security is also essential. The YDA's data platform meets the highest standards for secure data (e.g., not linked to the internet, only accessible from encrypted computers) and is operated and maintained by Stanford University. Other options include using a host partner's own server or purchasing external server space to store the data. The process of linking and analyzing data requires technical expertise, which may be available in-house at partner agencies.

Privacy and other legal restrictions pose another difficulty. Educational organizations, for example, are governed by the Family Educational Rights Privacy Act (FERPA), and health organizations are guided by the Health Insurance Portability and Accountability Act (HIPAA). The restrictions imposed by these or other regulations can be difficult to navigate, so partners should consider their options carefully when deciding how to proceed. Use of external research partners (or neutral third parties) can aid efforts considerably because regulations often allow for data exchange for research purposes if individual-level information is not shared publicly.[13]

Measuring Progress

How do partners in the youth sector know that their collaboration is making a difference for children and youth—and, ultimately, for the community? Progress can take time and can be difficult to assess. A key marker of success is the type of action—considerations or changes to policy or practice—that results from collective planning. Tracking the action resulting from the youth sector collaborative is critical, but our experience with the YDA suggests that community partners may not be able to act on findings immediately. The release of findings may not be timed to partners' decision-making cycles, acting may require additional funds, or partners may simply be busy with other pressing priorities. But there is no statute of limitations on action; partners may refer to research that is several years old to advance an agenda that was not possible when the research was performed.

CONCLUSION

We have made the case that collaboration among the youth-serving organizations in different sectors creates opportunities for enhancing the policies that govern programs and services for young people. The collaboration among typically siloed agencies can be greatly enhanced by shared data, allowing the collaboration members to examine and build on the synergies that exist among their varied efforts.

Research conducted using shared data allows members of a collaborative to see how well their service strategies align with those of other members in the community to support positive outcomes, or how they fall short of goals. It also allows collaborative members to see how families take advantage of multiple programs to support individual children and youth.

Private and public funders are beginning to recognize the importance of establishing youth sector collaboratives. To succeed, these collaboratives will need to embrace the essential role of linked, cross-institutional data

---

13 See McLaughlin and London, *From Data to Action*, appendix 1, for more information.

in supporting their goals. They will need to build internal capacity for asking cross-agency questions, use their data in new ways to answer them, and commit to using the analysis findings to create policy and programmatic improvements in support of positive youth outcomes.

■ ■ ■

REBECCA LONDON, *PhD, is assistant director of research and policy at the University of California–Santa Cruz Center for Collaborative Research for an Equitable California. Dr. London's research bridges academia and policy, focusing on the policies and programs intended to serve low-income or disadvantaged children, youth and families. She collaborates with community organizations and agencies to design and conduct actionable research that is relevant to the community's needs.*

■ ■ ■

MILBREY MCLAUGHLIN *is the David Jacks Professor of Education and Public Policy at Stanford University, Emerita. She is founding director of the John W. Gardner Center for Youth and Their Communities, which partners with communities and youth-serving agencies to support research and policies benefiting youth. McLaughlin also founded and co-directed Stanford's Center for Research on the Context of Teaching, an interdisciplinary research center engaged in analyses of how teachers' organizational, institutional, and social-cultural contexts shape practice.*

The linking and integration of large data sets offers a new dimension to the development, implementation, and evaluation of policy and program initiatives. Yet the ability to accomplish this often depends on identifying and confronting legal, political, and technical barriers. This essay discusses the potential benefits of linking large data sets. It also identifies some core barriers to doing so, focusing on legal, political, and technical issues. It also discusses potential solutions to overcoming those barriers and throughout identifies various resources that enable the reader to explore issues and solutions in more detail.

DATA INTEGRATION FOR SOCIAL POLICY: CHALLENGES AND OPPORTUNITIES

John Petrila
University of South Florida

Evolving technology has simplified and reduced the cost of creating and using linked data sets in ways that would have been unimaginable only two decades ago. Linked data sets are an increasingly important tool in marketing, in business decision making, and most relevant here, in shaping and evaluating public policy initiatives in health care, housing, and social services, among other domains. However, because these data sets often contain identifiable personal information, their creation and use can ignite broad and legitimate public concerns regarding the protection of personal privacy.

This essay discusses the tension between using linked data sets to inform policy and the privacy and other concerns that emerge from the use of such data. The United States Bureau of the Census defines a "data set" as "any permanently stored collection of information usually containing either case level data, aggregation of case level data, or statistical manipulations of either the case level or aggregated survey data, for multiple survey instances."[1] For purposes of this essay, "data sets" include but are not limited to data in electronic format such as health records, housing records, educational records, and child welfare records. "Linked data sets" refers to the ability to be able to work with and integrate information from one data set with that contained in another, for example, to "link" school discipline records with juvenile justice

---

1   United States Bureau of the Census, Software and Standards Management Branch, Systems Support Division, "Survey Design and Statistical Methodology Metadata," (Washington D.C.: August 1998), Section 3.3.7, page 14.

records to determine if individuals who appear in the juvenile justice system were more likely than those who did not to have a disciplinary record in school. The Early Childhood Data Collaborative defines "secure linking" of data sets as "the ability for state data systems to share unduplicated data about program participation, the services a child receives and developmental assessment data across programs and over time, while data are protected from inappropriate access or use."[2]

It seems inevitable that the use of such linked data sets will expand rapidly during the next few years, and that shared and linked data will become an essential tool of policymakers in every sphere. The reason for linked data's growing relevance is because policy initiatives in one area—for instance, housing—typically can affect individual and community outcomes in other areas such as health or education. As a result, analyzing data from only one system frequently results in a one dimensional perspective that misses myriad outcomes in other systems, and thus makes it more difficult to accurately diagnose a problem and develop a solution. Furthermore, linking data is necessary for understanding how interwoven systems affect individuals and communities over time. But in linking data, privacy concerns must be acknowledged and addressed. This essay provides examples of the use (and in some cases misuse) of linked data bases in developing and evaluating social policy, discusses political and legal challenges to using such data, and potential solutions to those challenges.

OPPORTUNITIES AND CHALLENGES

Linked data can help policymakers shed light on broad social issues in myriad ways. For example, Massachusetts created the Massachusetts Environmental Public Health Tracking Program in response to the lack of information on the impact of environmental factors on health.[3] The project provides prevalence and other information on the relationship between environmental factors and health issues such as birth defects, cancer, and heat stress. By providing this information, the project's web

---

2 The Early Childhood Data Collaborative. "2013 State of States' Early Childhood Data Systems" (2014). Available at http://www.ecedata.org/2013-national-results/.

3 For more information see, Massachusetts Department of Public Health, Bureau of Environmental Health, "The Massachusetts EPHT Program," available at https://matracking.ehs.state. ma.us/EPHT_Program/.

portal can provide common data to environmental and local and state public health officials interested in finding solutions to problems caused by the interaction between environment and health.

Although linked data is no guarantee of coordination among policymakers, it creates a tool and opportunities to do so, in part because it permits questions to be posed and answered empirically. In a paper urging states to more readily share data across state agencies, Rebecca Carson and Elizabeth Laird[4] assert that important questions about school progress can be addressed over time, for example:

- To what degree does participation in early childhood programs increase kindergarten readiness and do children sustain those gains through third grade?

- What indicators suggest that students may be at risk to drop out of school, or conversely may go onto college or careers?

- How many and what kind of high school graduates need assistance in their first year of postsecondary education?

The use of linked data for these purposes is not confined to the United States. In England, researchers linked health and social care (that is, social work, social support, personal care and related non-health services) data from disparate sources to create models that could predict which individuals aged 75 and older would require intensive social care in the subsequent 12 months. Although the models were less successful than hoped, the work points to further efforts to use linked administrative data to better target services.[5]

The type of data relevant to policy varies depending on context, situation, and source. For example, in health care, sources of data may be as disparate as social media and biometric data. "Big data" linking these various sources is enthusiastically discussed as a tool to control costs,

4   R. Carson and E. Laird, "Linking Data across Agencies: States That Are Making It Work" (Data Quality Campaign, March 2010), available at http://forumfyi.org/files/States.That.Are.Making.It.Work.pdf.

5   M. Bardsley et al., "Predicting Who Will Use Intensive Social Care: Case Finding Tools Based on Linked Health and Social Care Data," *Age and Ageing*, (Oxford University Press, Jan. 20, 2011): 1–5.

improve the quality and efficiency of care, address fraud, and detect disease earlier through advanced technology such as electronic sensors.[6] In other fields, such as community development, there is increasing interest on the part of international bodies such as the United Nations in using data "to gain insight into human well-being and development."[7] As promising as all these efforts might be, policymakers can anticipate political, legal, and technological challenges to using integrated data sets for policy purposes. Each is discussed briefly below with potential solutions.

Political Challenges

Public concern over personal privacy may create a barrier to data integration. It is unclear how deeply or broadly those concerns run. One poll regarding activities by the National Security Agency (NSA) to mine phone and other electronic data showed that a majority of Americans value privacy over security, while an earlier poll showed that a majority of Americans thought the NSA program was acceptable as a tool in combatting terrorism.[8] More influential in shaping public opinion are breaches of security that raise fears of identity theft on a mass scale, such as the Target data breach in late 2013. In addition, potential privacy issues emerging in geotagging (the process of adding geographical identification to a photograph or website) may add to the concern. The use of large data sets that might yield significant information about individuals without their express knowledge or consent may become more politically charged.[9]

There have also been multiple breaches involving health data, which may exacerbate fears over intrusions into privacy. For example, a health

---

6   See, e.g., Institute for Health Technology Information, "Transforming Health Care through Big Data: Strategies for Leveraging Big Data in the Health Care Industry" (New York: IHTI, 2013), available at http://ihealthtran.com/big-data-in-healthcare.

7   United Nations Global Pulse (2013). Big Data for Development: A Primer, available at http://www.unglobalpulse.org/bigdataprimer.

8   Associated Press, "Poll: Americans Value Privacy over Security," *Politico*, January 27, 2014, available at www.politico.com/story/2014/01/poll-americans-privacy-security-102663.html; and Pew Research Center for People and the Press, "Majority Views NSA Phone Tracking as Acceptable Anti-terror Tactic (Washington, DC: Pew, June 10, 2013), available at www.people-press.org/2013/06/10/majority-views-nsa-phone-tracking-as-acceptable-anti-terror-tactic/.

9   For a discussion, see A. Chawdhry, K. Paullet, and D. M. Douglas, "Raising Awareness: Are We Sharing Too Much Private Information?" *Issues in Information Systems*, 14(2) (2013): 375-381.

system in Texas revealed that records of up to 405,000 patients may have been compromised in December 2013 when one of its servers was hacked, potentially exposing names, dates of birth and Social Security numbers.[10] Data breaches involving health care records increased by 138 percent between 2009 and 2012, with nearly 30 million records compromised in that period.[11]

Political Solutions

Although there is no standard solution for addressing the politics of data sharing, there is little doubt that the issue has political salience and that privacy concerns must be balanced against the benefits of data use.[12] As the number and variety of examples of using integrated data in policy grow, the benefits and payoffs will emerge more clearly. Leaders of public agencies reluctant to share data to avoid the possibility of inappropriate disclosure or negative public perceptions may ultimately conclude that the benefits outweigh the risks. In addition, toolkits now exist for communicating the benefits of data integration and in the process ease doubts. Some excellent examples have been developed by the Data Quality Campaign and the National Neighborhood Indicators Partnership.[13] Ultimately, however, given that nearly all significant breaches of privacy have occurred because of insufficient security, the political issues regarding privacy can in part be addressed by improving data security.

---

10 D. Carr, "Texas Hospital Exposes Huge Breach," *Information Week*, Feb. 5, 2014, available at www.informationweek.com/healthcare/security-and-privacy/texas-hospital-discloses-huge-breach-/d/d-id/1113724).Names.

11 Erin McCann, "HIPPA Data Breaches Climb 138 Percent," *Health Care News*, Feb. 6, 2014, available at www.healthcareitnews.com/news/hipaa-data-breaches-climb-138-percent. The US Department of Health and Human Services, which now tracks breaches of health information affecting 500 or more individuals, reports scores of breaches. See www.hhs.gov/ocr/privacy/hipaa/administrative/breachnotificationrule/breachtool.html.

12 For example, in 2012, the Obama administration attempted to draw that balance in its release of "A Framework for Protecting Privacy and Promoting Innovation in a Networked World," available at http://www.whitehouse.gov/sites/default/files/privacy-final.pdf.

13 See Data Quality Campaign, "Let's Give Them Something to Talk About: Tool for Communicating the Data Message" (Washington, DC: DQC, Jan. 29, 2013), available at http://dataqualitycampaign.org/find-resources/tools-for-communicating-the-data-message; DQC, "Cheat Sheet: Data Privacy, Security, and Confidentiality" (Washington, DC: DQC, n.d.), available at http://dataqualitycampaign.org/files/Cheat%20Sheet%20Privacy.pdf; National Neighborhood Indicators Partnership, "Why Data Providers Say No...And Why They Should Say Yes," (Washington, DC: NNIP, Feb. 28, 2013), available at www.neighborhoodindicators.org/library/guides/why-data-providers-say-noand-why-they-should-say-yes.

Legal Challenges

Often those who do not want to share data believe the law does not permit it. Occasionally, this is true, but in many circumstances the claim that it is unlawful is a convenient reason to halt the conversation before it gets started. Confidentiality law in the United States is a patchwork of state and federal law. Some confidentiality laws (for example, many state health and mental health confidentiality statutes) were written long before the emergence of electronic data sets and therefore are increasingly antiquated. In other situations, such as confidentiality protection for those who are HIV positive, states wrote stringent special laws because of potential discrimination. Other laws, such as the federal Health Insurance Portability and Accountability Act (HIPAA) and the Family Educational Rights and Privacy Act (FERPA), are designed to create national standards. Courts have created other confidentiality rules. For example, the U.S. Supreme Court in 1996 ruled that clinical information created in psychotherapy sessions was privileged (that is, could not be accessed in legal proceedings).[14] But federal law does not always take precedence. For example, if a state law provides greater privacy protection to protected health information than HIPAA, then the state law applies. This complex web of overlapping and sometimes conflicting law can make negotiations over integration and use of data for policy purposes frustrating even for those fully committed to its use.

Before turning to potential solutions, it is worth noting why this complexity exists. First, each confidentiality law focuses primarily on a specific type of information created in the context addressed by the law. For example, HIPAA addresses "protected health information." FERPA primarily addresses educational records. As a result, standards for waiving confidentiality or accessing the information in question may vary by law, for information that identifies or may identify an individual and for such records in more aggregated form.

Second, although confidentiality is a core value, it is not absolute. Every confidentiality law provides for situations in which information subject to the law may or must be released. Sometimes information specific to an individual may be sought in a legal proceeding in which the court

---

14 *Jaffee v. Redmond*, 518 U.S. 1 (1996).

orders release of an individual's medical records. In other contexts, oversight agencies receive aggregated data on specific outcomes. For example, states must report child welfare data in seven categories to the U.S. Children's Bureau for an annual report to Congress. There are similar requirements for the reporting of homeless data to the U.S. Department of Housing and Urban Development.[15] While these data do not typically identify individuals, they rest on the collection of information from numerous individual cases.

Third, the real controversy that often arises in discussions about data sharing is whether the law permits access to *individually identifiable* information for the purpose of data integration and use. This can make access more complicated because of reluctance to release individually identifiable information. Yet information that identifies individuals may be essential for analyses most useful to policymakers.[16] For example, New York City staff reported the benefits of specific programs for the homeless. The reports were based on five years of "mortality surveillance" data of the city's homeless population.[17] The authors of the study noted the benefits of using real-time, individually identifiable data compared to aggregate data and it is worth quoting them at length:

*"Retrospective analyses of aggregate morbidity and mortality data from a specific study period can identify health problems such as multiple comorbid conditions, substance abuse, or mental illness that result in premature death in a homeless population. However, homeless mortality surveillance offers the advantage of ongoing, systematic, and timely data collection and dissemination that reflects the current health status of the homeless population. Ongoing surveillance can identify changing trends in illness and death...**in close to real time**, allowing faster implementation of preventive interventions."*

---

15 See http://www.hudhdx.info/.

16 Linking identifiable data to track cohorts is not only useful to policymakers. Linking cancer registry data to Medicare and Medicaid claims files enabled researchers to identify and track cancer patients over time to determine over time the effectiveness of care. See D. Schrag, B.A. Virnig, and J.L. Warren, "Linking Tumor Registry And Medicaid Claims To Evaluate Cancer Care Delivery," *Health Care Financing Review*, 30(4) (2009): 61–73.

17 M. Gambatese et al., "Programmatic Impact of 5 Years of Mortality Surveillance of New York City Homeless Populations," *American Journal of Public Health* 103 (2013):S193-198.

Legal Solutions

Despite these problems, policymakers are using integrated data, and there are good resources available for helping those who wish to take advantage of these data and techniques navigate the complexity. For example, the University of Pennsylvania leads the Actionable Intelligence for Social Policy initiative, which is developing and using large integrated data sets, many with individually identifiable information, for policy purposes.[18] They have commissioned a series of papers, including an overview I wrote of the "state of the law" on confidentiality and access.[19] Another example of a university-based initiative is the Information Sharing Certificate Program at Georgetown University, which teaches leaders in youth-serving agencies how to overcome information-sharing challenges while protecting the privacy of youth and their families.[20]

Other resources describe agreements that enable access and use of protected data. For example, HIPAA may require the use of a "business associate agreement" between a state agency and a party accessing protected health information for purposes of analysis. The US Department of Health and Human Services offers a description of the purpose and requirements of such a business associate agreement and also provides sample agreements that can be adopted.[21] The National Neighborhood Indicators Partnership devotes a web page to the "key elements of data sharing agreements."[22] The Data Resource Center for Child and Adolescent Health, which offers data sets based on interview data provided by the National Center for Health Statistics, provides a data use agreement with every request for data.[23] The State Data

18 See http://www.aisp.upenn.edu/.

19 John Petrila, "Legal Issues in the Use of Electronic Data Systems for Social Science Research," (Philadelphia: University of Pennsylvania, n.d.), available at: http://www.sp2.upenn.edu/aisp_test/wp-content/uploads/2012/12/0033_12_SP2_Legal_Issues_Data_Systems_000.pdf.

20 For more information, see http://cjjr.georgetown.edu/certprogs/informationsharing/certificateinformationsharing.html.

21 HHS, "Business Associate Contracts: Sample Business Associate Agreement Provisions" (Washington, DC: HHS, 2013), available at www.hhs.gov/ocr/privacy/hipaa/understanding/coveredentities/contractprov.html.

22 See "Key Elements of Data Sharing Agreements," available at www.neighborhoodindicators.org/library/guides/key-elements-data-sharing-agreements.

23 See data request form at http://childhealthdata.org/help/dataset.

Resource Center website of the Centers for Medicare and Medicaid Services provides information on the types of data available to state Medicaid agencies enrolled in both Medicare and Medicaid, including a Data Use Agreement.[24] In short, and in contrast to a few years ago, there is a wealth of information on using individually identifiable data for policy purposes. These resources make it easier to tend to the needs of all parties while overcoming barriers to the use of large data sets, including those which contain identifiable information.

Technical Challenges

Technical advances have made the development, integration and use of large data sets possible and have created a sense of promise about integrated data's potential. These advances include both vastly improved statistical and computational methods and the exponential growth in storage and computational capacity.

However, technical issues can also thwart the promise of the revolution in method and capacity. For example, a data set generated for one purpose (such as arrest data) may contain a different personal identifier than that contained in another (such as Medicaid data). This makes accurately linking the data sets difficult, and thus compromises the ability of analysts to perform the analyses that policymakers would like by complicating efforts to track individuals *across* data sets.

In 2011, 25 Semantic Web and Database researchers convened in Riga, Latvia to discuss opportunities and challenges of using "big data," including linked data. In a summary of the proceedings[25] one of the participants suggested that there were two "challenge classes" that must be met in order to use the data widely: the first, an engineering challenge of "efficiently managing data at unimaginable scale" and the requirement for advanced computing power and software that government agencies or nonprofits likely do not have. The other class of challenges is "semantics," that is, "finding and meaningfully combining information that is relevant to your concern."[26]

---

24 See State Data Resource Center site at http://www.statedataresourcecenter.com/.

25 C. Bizer, P. Boncz, M.L. Brodie, and O. Erling, "The Meaningful Use of Big Data: Four Perspectives—Four Challenges," *SIGMOD Record* 40 (4) (2011): 56–60.

26 Bizer, et al.

There are also resource and skills issues. The period of rapid advancements in data integration happened to coincide with cuts to the government workforce, limiting the number of staff available to work on data development. Therefore, whether a governmental agency has the intellectual capacity to engage in this work or develop the capacity to do so is an open question in some jurisdictions. In addition, this issue is not restricted to government. A 2012 survey of Fortune 500 executives revealed significant reservations about whether they had enough skilled workers to adequately use data in business planning, an issue exacerbated by staff and analytic capacity cuts during the recession.[27]

Technical Solutions

Solutions to some technical issues may be methodological. For example, one group of researchers interested in exploring clinical issues arising in pediatric cardiac care created a method that relied on "indirect identifiers" (date of birth, date of admission, date of discharge, and sex) that permitted the linking of administrative data (e.g. Medicare) to clinical registry data, thereby permitting better care for patients by permitting analysis of where various procedures were performed for patients over time.[28] Linked clinical and administrative data will become increasingly important in evaluating health policy questions, particularly around use and cost of services, so insight into methods that create this linkage are relevant to policymakers as well as clinicians.

Others have developed techniques based on probability theory that create unduplicated counts of individuals in data sets that do not contain unique person identifiers.[29] This permits policy analyses using individual data without having to find a common identifier for linking, thus reducing the barrier in linking individuals across data sets and providing privacy protection as well.

---

27 P. Barth and R. Bean, "There's No Panacea for the Big Data Talent Gap," Harvard Business Review blog, Nov. 29, 2012, available at http://blogs.hbr.org/2012/11/the-big-data-talent-gap-no-pan/.

28 S.K. Pasquall, et al., "Linking Clinical Registry Data with Administrative Data Using Indirect Identifiers: Implementation and Validation in the Congenital Heart Surgery Population," *American Heart Journal* 160(6) (2010): 1099–1104.

29 A description of the method can be found in S. Banks and J.A. Pandiani, "Probabilistic Population Estimation of the Size and Overlap of Data Sets Based on Date of Birth," *Statistics in Medicine* 20(2001): 1421–1430.

The capacity and resource issues might also resolve with better training of students. Business and government need employees who are more familiar with integrated data sets. Whether enough colleges and universities develop curricula to meet the needs of government and private business remains to be seen, but clearly private industry is interested in stimulating the movement. IBM, for example, has announced the creation of a "big data and analytics curriculum" in partnership with a number of academic institutions. The curriculum will prepare students for what it estimates to be the 4.4 million jobs worldwide that will be supporting "big data" by 2015.[30]

Finally, as government agencies, health care and social services providers, and educational institutions among others become more sophisticated about the issues involved in linking and using large data sets, they presumably will become more sophisticated about using their authority (often derived from their status as a contractor for services) to require the collection and transfer of relevant data from different vendors. As noted earlier, federal agencies already do this because they have reporting obligations to Congress or others, and one can anticipate that state and local governments will begin to do so more frequently to generate data more suited to later analyses. Therefore, if a county social welfare agency contracts for services with providers, it can contractually require the providers (consistent with various legal norms) to provide information, including individually identifiable information necessary to monitor outcomes that the county agency is purchasing.

OUTLOOK FOR THE FUTURE

Notwithstanding various challenges, the outlook for using integrated data for policy purposes is bright. The use of such data for policy is comparatively new, so it is not surprising that various political, legal, and technical challenges have arisen. Despite these challenges, it is difficult to imagine policymakers retreating from the use of linked data as these challenges are met. This is not to suggest that the development, implementation, and evaluation of all social policies will soon be informed by data. However, we do appear on the verge of an era

---

30 IBM Press release, "IBM Narrows Big Data Skills Gap By Partnering With More Than 1,000 Global Universities," (Armonk, NY: IBM, August 14, 2013), available at https://www-03.ibm.com/press/us/en/pressrelease/41733.wss.

when the use of such data for policy purposes will rapidly accelerate and expand.

On the political side, one promising development is a directive from the White House Office of Management and Budget (OMB) urging all federal agencies to set aside at least some program evaluation funding for evaluations that use integrated data. In a May 2012 memorandum, the acting director of OMB asked executive department and agency heads to "demonstrate the use of evidence" in their 2014 budget submissions. In addition, agencies proposing new evaluations were advised that "agencies can often use administrative data (such as data on wages, employment, emergency room visits or school attendance) to conduct rigorous evaluations, including evaluations that rely on random assignment, at low cost."[31] With time, this type of support should translate into more evaluations that rely on integrated data.

Technical and methodological advances will continue to open up exciting opportunities to supplement and enhance the power of administrative data. One of the most important is Geographic Information Systems (GIS). GIS permits users to collect, store, and analyze geographic data. GIS can be used to visually display the results of data analysis, but it can also be a complementary form of analysis itself, enabling analysts to build geographic data, such as the distribution of health centers or schools, into an analytic plan. Use of GIS is expanding very quickly. For example, the National Resource Center for Child Welfare Data and Technology describes how GIS can be used in the administration and planning of child welfare services.[32] A page on the U.S. Department of Housing and Urban Development website is devoted to the use of "geospatial data resources" in examining housing issues, including a large number of data sets.[33] NASA is increasingly using data it develops using GIS to examine health-related

---

31 Office of the President, "Memorandum to the Heads of Executive Departments and Agencies: Use of Evidence and Evaluation in the 2014 Budget" (Washington, DC: The White House, May 18, 2012), available at http://www.whitehouse.gov/sites/default/files/omb/memoranda/2012/m-12-14.pdf.

32 National Resource Center for Child Welfare Data and Technology, "Using GIS for Policy and Planning: New York City Example" (Washington, DC: NRCCWDT, n.d.), available at www.nrccwdt.org/2011/10/using-gis-for-policy-and-planning/).

33 See http://www.huduser.org/portal/datasets/gis.html.

issues alone and in partnership with agencies such as the Centers for Disease Control.[34]

Partnerships among the public, academic, and private sectors are another approach for driving innovation in the use of linked data. More colleges and universities are recognizing the potential for generating knowledge (and potential funding) through such partnerships. In addition to the IBM example and the Actionable Intelligence for Social Policy at the University of Pennsylvania, mentioned above, Harvard University has established the Institute for Quantitative Social Science as its home for social science research, with an emphasis on the use of quantitative data as a tool.[35]

Funders are stepping into this area as well. For example, the Annie E. Casey Foundation has funded a six-site project through the National Neighborhood Indicators Partnership titled "Connecting People and Place: Improving Communities through Integrated Data Systems."[36] The project spurs collaboration among universities, nonprofits, and public agencies to expand the use of integrated data systems (IDS) to generate neighborhood indicators and inform local policy issues. Seed money like this is important in enabling communities to begin using data to improve decision making and outcomes for individuals in particular neighborhoods.

The outlook for the use of integrated data for policy purposes in virtually any sphere seems boundless. Although there are challenges to meet, the use of integrated data can, with time, dramatically improve the public policy process. It can also help better ensure that initiatives in housing, child welfare, health, social supports, and education are grounded in evidence and, equally important, are evaluated using empirical data rather than anecdotal information.

---

34 Urban and Regional Information Systems Association, "Overview of NASA's GIS Leadership Role" (Des Plaines, IL, n.d.), available at www.urisa.org/awards/ national-aeronautics-and-space-administration-nasa/.

35 For more information see IQSS website at www.iq.harvard.edu/.

36 See National Neighborhood Indicators Partnership, "Connecting People and Places: Improving Communities through Integrated Data Systems," (Washington, DC: NNIP, June 2013), available at www.neighborhoodindicators.org/activities/projects/ connecting-people-and-place-improving-communities-through-integrated-d.

■ ■ ■

JOHN PETRILA *JD,LLM, is chair and professor in the Department of Health Policy & Management in the College of Public Health at the University of South Florida in Tampa Florida. He joined USF in 1992 as chair of the Department of Mental Health Law and Policy at the Florida Mental Health Institute and served as department chair from 1992–2004. He joined the College of Public Health in 2012. Before coming to USF he was General Counsel and Deputy Commissioner to the New York State Office of Mental Health. Mr. Petrila wrote the chapter on confidentiality in the 1999 Surgeon General's Report on Mental Health and works extensively with counties in Florida and elsewhere on the linking and integration of large data sets.*

The experience of mission-oriented housing providers is that affordable rental housing that connects low-income residents to educational resources, asset building tools, or health services can enable them to achieve a better quality of life. But efforts to weave together these types of disparate programs will not reach scale until there are sufficient data on outcomes to encourage providers to adopt new practices, persuade policymakers to redirect resources and eliminate regulatory barriers, and attract new investors. This essay focuses on an effort to build a systematic approach to measuring the effect of access to affordable housing enriched with supportive services on important life outcomes of residents.

AFFORDABLE HOUSING AS A PLATFORM FOR RESIDENT SUCCESS: BUILDING THE EVIDENCE BASE

Bill Kelly
SAHF

Fred Karnas
The Kresge Foundation

Low-income or disadvantaged people are often isolated in neighborhoods where affordable housing is not aligned with public transportation and where they are disconnected from employment opportunities, child care, education, recreation, health care, and quality food resources. For many, this disconnect has been devastating to personal well-being, life chances, and life expectancy.

However, a small number of housing providers are working to reverse these conditions by linking critical services to the physical place provided by affordable housing developments, and by fostering regular face-to-face interactions between residents and staff.

Their experiences are indicating that connecting residents of affordable housing with needed supports—such as educational resources, asset building tools, or health services—can enable low-income families, seniors, the chronically homeless, people with disabilities, and other vulnerable populations to achieve a better quality of life.

But these efforts to weave a range of related but distinct programs together with housing support will not reach scale until there are sufficient data and evidence of success to encourage providers to adopt proven practices and persuade policymakers to provide more resources and relax the housing, health care, and other regulatory restraints that make it so difficult to bring multiple programs together to enable residents to improve their lives.

There is as yet relatively little sound evidence that connecting housing to services results in positive outcomes for vulnerable populations. In an effort to strengthen the evidence base, Stewards of Affordable Housing for the Future (SAHF), with active support from The Kresge Foundation, has launched the Outcomes Initiative to gather consistent data across the housing portfolios of its members.[1] The data will measure the effect of access to supportive services on important life outcomes of affordable housing residents.

The members of SAHF expect that the initiative will enable them to engage and serve their residents in a more integrated, effective, and cost-effective way. Of equal importance, they anticipate that the data will help make the case for additional resources and, with time, move government policy toward more integrated approaches.

THE PROBLEM

Given the need for varied and integrated supports to improve quality of life for vulnerable populations, it is important to identify a place to bring various resources together in support of an individual or family. It seems intuitive to use the place where people live as a base for providing and connecting them with the array of resources they may need to improve their condition. A number of housing providers who have experimented with the approach are seeing that it makes a difference in people's lives. However, the evidence—and underlying data—needed to persuade policymakers to alter program design, resource allocation, and regulations to support this approach is currently very limited.

Numerous historical, political, programmatic, and regulatory reasons explain the lack of this evidence, not least of which is the relatively few

---

1 SAHF is a consortium of national affordable housing nonprofit organizations. Its members are BRIDGE Housing, Homes for America, Mercy Housing, National Church Residences, National Housing Trust/Enterprise, Preservation of Affordable Housing, Retirement Housing Foundation, The Community Builders, Evangelical Lutheran Good Samaritan Society, NHP Foundation, and Volunteers of America. The consortium serves more than 106,000 households (families, seniors, the formerly homeless, and people with serious disabilities) in affordable housing across the country. The Kresge Foundation determined early to invest in this effort because of its dual interests in identifying and applying evidence-based approaches for improving outcomes for vulnerable populations and in policy and systems change to facilitate the funding and implementation of proven practices.

integrated approaches from which to collect supporting data. Indeed, the design of public programs and regulatory frameworks is tied to old models or assumptions that are resistant to the funding and operating flexibility required to support better integration and service delivery. As result, the various programs and institutions charged with delivering services remain disconnected. Government housing subsidies, for example, seldom provide resources to address the additional health and human service needs of most families in subsidized housing. Likewise, health care Medicaid funds cannot generally be used to build housing or pay for its operating costs, even when it is clear that poor-quality housing can exacerbate health problems and even though health care subsidies routinely pay the far greater costs of room and board in nursing homes for the elderly than for aging in place.[2]

In the housing world, herculean efforts are required to move beyond providing basic shelter to enable residents to address the multiple other factors affecting their lives. To access and coordinate other, non-housing services, nonprofit housing owners typically must assemble limited, short-term funding from multiple local government and charitable sources. In some cases, owners can use the cash flow from property operations to fund some services, but often that cash flow is unreliable and its use for services risks starving the property of the resources needed for maintenance or weakening the financial sustainability of the owner.

Even where these efforts have been successful, the quantity and quality of available data are limited. Nonprofit owners generally lack resources to track how residents are faring. As a result, the data collected by providers are often simply the basic information required to satisfy funding sources. Too often, the data measure only activities rather than outcomes. Without measuring outcomes, property owners have no way to tell whether they are making a difference beyond providing shelter or how to change their approach if they are not. This void limits the utility of the data to support program design and policy change. Even if sufficient data are collected, there are few resources for data analysis.

---

2 J. Krieger et al., "Housing and Health: Time Again for Public Health Action," *American Journal of Public Health* 758 (May 2002). Also see R. Cohen, "The Impacts of Affordable Housing on Health: A Research Summary." *Insights from Housing Policy Research* (Washington DC: Center for Housing Policy, May 2011).

The data that exist vary in quality and consistency. Different reporting requirements from different funders result in a mishmash of data that make aggregation across owners nearly impossible. As a result, lessons are not transferrable. Moreover, isolated data have little or no impact on policy or social investment and are of limited use in demonstrating impact to potential partners in sectors important to resident success, such as health care and education.

As a result of these shortcomings, analyzing data collected from properties is difficult, even in the rare circumstances that providers have the necessary resources. Funders rarely aggregate or analyze data on the impact of housing connected to services in any methodologically sound manner, or regularly consider whether the data collected tell them what they need to know to improve policy and programs. The evidence that does exist supporting policy change and increased investment in the housing platform has come from a quite small base of studies often focused narrowly on particular populations (e.g., homeless people, seniors) or housing types (e.g., permanent supportive housing, public housing).[3]

THE SAHF OUTCOMES INITIATIVE

The dearth of data on how residents fare in settings where housing is linked to services prompted SAHF and its members to embark on an effort to gather consistent, aggregated data across members. The Outcomes Initiative aims to:

- Develop baseline data on the impact that having stable, affordable housing has on the lives of residents;

- Develop baseline data on housing connected to services (e.g., key services, the commonly accepted definitions of those services);

- Show which program-delivery mechanisms have the greatest effect on an individual's quality of life;

---

3 D.J. Rog et al., "Permanent Supportive Housing: Assessing the Evidence," *Psychiatric Services*, 65(3) (March 2014). Also, see wide-ranging research on impact of housing and services funded by the John D. and Catherine T. MacArthur Foundation at http://www.macfdn.org/press/article/how-housing-matters-research-briefs/.

- Develop measures that matter to social investors, foundations, and those who control the resources in related fields such as health and wellness and education;

- Gather evidence to make the case with policymakers for additional resources to support integrated housing and services efforts, and to create a public policy environment that can stimulate more extensive private grantmaking and investment.

A planning group of SAHF and four of its members began by sorting through current approaches and identifying common outcome measures across five areas important to residents:

1 Health and wellness;

2 Work, income, and assets;

3 Housing stability;

4 Children, youth, and education; and

5 Community engagement.

The planning group began by reaching consensus on a list of interim outcome measures across all five fields. Through this process, the group worked to balance the desire for standardization with the competing reality that each member has its own internal structure and is at a different point in its data collection efforts. The members were able to agree on 30 measures that they either were already collecting or would be willing to begin collecting. The measures include, for example, the percentage of students who advance to the next grade level, percentage of households with a checking or savings account, number of lease violations, and number of emergency room visits in the prior year.

The group also worked to develop an aggregation process that would allow members to use their current collection methods (such as annual resident surveys) while still achieving the consistency needed for aggregation. In the end, the measures adopted are clearly defined, flexible for different staff resources and resident populations, and of high value to residents, members, and potential funding partners.

This is an ongoing process. These measures may well be adjusted following the deeper dives described below. Members will move forward with collecting and aggregating data across their portfolios to the extent feasible in early 2015.

DIVING DEEPER

SAHF is drawing on specialized expertise to inform the continued outcomes data work and to explore effective strategies to serve residents in each of the five domains noted above. These "deeper dives" into specific focus areas enable the group to better understand the evolving landscape in each of these fields and understand the types of metrics that would resonate with and assist in bridging to potential partners. The planning group chose health and wellness as the first area of focus because of its promise for housing-based approaches that both improve health and reduce costs, especially in the Medicare and Medicaid programs.

The Affordable Care Act's Medicaid expansion, the act's funding for innovation, and health care reform more generally are changing health care quickly. SAHF retained Health Management Associates (HMA), a national health care consulting firm, to help navigate the complex health care landscape. HMA determined which outcome data are substantiating in the health care field and how to agree on a common set of measures, and identified the opportunities for accessing funding for services or capital from health care payers such as state Medicaid programs, managed care organizations, and insurance companies. The firm strongly recommended that SAHF: 1) pay close attention to indicators that are used to evaluate the performance of health care providers and payers, and 2) build a business case that supporting housing with services can help them meet industry and regulatory quality standards more effectively and cost-effectively than they can by providing all services themselves.

Following this planning effort, SAHF engaged all interested SAHF members in the discussion. The larger group identified services of high value to health care payers and target properties where members could document value. SAHF also undertook an initial exploration of a second area of focus: children, youth, and education. Specifically, it identified: 1) the outcome measures educators and others in the child development field find useful, and 2) evidence-based programs supporting these outcomes that are based in or linked with affordable housing.[4] The initiative will later focus on work, income, and assets; community engagement; and housing stability.

CHALLENGES AND SOLUTIONS

Even among motivated housing providers, determining how to collect outcome data in a consistent manner posed challenges.

First, each SAHF member had its own starting point. The populations SAHF members serve are diverse in their needs and aspirations, ranging from seniors and families with children to people with disabilities and formerly homeless individuals. Some members had collected only data about participation in activities—logging attendance at meetings or classes and contacts with residents. Others had tracked only information relating to specific services they have offered, often in a format designed to satisfy a government funder or foundation. Even when members measured the same concept, some collected information at the household level while others collected it at the individual level. Similarly, some members collected information only about adults; others, about children as well. In some cases, groups asked the same question, but response categories differed. For example, all members measured "type of lease violation," but grouped the responses in different categories. Finally, most members had not aggregated any data across properties.

Working together requires not only a commitment to outcomes and consistency, but also a willingness to surrender approaches that have been developed at significant expense in staff time and consulting fees. It also requires engaging with staff at sites across a member's portfolio. With sustained discussion and negotiation, the participating SAHF members came together around a tentative list of outcome indicators across the five areas, all to be tested and honed based on experience.

To ensure consistency in the data, the planning group created a data "dictionary." With respect to lease violations, for example, they agreed

---

4   SAHF retained the Urban Institute, a national nonpartisan research organization, to explore the education landscape and build the connection to affordable housing.

to disaggregate response categories and added "damage to property" and "criminal activity" to "nonpayment of rent" as separate categories.

A second challenge in improving data collection is competing demands on already busy senior staff to engage in the design process and property staff to gather and record the data. Both groups already have more than a full array of responsibilities. Properties owned by mission-driven nonprofits often operate in the red or with limited or no operating margins, making it almost impossible to hire staff to focus on data collection and analysis. Although some large properties have significant staff, and many properties, especially senior properties, have service coordinators, most SAHF member properties have only a property manager and janitorial staff. The average property size is small, in the range of 65 apartments, and many have only 20 or 30 apartments.

Accordingly, it made sense to start the data collection process by looking at what data could be gleaned from the annual income recertifications required for residents of HUD-assisted housing, expand somewhat the information gathered in that process, and supplement that data with resident surveys. But even this level of data collection requires significant training and staff time, and therefore was not feasible for understaffed properties. Rather than await additional resources, the initiative focused first on properties with service coordinators.

A third challenge is the time and expense required to aggregate and analyze data. In a perfect world, an external IT vendor would provide an inexpensive platform for aggregation. As it turns out, the available vendor technology is expensive, having been designed for intensive assessment of specific programs at properties rather than the overall life success of residents. Rental-assistance programs do not provide resources for this work, and one-time funding could create a data strategy that would turn out to be unsustainable. To address the aggregation problem, the team adopted the interim solution of using common Excel spreadsheets that can easily be aggregated across members. Using this simple approach will likely help build toward the next stage of technology.

Other challenges are institutional barriers to existing data. Institutions in other sectors, such as managed-care organizations, hospital systems, community clinics and school systems, gather and often analyze extensive data about residents of affordable housing. Health care payers, for example, often know who are the high-cost users of health care and why. The data they collect would provide a richer sense of how an individual is faring in terms of health. Similarly, school systems have data about school attendance, grade progression and, often, personal development.

But the institutional barriers to accessing those data for the residents of even one property, much less across a portfolio, are daunting. They begin with the difficulty of getting the attention of senior officials in the other sectors. Privacy laws compound the problem and often provide an excuse for inaction. The team is addressing these issues first through dialogue with "coalitions of the willing" in the other sectors. Owners can request that residents waive their rights so that data can be shared with their housing members, and schools and health care systems can share data that have removed individual identifiers. Over the longer term, as it becomes clearer that well-intended restrictions can defeat efforts to serve the "whole" person, policy change will likely be required to facilitate data sharing.

A final challenge in collecting and using data is that even data collected widely and consistently may not always meet academic or "evidence-based" government standards. Moreover, outcome data alone are generally not sufficient to establish cause and effect; the housing provider cannot control all the factors that affect resident well-being.

Nonetheless, the data will enable better decisions, and housing owners and managers can craft stronger programs. Moreover, institutions in related sectors, such as health care payers, are not bound by academic standards of evidence and will instead be able to use their business judgment to engage housing providers based on a combination of these data and their own data. Social impact investors may conclude that the data are strong enough to warrant investment. Finally, the data may persuade policymakers to redesign existing programs that lack data support. More methodologically sound data, even though short of academic standards, may be sufficient to support changes in programs or policies.

Broad-scale data collection can also spawn pilots and demonstrations to test the effectiveness and cost-effectiveness of specific interventions, and the evaluator of those demonstrations will collect and analyze more detailed data. For example, a demonstration of the ability of housing providers to increase access to primary care or improve chronic disease management will generate detailed data on health impact and cost. Potentially, basic outcome data can be correlated with in-depth data and the basic indicators, possibly modified with experience, can become affordable proxies for the in-depth data.

SPREADING THE IDEA

This SAHF initiative was launched at an opportune time for both its focus on data-driven approaches to social problems and its ultimate goal of enhancing resident success.

In 2013, the Bipartisan Policy Center's Housing Commission released "Housing America's Future: New Directions for National Policy." The report's recommendations were the culmination of a 16-month process of roundtable discussions and regional housing forums.

The report included a focus on outcomes-based performance, recommending:

[A] focus on outcomes, rather than process. We propose establishment of a performance-management system that measures resident outcomes across all rental-assistance programs, focused on creating incentives for greater efficiency and improved housing quality, as well as ensuring that rental assistance meets its full potential to serve as a platform for the achievement of other social outcomes.[5]

Of even greater significance is that the public sector was beginning to appear receptive to integrated services. In 2010, when HUD released its 2010–2015 strategic plan, it included a new goal: to "utilize housing

---

5 Bipartisan Policy Center, "Housing America's Future: New Directions for National Policy" (Washington, DC: Bipartisan Policy Center, February 2013), p. 97, available at http://bipartisanpolicy. org/library/report/housing-america%E2%80%99s-future-new-directions-national-policy. The report also noted SAHF's efforts in this area (p.98), ensuring that affordable housing is a platform for delivering services.

as a platform for improving quality of life."[6] For those in the housing field who have been connecting housing and services for years, this was by no means a new idea. But the fact that HUD elevated this concept to one of its five strategic goals signaled new attention to this important link between housing and services and how the physical "place" of housing can serve as a hub for needed services. The secretaries of HUD and Health and Human Services have recognized that their departments are serving essentially the same people and have sought to work together to better connect their programs and policies.[7]

Building momentum will require enlisting other affordable-housing owners in the effort. With that in mind, SAHF and the Council of Large Public Housing Authorities convened a meeting at which SAHF presented its tentative list of outcome measures and the council, the Housing Partnership Network, and NeighborWorks® America outlined their own approaches.

THE END GAME

Accessing resources from multiple systems (e.g., housing, health and human services) can be a challenge for even the most committed and knowledgeable providers. As noted, the challenges include the absence of direct funding for services in assisted housing, inadequate space for on-site services in assisted housing, regulatory limits that create barriers to accessing or aligning certain services, and lack of resources for service coordination.

Not every individual or family needs a full range of services; nor does every housing provider need to provide comprehensive supports. But where needed, access to the right services at the right time can make all the difference in creating stability and fostering a path to the economic mainstream.

---

6   U.S. Department of Housing and Urban Development, "HUD Strategic Plan FY 2010–15" (Washington, DC: HUD, May 2010), p. 11, available at http://portal.hud.gov/hudportal/HUD?src=/program_offices/cfo/stratplan.

7   U.S. Department of Housing and Urban Development, "HUD Secretary Donovan, HHS Secretary Sebelius Discuss Housing, Health, Education, Economic Outcomes of Low-Income Families,. HUD No. 11–259. (Washington, DC: HUD, 2011), available at http://portal.hud.gov/hudportal/HUD?src=/press/press_releases_media_advisories/2011/HUDNo.11-259.

Kresge and SAHF anticipate that the Outcomes Initiative will identify services that have the most impact on improving well-being and could open up opportunities for approaches that provide a payback over time. That payback would come through reduced system costs stemming, for example, from less use of the emergency medical system, improved academic performance, increased employment in living-wage jobs, and improved health.

Once positive effects are identified, the policy and systems barriers to integrating these services with housing can be addressed. The Kresge Foundation and SAHF further expect that the initiative will uncover opportunities for third-party "pay for performance" investments that enable residents to achieve improved outcomes and control or even reduce costs. These have the potential to lead to significant policy changes once results are proved.

SAHF and its members, with active support from Kresge, have embarked on a long journey, but a journey that will enable them both to serve residents better and to work effectively with new partners using approaches shown to make a difference.

■ ■ ■

BILL KELLY *was president and co-founder of Stewards of Affordable Housing for the Future (SAHF) and is now its strategic adviser. Prior to SAHF's launch, he was a partner in the law firm of Latham & Watkins and earlier served as a law clerk to U.S. Court of Appeals Judge Frank M. Coffin and Supreme Court Justice Lewis F. Powell, Jr. and as Executive Assistant to the HUD Secretary. He is a director of Ashoka Innovators for the Public, the International Senior Lawyers Project, and the Governance Institute.*

■ ■ ■

FRED KARNAS *is a senior fellow at The Kresge Foundation. Previously, he served as a liaison between HUD and HHS in his role a senior advisor to the HUD Secretary in the Obama administration. He also served as Deputy Assistant Secretary for Special Needs at HUD in the Clinton administration and in Arizona Governor Janet Napolitano's cabinet as director of the state Department of Housing. Karnas has a PhD in Environmental Design and Planning from Virginia Tech.*

Social enterprises can more effectively unlock the power of performance metrics by collaborating with peers to share and compare data. In this essay, we use two case studies to illustrate how comparable organizations can work together to make the collection and analysis of social and financial performance data easier and more useful. CoMetrics helps cohorts of nonprofits and cooperative businesses compare complex financial performance data on a common chart of accounts. HomeKeeper enables affordable homeownership programs to understand their social impact by comparing it to their peers. By providing context to otherwise abstract numbers, these kinds of peer benchmarking tools make performance data more concrete and actionable.

THE TRANSFORMATIVE POWER OF SHARED DATA

Annie Donovan and Rick Jacobus
CoMetrics

There is tremendous power in data; it enables better decision making and wiser resource allocation. There is good reason that we're having a national conversation about how the social sector can become more data driven. Much is at stake. Many believe that billions of "impact" dollars might be unleashed if social enterprises—whether they are for-profit, nonprofit, cooperatives (co-ops), or B Corps—can better demonstrate their performance and impact. The public sector is aiming increasing resources at programs that provide "evidence" of effectiveness. Programs such as the Social Innovation Fund (SIF), and the Department of Education's Investing in Innovation (i3) Fund, reward evidence-based programs with higher funding levels.

However, progress is slow. Our conversations are bogged down by seeking agreement on things such as top-down industry standards that might apply to vastly different types of organizations and efforts. Standardization sounds good, but the social sector is full of diversity. We create tools that require organizations to fill out survey forms with self-reported data that never result in any real benefits to the submitters of data. Many times, their data never makes its way back to them, let alone in a form that can lead to actionable insights. Is there any wonder that these databases are hard to populate?

Topics such as "big data," although thrilling us with their potential for breakthrough insights, do not help us focus on the building blocks of a desperately needed data infrastructure. The road to building data infrastructure for the social sector is through tools that create tangible benefits for enterprises and, we would argue, for whole sectors as well. The data must enable better decisions and unleash resources, either through cost savings or by attracting more capital to worthy programs.

These tangible benefits will drive the culture change inside organizations that is necessary for data to become a strategic driver of performance in the social economy. In the end, being data driven is all about culture.

Organizations around the country have begun experimenting with "bottom-up" approaches that unlock the more tangible and immediate benefits of better performance data. Here we discuss two such systems, CoMetrics (formerly CoopMetrics) and HomeKeeper, and although we are still learning what it takes to make these tools sustainable, we think that they illustrate an important approach for using data to drive both social and financial performance in the social sector.

COMETRICS

In the late 1990s, Whole Foods Market was growing very fast. This growth was, in many ways, a triumph for a retail sector that had been promoting healthier food for decades, but many of the neighborhood-based, community-owned co-op stores that pioneered the sector were now struggling to compete with this well-capitalized and centrally managed chain. Leaders in the co-op grocery sector realized that they would have to change to keep their social enterprises alive.

The food co-ops came together to create a new financial data platform, now called CoMetrics, which allowed them to work together to improve the financial health of their individual businesses and their sector as a whole. The new tool allowed each store to track its own financial performance on a set of standard metrics and to see the detailed performance of their peers. Sharing data in this way made it possible for the co-ops to create a shared purchasing program based on shared financial risk. The program gave them access to goods and credit on terms that made them competitive with a national chain.

CoMetrics has grown beyond the natural foods sector and built a suite of tools for organizations ranging from ethanol producers to affordable housing developers that want to better understand their own performance, and measure that against a set of peers. CoMetrics pulls financial information from disparate accounting systems and maps it to a common chart of accounts. To submit their data, participants only have to export existing files. There are no spreadsheets to fill in and no separate forms to keep track of. In fact, some accounting programs automatically send trial balances straight to CoMetrics with the click of button. The common chart standardizes the data, which is stored in a multidimensional database for ease of analysis. The initial work of agreeing on the common chart, and mapping the data the first time takes some effort, but once that is done, quarterly uploads of the data become routine. Furthermore, the process forces issues of common definitions and accounting best practices to the forefront. When successfully resolved, greater standardization of terms and practices will benefit the whole sector.

CoMetrics creates interactive reports that provide a standardized view of the financial performance of each participating business and enables companies to gauge their performance against their closest peers. In addition, this sector-wide data platform allows networks, trade associations, and funders to gain a high-level overview of the financial strengths (and weaknesses) in a sector.

The tools created by CoMetrics are being used to create data cultures that improve the financial performance of enterprises and sectors. It goes without saying that creating tools for financial data is easier than creating tools for impact data, but the same principles can apply to both types. The next example, HomeKeeper Project, demonstrates that a very similar approach can be used to unlock the power of social impact data.

HOMEKEEPER

HomeKeeper is a data system created by Cornerstone Partnership, a program of Capital Impact Partners, with key support from the Ford Foundation. Cornerstone Partnership is working to build and strengthen the field of nonprofit and government agencies that help lower-income families to purchase homes while preserving lasting affordability of those homes for future generations of homebuyers.

The HomeKeeper application helps manage the day-to-day tasks of running an affordable homeownership program. It is built on the Salesforce.com platform and available on the Salesforce AppExchange. For most users, the HomeKeeper app replaces half a dozen or more different spreadsheets users previously maintained to keep track of all the moving parts in their programs. However, unlike other administrative data systems, HomeKeeper was built from the ground up to answer key questions about the long-term social impact of these programs. Each instance of the HomeKeeper application automatically submits anonymous transaction-level data on each home sale to the HomeKeeper National Data Hub. The data that is shared includes household demographic data (stripped of identifying information); the size and age of the home purchased; the purchase price; and detailed information about financing and public subsidy sources (again, stripped of identifying information). Cornerstone uses the aggregated data to produce standardized and accessible social impact reports that help individual programs understand their social performance relative to other participating organizations. At the same time, by standardizing data among many organizations, Cornerstone is able to understand and analyze the impact of the sector as a whole.

HomeKeeper and CoMetrics are different in many ways but they share an underlying approach that has proved powerful in both cases and has the potential to be truly transformative.

PERFORMANCE MANAGEMENT FOR A WHOLE SECTOR

These two systems grew in response to two problems common to social enterprises. First, small organizations have as much to gain from the use of performance data as large corporations do, but small organizations generally cannot afford to build the kinds of systems necessary to address their most important performance business needs. Second, to bring in new resources to expand a sector, it is helpful to have better data on the overall performance of the sector; however, it is almost impossible to compare and consolidate data from many small organizations that each track different metrics.

CoMetrics and HomeKeeper both grew from a common recognition that these two problems are easier solved together than alone. That is, the way to solve the second problem and obtain quality standardized data on the performance of a whole sector is to help individual social enterprises work together on a shared solution to the first problem so that they can each gather better data to manage their performance internally.

Teaming Up to Capture Enterprise Performance Data

The Champlain Housing Trust (CHT) in Burlington, Vermont, sells homes at deeply discounted prices to lower-income families that would otherwise be priced out of homeownership. However, they make an agreement with those families that is becoming increasingly more common as homeownership subsidy sources run scarce; in exchange for help in buying a home, CHT maintains an equity stake in the property, the value of which is passed to the next family that needs help to purchase the unit when it is sold. When the organization was founded in 1984, this was still a very new idea and no one knew how well it would work. For example, could homeowners build meaningful wealth while the program preserved affordability?

By 2008, when CHT had sold more than 400 houses and seen 200 of those homes resold by the original buyer to another lower-income buyer, they decided that they had enough experience to finally ask hard questions about whether the experiment was working. CHT dedicated significant resources for an entire year to tracking down its paper files on each home sale, entering the relevant data into a spreadsheet and analyzing the results. The resulting report focused on whether the program had delivered on its initial promises: Did owners build wealth, did the program preserve affordability, were subsequent buyers able to purchase without any new public assistance, and other similar questions.[1] They found that the homes became slightly more affordable with time (reselling at prices that were affordable to a lower-income group than the initial buyers) whereas the sellers realized enough equity gain that 70 percent were able to purchase market-rate homes with no public assistance. These results were encouraging but also quite surprising. Because the work of compiling the performance data was so daunting, they had operated for decades without really knowing if their program was doing what it was designed to do.

CHT is not alone in facing this driving-in-the-dark dilemma and, in fact, they are unique among comparable homeownership programs because they made the resources available to answer these big questions.

---

1 J. E. Davis and A. Stokes, *Lands in Trust, Homes That Last: A Performance Evaluation of the Champlain Housing Trust* (Burlington, VT: Champlain Housing Trust, 2009).

There is a trend in philanthropy to provide nonprofit staff with training in designing systems for data collection and evaluation and then expecting each organization to manage an ongoing research effort on its own. For the smaller organizations that constitute the bulk of the sector, this is an unrealistic expectation given limited resources and the lack of data cultures. When Cornerstone Partnership was formed, we realized that it was not practical to expect every homeownership program to undertake the kind of research project that CHT had, but we wanted every organization to be able to see its performance in the same way.[2]

Rather than asking each organization to construct its own "theory of change" and related impact metrics, and then build a unique data collection program, Cornerstone convened stakeholders from more than 100 organizations to identify shared values and common social impact goals. Cornerstone then constructed a set of social impact metrics focused on the social goals shared by most of these programs. These standardized measures are specific to this particular type of housing program and most would not be relevant to any other type of program. At the same time, they surely do not capture every impact that is important to every participating organization. Just as the food co-ops did through CoMetrics, by bringing together a large number of programs that were similar enough, we were able to spread costs in a way that made it practical to undertake the kind of thoughtful and robust data collection project that would have been entirely impractical for any organization to undertake alone.

Understanding Sector Performance

At the launch of Cornerstone Partnership it was clear that growth in the sector would require better long-term performance data—not just in one community but across the country. Cornerstone commissioned the Urban Institute to conduct a formal evaluation of seven shared equity programs that concluded that other programs could have similar results in very different housing markets and using different affordability mechanisms.[3] However, the process took a full year and thousands of

---

2 At the time, Rick Jacobus was Director of Cornerstone Partnership and Annie Donovan was Chief Operating Officer of Capital Impact Partners.

3 K. Temkin, B. Theodos, and D. Price, *Balancing Affordability and Opportunity: An Evaluation of Affordable Homeownership Programs with Long-term Affordability Controls* (Washington, DC: Urban Institute, 2010).

hours of staff time. Although this kind of formal evaluation is essential, HomeKeeper was born out of the recognition that we needed a more everyday approach to performance measurement.

To obtain relevant data about long-term outcomes, we needed all the programs to collect a standardized set of data at the time that they were providing service. Cornerstone convened a working group to define metrics and design a data system that would consolidate outcome data from the entire sector. Most of the participating organizations reported that they already collected the key data necessary to track the common impact metrics, and we initially assumed that the primary challenge would be to convince participating organizations to change their existing databases to collect the data in a more standardized format. However, as we looked more closely, we found that none of the organizations had anything approaching a formal data system. They were tracking different data in different systems and, in many cases, key information was not tracked in any electronic system. If we wanted impact data, we would have to help our members build better administrative data systems. At the time, this seemed like a setback, but in hindsight, it was a lucky break. We wanted a top-down view of the sector, but to find a useful view we had to start from the bottom.

Although HomeKeeper is still under revision, the users consistently mention how much they love it. It has yet to develop the bells and whistles that people have come to expect from slick software, but it is designed from the ground up around the very specific tasks that an administrator of a homeownership program has to complete every day. It makes people's jobs easier. Putting all of their data in one place makes it possible to answer questions in seconds that previously took hours to answer—if they could be answered at all.

Each HomeKeeper user has his or her own version of HomeKeeper, which can be customized and modified as needed. Only the relatively small number of fields that are used in calculating the social impact metrics cannot be modified by users. HomeKeeper was built so that as programs sell homes, the system continuously submits transaction data to the national data hub. Users have the ability to see and correct data that is being submitted, but they don't have to take any special action to submit it.

In the HomeKeeper National Data Hub, data are aggregated from all the participating programs and standardized social impact reports are produced. These reports help people see how their programs are doing on the common impact metrics and benchmark their performance against the results from their peers.

On the strength of the Urban Institute research and the initial investment in HomeKeeper, Cornerstone was able to secure a $5 million competitive grant from the federal Social Innovation Fund (SIF). The SIF was designed to support social program innovations that are backed by evidence of effectiveness. Cornerstone Partnership is working with the Urban Institute to complete a formal evaluation of its SIF investments, and HomeKeeper is providing a ready platform for data collection for that study. Although most HomeKeeper users are not involved in the SIF grant program, the Urban Institute is able to access data collected through HomeKeeper by the SIF grantees to conduct its evaluation.

In the food sector, which operates on notoriously slim margins, the national organization that sponsors CoMetrics, National Cooperative Grocers Association (NCGA), has created a $1.6 billion shared purchasing program that delivers an increase of more than 1 percentage point in gross margin, on average, for its members. Because the organizations share risk to gain this kind of value, NCGA must regularly take the pulse of members' financial performance. CoMetrics creates a quarterly risk matrix report (Figure 1), which gives a snapshot of performance and an easy, faster way to identify potential trouble.

SOME LESSONS

Although both of these experiments in shared data are relatively new, they point in a very promising direction. These two projects have developed some practices that seem worthy of widespread implementation in any shared data project.

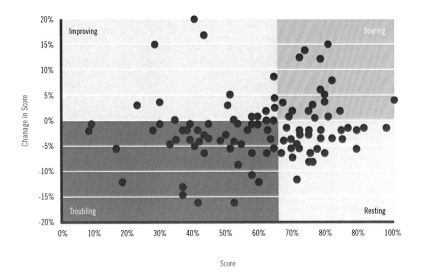

Figure 1. Sample Risk Matrix Report. This visualization makes it easy to pinpoint underperformers, who are then given technical assistance to improve their performance. The multidimensional database underlying the presentation of the data is used for deeper analysis of problems and can point to resolutions. Throughout the Great Recession, no defaults occurred under the national purchasing agreement. This outcome was possible only because co-ops had access to data in an actionable form and the ability to respond quickly to problems.

Telling a Story with the Data

As hard as it is to collect useful data, it is even harder to put the data to work to change policy or practice. People want to use data but, when confronted by complex tables and charts, meaning can be elusive. The human mind processes stories more readily. A key challenge for data projects such as these is to assemble data into a narrative that is relevant and actionable. This is easier said than done because with most data there is no obvious narrative.

This challenge can be addressed in two important ways. First, organize data analysis around specific, plain-language questions that practitioners have identified as important. Second, provide peer benchmarks, which put these answers in context, make them more concrete, and provide a natural narrative framework that makes it easier for people to understand and act on the data.

Leading With Questions That Matter

Before building the HomeKeeper data system or designing the Social Impact Report, Cornerstone convened more than 100 industry stakeholders in three different daylong meetings to discuss what success looks like for an affordable homeownership program.[4] Furthermore, although they ultimately developed mathematical formulas that produce standardized "metrics," Cornerstone started with plain language statements about what an ideal program "should" accomplish. For example, everyone seemed to agree that a successful program should serve families that were otherwise underserved and should have a low foreclosure rate.

For each of these "should" statements, there is a corresponding performance question (e.g., "Who did you serve?" or "How many foreclosures were there?"). To build the HomeKeeper system, Cornerstone identified the data that organizations currently were or easily could be collecting that were relevant to these questions. Next came intensive technical work to develop metrics with precise definitions for each of the elements. However, when we designed the HomeKeeper Social Impact Report, we returned to the big-picture questions. The HomeKeeper reports are structured around 27 plain-language questions. For each question, there are one to three charts or metrics that are meant to answer the question. (Figure 2)

The questions include:

- What are the income levels of homebuyers?

- Are buyers paying more than they can afford?

- Is the program preserving affordability?

- How often were homes sold?

- What return on investment did sellers receive at resale?

- How many buyers still own a home after five years?

- Are foreclosures common?

---

4 Cornerstone Partnership, "Stewardship Principles for Affordable Homeownership." http://affordable-ownership.org/principles/.

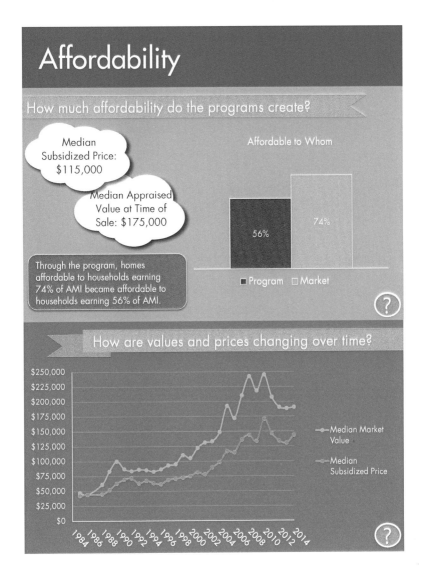

Figure 2. Sample HomeKeeper Report

These reports are automatically generated by our data system with little or no human editing, but they were designed to follow a clear storyline as much as possible. In many cases, in addition to charts and graphs with the relevant metrics, the report includes a plain-language restatement of the finding in the chart so that the "answer" appears twice— once as a chart and once in a sentence. The hope is that by structuring the meaning into the presentation in this way, the data becomes more accessible and ultimately easier for people to use to improve their work.

Finding Common Cause

The power of sharing performance data is not always immediately obvious. At one point, CoMetrics founder, Walden Swanson, was conducting a data dive with a peer group of produce managers from dozens of retailers from the Northeast. To Swanson's surprise, a general manager (GM) of one of the stores walked into the meeting.

The GM pulled Swanson aside to let him know why he was there. The reports generated by CoMetrics showed a decline in performance of his store's produce department. He wanted to fire his produce manager, and he was there to find and recruit the best performing produce manager in the region.

As the GM watched from the back of the room, Swanson led the produce managers through their numbers. Because results are standardized, individual store performance can easily be compared with the peer group. It did not take long to discover that *everyone's* produce department performance was down. The group grappled with the reasons why and concluded that there was a common cause: it was an El Niño weather year and rising produce prices had pushed everyone's margins down.

The store the GM managed was performing in the top quartile. As it turns out, the GM already had one of the highest performers. The problem was that without this kind of comparative benchmark, it is impossible to understand what is driving overall performance.

Closing the Loop: Taking Data in a Full Circle

Too much of the social sector's data flows in one direction only—away from the people doing the work and toward the people funding the work. Obviously funders have a legitimate need for data. However, there is a concern that some funders cannot make real use of the data that they collect because neither the funder nor the grantees has any confidence that the data accurately reflect what is happening on the ground.

There are many reasons for this lack of confidence. Whenever we try to aggregate data from multiple organizations, real work is involved in translating the way each organization codes its information into whatever the standard is. In the worst cases, grantees are left to their own devices to struggle with this problem and, in the face of limited resources, they do whatever is easiest even though that might generate misleading data. However, even in the best cases in which grantees diligently attempt to fit their square-peg data into the funder's round holes, they have to make many assumptions just to make things work. The grantees never know if they are doing it "right." Whoever receives and attempts to analyze the resulting data cannot know what those assumptions were and, in all likelihood, different grantees made differing assumptions. The result is that the aggregate data are less and less useful to the funder. This is an inherent challenge facing any data aggregation project, no matter how well designed and executed.

HomeKeeper and CoMetrics have developed a similar response to this challenge. Rather than pull data one way only, we take the data around a full circle; after being aggregated and analyzed, the data return to the hands of the very people who created it. Sometimes what they see makes sense to them and sometimes the results look very wrong and they speak up. Sometimes we have to change the way we interpret the data that they are providing and sometimes they have to change the way they enter the data in the first place. Either way, we both end up with greater confidence that the end analysis is "right."

When the data makes a round trip, end users often discover outcomes previously unrealized. There was wide agreement among HomeKeeper users that all homeownership programs should be ensuring that their homeowners were paying no more than an "affordable" share of their monthly income for housing costs. The Department of Housing and Urban Development (HUD) considers any household that pays more than 30 percent of its income for housing to be "cost burdened," but most HUD programs do not strictly prohibit selling to buyers who will be cost burdened so long as they meet other standards. Although many of our stakeholders believed that 33 percent or even 35 percent might be a more appropriate standard, they agreed that this measure was a key part of evaluating a programs performance. Therefore, when data started flowing into the HomeKeeper hub, we were surprised to see that nearly 20 percent of homebuyers were paying housing costs that initially represented more than 33 percent of their income.

Because the program administrators themselves are a key audience for the HomeKeeper Social Impact Reports, we were able to receive quick and clear responses to this finding. Users viewing the HomeKeeper report can click on individual data points and "drill down" to the underlying transaction data, and one further click will open their Salesforce account to the relevant homebuyer's record so that they can make changes or explore further. Users confronted with this unexpected outcome could easily perform a "reality check" on the average and tell us if we were doing something wrong or if they were.

What we learned was that the problem resulted from a number of different situations that fell into three general categories:

1 Some programs were delegating the job to mortgage lenders of ensuring that purchases were affordable. In the past, lenders had been unwilling to lend to buyers who would be cost burdened, but like so many other lending standards, this one was relaxed significantly in the early 2000s. In these cases, the impact report was doing its job and pointing out a failure on the part of the programs.

2 Just as often, we found that complexities related to the entry of a household's income (particularly related to income sources such as Social Security or child support) made buyers who actually were not cost burdened appear to our report to be paying a higher share of income than they really were. This was a failure of our data system to consistently capture all the relevant information.

3 But after accounting for both of these cases, a large number remained in which programs had knowingly allowed buyers to purchase even when their total housing costs exceeded the cost-burden standard. Most frequently, this occurred because the families had been facing an even higher cost burden in their prior housing situation. HUD rules generally allow this kind of exception but we were surprised by how many buyers fell into this category. This is a failure of the standard itself. As housing costs have risen, families have become accustomed

to paying far more than one-third of their income for housing, and what was once a rare exception has become something of the norm.

Without this kind of open-ended exploration of the data directly along-side the end users, we could never have made sense of this result. We would have had to choose between *wrongly* concluding that the data pointed to an enormous failure of our programs to meet an appropriate standard or *wrongly* concluding that there was no cause for concern because our data was flawed. As it turned out, there was some cause for concern. The data called out a practice that was leading some programs to sell to buyers who might be in over their heads, but the practice was nowhere near as widespread as it looked at first. Only by bringing the data full circle back to the ground level data providers could we have developed enough confidence in the results to call attention to the real problem.

The F. B. Heron Foundation appreciates how interacting around the data can contribute to better performance management of its investees. It has broken from the pack by investing in CoMetrics to create a common platform through which recipients of its newest investment product, Philanthropic Equity (PE), will report their results. PE is funding targeted to the growth of enterprises (nonprofit, for-profit, or other legal forms) and not to specific projects. CoMetrics has created a common chart of accounts onto which each investee has been mapped. Each quarter, investees will submit both financial and social impact data, which can be standardized, reported to Heron through an interactive web interface, and then returned to investees for their own analysis.

CONCLUSION

Everyone wants better data, but it is hard to justify taking scarce resources away from *delivering* social impact and putting it into *measuring* social impact. In the private sector, data has already won this rhetorical battle: There is a widespread recognition that companies that have invested in better data have frequently been able to use that data to drive improvements in financial performance that more than justify even very significant data system costs. Better data helps companies do everything else more effectively and efficiently.

But in the social sector, we have not yet proven this point. HomeKeeper and CoMetrics show that by working together, social enterprises can marshal data to drive meaningful insights, but we have yet to fully see those insights consistently hitting the (social) bottom lines of participating organizations. Data projects such as these will be fully sustainable only when participating organizations tap the power of the data to drive regular and ongoing incremental improvements in how they deliver social impact. Unless organizations can use better data to make more of a difference, better data will be an expensive luxury both for organizations and their funders.

■ ■ ■

ANNIE DONOVAN *is CEO of CoMetrics. She was formerly senior advisor to the White House Office of Social Innovation and Civic Participation and chief operating officer of Capital Impact Partners.*

■ ■ ■

RICK JACOBUS *is a consultant specializing in strategies for creating and preserving mixed income communities. He is currently F.B. Heron Foundation joint practice fellow at CoMetrics. He previously served as director of Cornerstone Partnership where he led the team that created HomeKeeper, a tool for managing affordable homeownership programs and tracking their long-term social impact.*

DATA TRANSPARENCY AND STANDARDIZATION

Paige Chapel
Aeris (formerly CARS Inc.)

Ten years ago, community development loan funds, led by Opportunity Finance Network, tasked themselves with increasing transparency, accountability, and standardization in their industry to strengthen performance and attract increased capital. The result was CARS, the Community Development Financial Institution (CDFI) Assessment and Ratings System, which over the past decade has led to the collection of an unprecedented amount of data and information on individual CDFIs. The CARS methodology is used by Aeris (www.aerisinsight.com) to analyze and rate CDFIs' impact performance and creditworthiness. Back in 2004, being rated was an unsettling proposition for many CDFI leaders, who worried that capital would flee to only the highest-rated institutions and that CDFIs would be pitted against each other. Ten years later, those fears have not materialized. Instead, ratings have brought more standardization and transparency to CDFIs' financial and portfolio performance reporting. Some CDFIs have used the ratings as a management tool for strengthening organizational effectiveness. For others, the ratings have sped up the underwriting process for their investors and, for a small but increasing number, attracted capital from new investors.

Aeris ratings sit atop a deep foundation of highly standardized data, but until recently those data were not available to the general investor market. As the number of rated institutions has increased, investors new to the CDFI sector approached us about accessing CDFI data. Investors recognize that CDFIs are one of the few mission-driven, fixed-income investment opportunities in the social investment space. But without timely, standardized data, it was nearly impossible to understand the performance of CDFIs as an investment class. Aeris had much of the data investors sought, but not in a format that would serve as a due diligence vehicle for investors and a useful management tool for CDFIs.

With significant support from the Citi Foundation and the Ford Foundation, Aeris built a cloud-based data collection and analytic system—the Aeris Cloud—that allows both Aeris-rated and non-rated CDFIs to easily upload quarterly financial and portfolio performance data and annual impact metrics. The Aeris Cloud provides both CDFIs and investors access to standardized quarterly performance data—including all the ratios, tables, and graphs used in Aeris ratings analyses, as well as real-time peer and industry trend analytics drawing from CDFIs' audited annual and internally reported quarterly data.

We created the Aeris Cloud as a central repository of standardized data that would: (1) help position CDFI debt as part of a recognized asset class in mainstream financial markets; (2) reduce reporting redundancies that divert CDFI resources from creating opportunities in underserved, low-income, and marginalized communities; and (3) serve as a useful tool for CDFI managers and boards. The challenge was building a system that could capture the complexity of these diverse institutions without adding burden to their reporting process.

Surveys had shown that CDFIs supported creation of a central repository and saw value in quarterly reporting, but only if it required fewer than 30 minutes each quarter to input data. To ensure the system's responsiveness to CDFI needs, Aeris assembled 10 chief financial officers (CFOs) from a diverse group of loan funds. The CFOs emphasized that data input had to be easy, but also that they wanted to be able to access the data to both ensure the data were correct and to track their own performance. Accordingly, uploading data requires as few as five minutes each quarter. The only requirement is that the upload must be in a single Microsoft Excel file in whichever format the CDFI uses. Once the data are uploaded, the CDFIs can click on their standardized financial statements to check for accuracy and review multiple years (or quarters) of data, performance ratios, and analytic trends. The process for submitting data corrections to Aeris is interactive, electronic, and tracked in perpetuity to create an audit history. Once the CDFI's financial audit is available, Aeris staff "true-up" internally reported year-end data to reflect audited results.

The Aeris Cloud also allows CDFIs and investors to track a variety of performance metrics (annually or quarterly) against an Aeris-established or user-defined peer group. It supports trend analysis for all reporting CDFIs, specific lending sectors, or a user-defined set of loan funds. CDFIs can compare their own performance with that of their peers, and investors have the tools they need to better understand and assess industry and enterprise risk and performance.

Standardized financial performance data and analytics are one piece of the investment puzzle—impact data are another. CDFI loan funds collect and report myriad impact metrics based on funder and investor requirements and the CDFI's own internal assessment of progress against its mission. But these data are not in forms that can be aggregated to support an under-standing of the industry's impact on the nation's low-income populations or communities. As a future project, Aeris will work with CDFIs and investors to define a set of standardized impact metrics that apply to specific CDFI sectors and can be easily collected, reported, and aggregated.

Reliable data are important for positioning CDFI loan fund debt as part of a recognized investment class. The Aeris Cloud is a major advancement, but more is needed. At a minimum, the following must be achieved:

- More CDFIs must join the early adopters who embrace the greater transparency and standardization that mainstream financial markets expect. Although financial data are publicly available for nonprofit loan funds via the Internal Revenue Service (IRS), some CDFIs are hesitant to share their data. Unfortunately, IRS data, which do not capture the complexity of CDFIs, can be easily misinterpreted. The Aeris Cloud allows CDFIs to share their financial data in a format appropriate for a financial institution.

- CDFIs must make transaction-level performance data more transparent to support development of new capital vehicles and to open investment management platforms to CDFIs. These data could be used to: (1) chal-lenge the convention that CDFIs must maintain high net-asset levels to protect investors from loss (capitalization ratios for CDFI loan funds are at least double the level for regulated depositories); (2) help overcome misperceptions about loan performance that prevent CDFIs from being listed on trading platforms; and (3) support development of investment vehicles that provide access to new sources of capital.

It may take a decade or longer, but with the infrastructure Aeris has built, the CDFI industry is closer to meeting the data and information needs of the capital markets and realizing improved efficiencies through standard-ized reporting. The ultimate beneficiaries will be underserved communities throughout the United States that will gain access to more capital and more opportunity as CDFIs thrive and expand.

■ ■ ■

PAIGE CHAPEL *is President & CEO of Aeris (www.aerisinsight.com), the information service for community investors. Paige has been a leader in community development finance for more than three decades, and is one of the foremost experts on community development financial institution (CDFI) loan funds. Presently, her career is devoted to connecting CDFIs with financial markets to increase the flow of capital to disadvantaged communities in the U.S.*

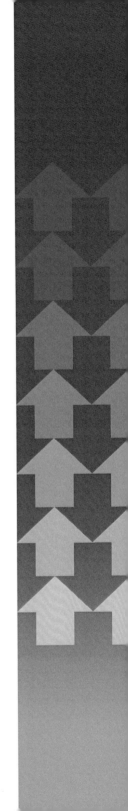

4

STRENGTHENING THE VALIDITY AND USE OF DATA

Community-based participatory research (CBPR), which uses a community-centered approach to data gathering and translation, can significantly improve the "relevance, rigor and reach" of data-driven practices. Engaging community members in problem definition, data collection, analysis, and design of interventions can ensure that data-driven practices are culturally meaningful, valid, and appropriate. It can also help build the capacity of both individuals and the community to study and address health and social issues of local concern. While not without challenges, CBPR is a critically important approach to use when working in historically marginalized and vulnerable communities.

ENHANCING DATA QUALITY, RELEVANCE, AND USE THROUGH COMMUNITY-BASED PARTICIPATORY RESEARCH

Meredith Minkler
University of California, Berkeley

The past two decades have witnessed growing calls for research conducted with—rather than on—communities. Researchers themselves have often voiced frustration with the limitations of traditional "outside expert–driven" research for gathering data and developing evidence-based interventions to address complex health and social problems. Meanwhile, calls from National Institutes of Health (NIH), the Institute of Medicine, and other government bodies, foundations, and communities for research that is "community *based*," not simply "community *placed*," have stimulated the movement toward new, community-engaged approaches to data gathering and translation. Long-standing distrust of outside researchers doing "parachute research"—dropping in , collecting data, disappearing, and leaving nothing behind—has also necessitated a new, more culturally sensitive orientation to research.[1] This is the case particularly in low-income communities of color, which sometimes refer to academic researchers as "the real undocumented workers."

Yet another reason exists for the increasing attention to research that actively engages local residents and other partners: Communities often have sophisticated insider knowledge and understanding that allow researchers to ask the right questions and gather data in ways that will increase the "relevance, rigor and reach" of the findings to effect change.[2]

---

1   V. Deloria, *God is Red: A Native View of Religion.* (Golden, CO: North American Press, 1992).

2   C. L. Balazs and R. Morello-Frosch, "The Three Rs: How Community-Based Research Strengthens the Rigor, Relevance, and Reach of Science," *Environmental Justice* 6 (1) (2012): 9–16.

DEFINITION AND CORE PRINCIPLES

Community-based participatory research (CBPR) is concisely defined as "systematic investigation, with the collaboration of those affected by the issue being studied, for the purposes of education and taking action or effecting change."[3] Drawing on the work of Barbara Israel at the University of Michigan and her community and academic partners, the core principles of CBPR include (1) recognizing the community as a unit of identity; (2) emphasizing community strengths; (3) ensuring the research topic is important to the community; (4) engaging community members throughout the research process; (5) facilitating community capacity building and systems change; and (6) balancing research and action.[4] In addition, CBPR should explicitly include attention to gender, race, class, and culture. These factors interlock and influence every aspect of the research enterprise.[5] The concept of "cultural humility" is particularly useful for recognizing and helping address the privilege and unintentional biases researchers may bring to a CBPR effort. Developed by Melanie Tervalon and Jane Garcia, cultural humility suggests that while researchers can never be "competent" in another's culture, they can demonstrate openness to learning about other cultures while examining their own biases, addressing power dynamics, and committing to authentic partnership.[6]

CBPR occurs on a continuum. Applications range from the use of community advisory boards (CABs) to help with sample recruitment or other specific tasks, to the more emancipatory end of the continuum with its emphasis on community engagement throughout the processes

---

3   L. W. Green et al., "Study of Participatory Research in Health Promotion: Review and Recommendations for the Development of Participatory Research in Health Promotion in Canada" (Vancouver, British Columbia: Royal Society of Canada, 1994).

4   B. A. Israel et al., "Review of Community-Based Research: Assessing Partnership Approaches to Improve Public Health," *Annual Review of Public Health* 19 (1) (1998): 173–202. Also see B. A. Israel et al., "Introduction to Methods for CBPR for Health." In *Methods in Community-Based Participatory Research for Health*, 2nd ed., edited by BA Israel et al. (San Francisco: Jossey-Bass, 2013).

5   M. Minkler and N. Wallerstein, "Introduction to Community-Based Participatory Research: New Issues and Emphases." In *Community-Based Participatory Research for Health: From Process to Outcomes*, 2nd ed., edited by M. Minkler and N. Wallerstein (San Francisco, CA: Jossey-Bass, 2008).

6   M. Tervalon and J. Garcia, "Cultural Humility Versus Cultural Competence: A Critical Distinction in Defining Physician Training Outcomes in Multicultural Education," *Journal of Healthcare for the Poor and Underserved* 9 (2) (1998): 117–125.

of data collection, data interpretation, and data-based action for change.[7] Increasing efforts are made in both government-and philanthropic-funded university partnerships and grassroots community-led partnerships to meet the gold standard of CBPR, with genuine, high-level community engagement occurring throughout the process.

HOW COMMUNITY-BASED PARTICIPATORY RESEARCH IMPROVES DATA COLLECTION, ANALYSIS, AND USE

CBPR can add value to data collection, relevance, and use in multiple ways. Here, I examine specific advantages of this community-partnered approach for improving data and research, using "real world" examples to illustrate each point.

Source and Relevance of Research Questions

CBPR helps ensure that the research question comes from—or is of genuine concern to—the community. When funding sources mandate research on particular health or social problems, or when researchers in academia, government, or the private sector decide in advance the topic to be studied as it relates to a particular community, valuable data may be produced. But that data may be irrelevant to genuine concerns of community residents. Consequently, the findings may be used to develop and deploy interventions that achieve modest results at best, partly because of lack of community interest or uptake.[8] In contrast, when communities are actively engaged in identifying a problem they believe is relevant, their involvement with the study will be greatly improved. Furthermore, community engagement ensures greater likelihood that the findings will be both useful and translatable into changes in programs, practices, and policies that benefit the community.

Getting it right. In the early 1990s, residents of Harlem strongly suspected a link between the area's high rates of childhood asthma and the presence of seven of the eight city bus depots, in addition to

---

7 Minkler and Wallerstein, "Introduction to Community-Based Participatory Research." Also see E. J. Trickett, "Community-Based Participatory Research as Worldview or Instrumental Strategy: Is it Lost in Translation(al) Research?" *American Journal of Public Health* 101 (8) (2011): 1353–1354, available at http://health-equity.pitt.edu/2614/.

8 S. L. Syme, "Social Determinants of Health: The Community as an Empowered Partner," *Preventing Chronic Disease* 1 (1) (2004): 1–5.

numerous other polluting facilities.[9] A local organization, West Harlem Environmental Action (WE ACT; www.weact.org) reached out to an epidemiologist at the Mailman School of Public Health at Columbia University to study this problem. The resulting partnership used air monitoring and geographic information systems (GIS) mapping as key data collection methods. Their studies, conducted in part with WE ACT's high school-aged "Earth Crew" youth, led to high-quality data. These data helped achieve a number of important policy outcomes, including stricter air quality standards, which withstood all legal appeals, and the conversion of all city buses to clean diesel.[10] The respect shown for community identification of need also formed the basis of a long-term collaboration. After more than 16 years, partnership continues and the community partner has occasionally been the recipient of federal grants, which are subcontracted to the university partner. Had the researcher at Columbia failed to acknowledge the wisdom of the community's concern with asthma and diesel pollution, this long and highly successful partnership would likely never have taken shape.

Acceptability of Data and Data Collection Tools

CBPR can improve the cultural acceptability of data collection tools, often enhancing their validity and the utility of the data collected. Data collection instruments that reflect lack of familiarity with acceptable terms and local concerns often result in lower participation rates and data of questionable value. For example, although the notion of empowerment is central to CBPR, no single word in Spanish captures this concept and, indeed, many Spanish terms with power at their center refer to "power over," not "power to" or "power with," and thus completely miss the true meaning of this term. Similarly, data instruments referring to a community by its official name may miss the common and deeply valued local designations of a neighborhood and reinforce the lack of cultural and social familiarity of outside researchers. We can learn from community partners for more successful and effective data gathering and use. Community partners teach us how

9 P. Shepard, V. B. Vasquez, and M. Minkler, "Using CBPR to Promote Environmental Justice Policy: A Case Study from Harlem, New York." In *Community-Based Participatory Research for Health: From Process to Outcomes*, 2nd ed., edited by M. Minkler and N. Wallerstein (San Francisco, CA: Jossey-Bass, 2008).

10 Ibid.

to refer to particular health or social conditions in a local community. In addition, they teach us whether individual interviews, focus groups, secondary data analysis, air monitoring, or other data collection methods may be most acceptable and useful.

Getting it right. Partnering with the local Chinese Progressive Association and the hiring and training of six immigrant restaurant workers in the Chinatown Restaurant Worker Health and Safety Study in San Francisco resulted in substantial improvements to both a detailed survey instrument and a new restaurant observational tool that the health department partner used to assess restaurant health and safety from a worker perspective, and not merely that of a customer. The final data collection instruments enabled the gathering of detailed data from 433 individual workers and all but two of Chinatown's 108 restaurants. Policymakers later credited the data as contributing substantially to the city's passage and implementation of one of the nation's first wage theft ordinances.[11]

"Ground-Truthing"

Community members can also play a key role in "ground-truthing," or checking the validity of existing government or other data sets.[12] Although many scientists rely on government data sets and conduct secondary data analysis on problems such as air or water pollution, these data sources are often dated and flawed. The quality and utility of data sets can be improved with assistance from the community in checking the accuracy of the data sets and using area "walk-throughs" with maps and/or tablets and GIS devices.

Getting it right. Using government GIS maps of stationary toxic pollution emitters and "sensitive receptor land uses" (e.g., schools, day care centers, and other places where residents are likely to be particularly sensitive to such emissions), residents in California's San Fernando

---

11 C. C. Chang et al., "Popular Education, Participatory Research, and Community Organizing with Immigrant Restaurant Workers in San Francisco's Chinatown: A Case Study." In *Community Organizing and Community Building for Health and Welfare*, 2nd ed., edited by M. Minkler (Piscataway, NJ: Rutgers University Press, 2012). Also see M. Minkler et al., "Wage Theft as a Neglected Public Health Problem: An Overview and Case Study From San Francisco's Chinatown District," *American Journal of Public Health*, 104(6)(2014), 1010–1020.

12 P. Brown et al., *Contested Illnesses: Citizens, Science, and Health Social Movements* (Berkeley: University of California Press, 2012).

Valley and other areas have successfully "ground-truthed." They performed the process by walking through neighborhoods with existing data sets and using their observations "on the ground," in addition to their lay knowledge of new facility closings or openings, etc., to provide substantially better and more up-to-date data than the data on which government offices and decision makers had previously relied. In the San Fernando case study, residents also found a number of previously unnoted sensitive receptor land uses, which they added to what is now a much more accurate data set.[13]

Design and Implementation of Data-Driven Interventions

Community engagement can improve the design and implementation of data-driven interventions, increasing the likelihood of success. Outside expert-designed interventions often reflect little knowledge of local customs and beliefs. Resulting interventions may be doomed to fail, often at substantial cost. Numerous multiyear, multimillion dollar research efforts to address problems such as tobacco control in low-income communities have attempted community engagement. However, these efforts were largely designed and implemented by outside experts. As public health leader S. Leonard Syme and others have noted, the results have tended to be disappointing, and community distrust of outside researchers has often been reinforced in the process.[14]

Getting it right. A cluster-randomized, controlled trial was conducted in California's Salinas Valley to test interventions aimed at reducing children's exposure to pesticide residue brought home on the clothing etc. of their farmworker parents.[15] Yet two of the interventions never would have succeeded had it not been for the input of farmworker members of the project's Community Advisory Board (CAB). For example, when CAB members were asked about the proposed addition of hand washing stations in the fields, they pointed out that in their Mexican culture, washing hands in cold water was believed to cause arthritis. With that

---

13 Ibid.

14 Syme, "Social Determinants of Health." Also see N. B. Wallerstein, I. H. Yen, S. L. Syme, "Integration of Social Epidemiology and Community-Engaged Interventions to Improve Health Equity," *American Journal of Public Health* 101 (5) (2011): 822–830.

15 A. L. Salvatore et al., "A Community-Based Participatory Worksite Intervention to Reduce Pesticide Exposures to Farmworkers and their Families," *American Journal of Public Health* 99 (S53) (2009): S578–S581.

information, the proposed intervention was redesigned to include water heaters, and hand washing rates at lunch time and before going home significantly improved.[16] Respect for community wisdom also helped build the trust that has enabled more than a decade of additional data gathering from this community, including current policy-focused interventions and an environmental health youth leadership program.[17]

Data Interpretation

Community-engaged research can improve data interpretation. Outside researcher interpretation of data based solely on scientific approaches, and lack of familiarity with local cultures and contexts, can lead to misunderstanding of the data, decreasing its usefulness and sometimes leading to flawed program recommendations and policy.

Getting it right. The East Side Village Health Worker Project, a partnership between Detroit community-based organizations and academic partners at the University of Michigan, Ann Arbor, trained and actively engaged village health workers (VHWs) in collecting and interpreting data from a random household sample of more than 700 residents.[18] Although the academic partners were surprised to find overall resident satisfaction with access to care, the VHWs quickly explained that quality of care was a far greater concern than access to care in this low-income neighborhood, whose members sometimes had access to government programs or clinics for the poor, but of less-than-adequate quality. Similarly, in the Chinatown study, trained worker partners participated in weekly data interpretation workshops. Their many contributions included pointing out that the high proportion of workers reporting that they received "paid sick leave" (42 percent) was likely inflated. This figure reflects the fact that for many in this community, paid sick leave simply means having the ability to take a day off when ill or caring for a sick relative and making it up later with an extra day's work without pay.[19]

16 Ibid.

17 D. Madrigal et al., "Health in My Community: Conducting and Evaluating Photovoice as a Tool to Promote Environmental Health and Leadership among Latino/a Youth," *Progress in Community Health Partnerships: Research, Education, and Action (in press).*

18 A. J. Schulz et al., "The East Side Village Health Worker Partnership: Integrating Research with Action to Reduce Health Disparities," *Public Health Report* 116 (6) (2001): 548–557.

19 Chang et al., "Popular Education," Minkler et al. "Wage Theft."

New Channels for Data Dissemination

Engaging community partners in research can help identify and use new channels for data dissemination. Canadian scholar and activist Dennis Raphael is fond of asking, "If an article is published in *Social Science and Medicine* but nobody reads it, does it exist?" Although the importance of traditional academic and professional vehicles for disseminating findings cannot be minimized, community partners can play an important role in determining how best to reach the community "end users" of data, relevant organizations, and policymakers.

Getting it right. In the Harlem case study mentioned earlier, the data generated on asthma and diesel exposure were both scientifically sound and deeply troubling. Although the academic partner took the lead in submitting jointly authored articles to peer-reviewed journals, the community partner used numerous other avenues to "get the word out" to the local community and policymakers. Seventy-five bus shelter ads, an alternative fuels summit, legislative briefings and testimony, and articles in a community newspaper were among the methods used. WE ACT also conducted "toxic and treasure tours" for local policymakers—highlighting not only toxic exposures but also the rich cultural heritage of the neighborhood, with landmarks such as the Apollo Theater and its pivotal role in the history of jazz.[20] This dissemination of findings did not preclude subsequent publication of more detailed analysis. But it did help jump start the process of data-driven community organizing and advocacy and helped effect many significant policy changes.

Improving Public Policy

Community-engaged research can help in the use of data to improve public policy. Many academic and other researchers develop reliable data with substantial policy and practice relevance but believe that using that data to help inform action for change is outside their purview. With its emphasis on action as part of the research process, and the credibility it has achieved with numerous public and private sector sources, CBPR can help legitimize the role of researchers, as part of a

---

20 Shepard et al., "Using CBPR to Promote Environmental Justice."

partnership, in ensuring that data are used to effect positive community and social changes.

Getting it right. For many incarcerated men, leaving jail or prison is a "round trip," and in some areas, close to one-half of newly released prisoners are back in custody within a year.[21] A community-academic partnership in New York City collected extensive data on this situation through multiple methods, including secondary data analysis, public opinion polls, focus groups, policy analysis, and interviews with social service providers and recently incarcerated men. Through these multiple means, they uncovered 11 state policies that worked against staying out of jail. These included the common practice of releasing men after midnight with a bus ticket back to the community where they were arrested in the first place. In addition, policy included terminating rather than temporarily suspending, their access to Medicaid, meaning that those with substance abuse, other mental health problems, or physical conditions such as HIV/AIDS, were unable to receive the help they needed on release. By working together beyond the funded project period, academic/activist Nicholas Freudenberg, his community, and other partners used these data to help change these and other policies citywide.[22] Other communities have followed their example.

Building Individual and Community Capacities

Engaging community partners in research can help build individual and community capacities, leaving behind a community more able to study and address other health and social issues of local concern. One of the greatest benefits of CBPR is, arguably, its contributions to increasing critical thinking, individual and collective problem-solving abilities, civic engagement, and future orientation among partici-pants—particularly those from marginalized communities. Sometimes called "street science," CBPR is a means of democratizing the collection and use of data and in the process increasing active citizenship and local leadership.[23]

---

21 A. G. Blackwell et al., "Using Community Organizing and Community Building to Influence Public Policy." In *Community-Based Participatory Research for Health: From Process to Outcomes*, 2nd ed., edited by M. Minkler and N. Wallerstein (San Francisco, CA: Jossey-Bass, 2008).

22 Blackwell et al., "Using Community Organizing and Community Building to Influence Public Policy."

23 J. Corburn, *Street Science: Community Knowledge and Environmental Health Justice* (Cambridge, MA: MIT Press, 2005).

Getting it right. In Old Town National City, a once-vibrant heart of the Latino community in San Diego County, California, rezoning as a mixe use neighborhood led to skyrocketing asthma rates as the community was overrun by auto body and paint shops and other polluting businesses.[24] The local Environmental Health Coalition (EHC) hired and trained Latinas as lay health advocates, or *promotoras*, to help study and address this problem. The promotoras learned to do door-to-door surveys and to measure ultrafine particulate matter, which academic colleagues recently had shown to be related to adverse lung development in children.[25] At the same time, the promotoras also learned public speaking, media advocacy, and "data language," including how to present both their findings and those from GIS–based "visual foot prints" developed by EHC staff, to capture the huge disparities in toxic emissions exposure between their community and three adjacent footprints. The promotoras used role playing and follow-up debriefings to improve their presentations before City Council hearings and in private testimony. They learned to do base building, recruiting many other local residents to become civically active. The work of the promotoras and their partners was given much of the credit for helping pass a Specific Plan in 2010, restoring the community to resident-friendly uses Additionally, many of the promotoras continued their high-level civic engagement in other issues of concern. One of these women not only successfully ran for city council but became Old Town National City's vice mayor, a position she continues to hold at this writing.[26]

CHALLENGES AND LIMITATIONS IN COMMUNITY-BASED PARTICIPATORY RESEARCH

Although I have stressed the many ways in which CBPR can improve data collection, interpretation, and use to effect change, this approach can be messy, time consuming, and fraught with challenges.

---

24 M. Minkler et al., "Si Se Puede: Using Participatory Research to Promote Environmental Justice in a Latino Community in San Diego, California," *Journal of Urban Health* 87 (5) (2010): 796–812.

25 W. J. Guaderman et al., "The Effect of Air Pollution on Lung Development from 10–18 Years of Age," *New England Journal of Medicine* 351 (11)(2004): 1057–1067.

26 M. Minkler et al., "Community-Based Participatory Research: A Strategy for Building Healthy Communities and Promoting Health Through Policy Change: A Report for the California Endowment" (Oakland, CA: PolicyLink, 2012). http://www.policylink.org/sites/default/files/CBPR.pdf.

Time and Labor-Intensive Nature of the Work

Building and maintaining partnerships take substantial time both early on and throughout the research and action processes. This often is compounded when working with youth, low-literacy groups, or immigrant workers who frequently work long hours and return home to serve as primary caregivers across generations. Translation costs and time delays, and the extra training time needed when working with partnerships that vary dramatically in education, social class, and racial/ethnic background add to the time and costs incurred. Finally, as highlighted earlier, the call to include action as part of the research process itself often requires the engagement of outside researchers and their partners well beyond the funded project period.

In the community reentry project for men recently released from incarceration in New York City, many of the most significant policy victories occurred after the funded project period had ended.[27] Similarly, in the Chinatown case study, policy-level change to address rampant wage theft among restaurant workers took place, in part, because project partners continued to work with policy allies at city hall to help craft and achieve passage of two new pieces of legislation after the project funding had ended. This work, and the resulting wage-theft ban and enforcement measure, contributed substantially to the subsequent record levels of recovered wages in Chinatown and other parts of the city as well.[28]

Conflicts and Power Dynamics

Conflicts and power dynamics are a challenging but necessary part of community-engaged research. Civil rights leader Bernice Regan once remarked that if a coalition is too comfortable, you probably do not have a very good coalition. Similarly, in CBPR, partners should include groups that do not see eye-to-eye on all issues but who share a commitment to the topic being studied and are willing to deal with conflict. Struggles for power, the just allocation of resources, and elements of the study design and implementation are parts of the process itself. Developing initial ground rules, principles of engagement, and

---

27 Blackwell et al., "Using Community Organizing and Community Building to Influence Public Policy."

28 Chang et al., "Popular Education"; Minkler et al., "Wage Theft."

memorandums of understanding (MOUs), as well as ongoing evaluation and feedback, may help address these concerns early. Having a partnership evaluator or evaluation subcommittee, and using guiding criteria and rating scales to assess partnership adherence to CBPR principles and best practices, may also help the partnership stay on track and confront and address difficult issues as they arise.[29]

Ethics Committees and Institutional Review Boards

Ethics or institutional review board (IRB) processes and criteria typically are not well aligned with the principles and processes of community-engaged research. Requirements that the principal investigator (typically a university-based partner) assume overall responsibility for major project-related decision-making is antithetical to CBPR, with its emphasis on shared power and equitable participation of all partners in project-related decision-making. Similarly, IRBs seldom are comfortable with the extensive ongoing community involvement in data collection and use that CBPR projects can entail—a problem that commonly can lead to long delays in IRB clearance.[30]

Educating IRBs on CBPR can help address this process, and a small but growing number of universities have created IRB subcommittees specifically trained to evaluate community-engaged research proposals. Yet the continued mix-match between principles of CBPR and the requirements for IRB approval often remains a substantial hurdle. Sarah Flicker at York University and her colleagues in Toronto[40] have developed a helpful set of guidelines for IRBs as they review community-engaged research projects.[31] These criteria stress community, not only individual-level risks and benefits of research proposals. Included among their guidelines are questions such as: How was the community involved or

29 Chang et al., "Popular Education." Also see S. L. Mercer et al., "Reliability-Tested Guidelines for Assessing Participatory Research Projects." In *Community-Based Participatory Research for Health: From Process to Outcomes*, 2nd ed., edited by M. Minkler and N. Wallerstein (San Francisco, CA: Jossey-Bass, 2008).

30 D. Buchanan, F. Miller, and N. Wallerstein, "Ethical Issues in Community Based Participatory Research: Balancing Rigorous Research with Community Participation in Community Intervention Studies," *Progress in Community Health Partnerships* 1 (2) (2007): 153–160. Also see P. Brown et al., "Institutional Review Board Challenges Related to Community-Based Participatory Research on Human Exposure to Environmental Toxins: A Case Study," *Environmental Health* 9(39) (2010): 1–12.

31 S. Flicker et al., "Ethical Dilemmas in Community-Based Participatory Research: Recommendations for Institutional Review Boards," *Journal of Urban Health* 84 (4) (2007): 478–493.

consulted in defining the need?; How will the project balance scientific rigor and accessibility?; and, Are there built-in mechanisms for dealing appropriately with unflattering results? Partnerships themselves can also benefit from using these tools and discussing these issues well in advance of data collection, which brings up a related question: What will be done if findings do not support the action agenda, which the community partner may be hoping to pursue?

In a CBPR project between academic partners and hotel workers and their union in San Francisco, a preliminary agreement was made that findings would be published, even if the findings did not support the workers who hoped to show that lean staffing and pressure to work more quickly had adversely affected their health. Fortunately in this case, the data strongly supported their position and were successfully used in contract negotiations, with the outside researcher and worker partners at the bargaining table to help make the case for reductions in work load.[32] But the opposite could have happened, and having agreements in place early on about how data will be used can help avoid tensions later.

Scientific and Community Concerns Regarding Data Collection and Interventions

Tradeoffs exist between scientific priorities and community concerns regarding data collection and data-driven interventions. The enhanced cultural sensitivity and relevance of research instruments made possible by high-level community collaboration may also, at times, conflict with outside research partners' desires for the most rigorous possible research designs and study instruments. Community partners may question the relevance of certain validated scales or may oppose, on the grounds of fairness, a randomized controlled study, given that not all participants stand to gain from a potentially useful intervention. Approaches such as a staggered research design, in which control group members do receive the intervention, albeit not as early as the treatment group, may help address these concerns but may not fully satisfy some community partners who are anxious to see widespread local benefit from their participation.

---

32 P. T. Lee and N. Krause, "The Impact of a Worker Health Study on Working Conditions," *Journal of Public Health Policy* 23 (3) (2002): 268–285.

Timelines for Data Sharing

Tensions exist between the "necessary skepticism of science" and the "action imperative of the community" with regard to data sharing and use.[33] Public health leader Richard Hofrichter points out the mixed messages frequently given by academic researchers: "What do we want? Evidence-based policy! When do we want it? After peer review!" Community partners may wish to move more quickly from findings to action, including advocating for change, whereas research partners may wish to move more slowly, conducting further data checks to ensure the accuracy of any findings put forward and, in some cases, waiting for peer review and publication of findings. Moreover, some scientific journals require that results not be shared before their publication. Yet asking community partners to wait for what may often be two to three years before sharing data that could help move programs, policies, and practices does not keep with the fundamental commitments of CBPR. A growing number of top-quality journals now publish CBPR and understand that some key findings may indeed have been shared with primary stakeholders in advance to help promote change. Although some journals continue to have editorial policies stating that recommendations for policy and other changes should be omitted and placed instead in commentaries and letters to the editor, these are not appropriate venues for the publication of community-engaged work.

As noted earlier, data also may emerge, which could show the community in an unflattering light and which community partners do not want to have "go public." Continued dialogue and MOUs may be helpful in anticipating these uncertainties and deciding on ways to deal with them early on, but these methods are not likely to preclude unanticipated issues regarding data ownership and use from arising. Such issues will require the utmost care as they are addressed.

SUMMARY AND CONCLUSIONS

CBPR involves many challenges, from the substantial time and labor involved through the compromises that must sometimes be reached regarding data collection methods and other key aspects of the work.

---

33 R. Price and T. Behrens, "Working Pasteur's Quadrant: Harnessing Science and Action for Community Change," *American Journal of Community Psychology* 31 (3/4) (2003): 219–223.

These challenges may be intensified when partnering with marginalized groups, often with low educational levels, limited command of the dominant language, and severe time and income constraints. Yet, the potential of CBPR for improving the "relevance, rigor and reach" of data, and for building individual and community capacity, is increasingly seen as outweighing the challenges involved.[34] Community engagement clearly is not appropriate for all forms of research. However, when it is appropriate, working collaboratively with community partners in the research process can improve a particular research endeavor. It can also help to further increase the democratization of data collection and use as we continue progressing into the 21st century information age.

■ ■ ■

MEREDITH MINKLER, DrPH, MPH, is a professor of health and behavior at the School of Public Health, University of California, Berkeley, and the founding director of the university's Center on Aging. She co-edited the first major book on community based participatory research in the health field and has more than 30 years of experience in developing and implementing community partnerships, community organizing and community-based participatory research that engages with diverse community groups including the low-income elderly, people with disabilities, youth and women of color.

---

34 Balazs and Morello-Frosch, ,"The Three Rs."

Residential mobility is one of the primary factors driving neighborhood change and can have an important effect on social conditions and quality of life in an area. Community organizations need data on residential mobility to guide strategic decisions about their work with people and places and accurately evaluate the effect of their efforts. However, measuring residential mobility is not a simple matter. This essay discusses the range of indicators that are needed to capture different aspects of the process: residential mobility, residential instability, housing unit turnover, and the components of neighborhood change. Use of a mosaic of data sources is recommended for calibrating the understanding of how mobility affects neighborhood progress.

USING DATA TO UNDERSTAND RESIDENTIAL MOBILITY AND NEIGHBORHOOD CHANGE

Claudia J. Coulton
Case Western Reserve University

Residential mobility shapes both the experiences of individuals and the characteristics of neighborhoods. Approximately 12 percent of U.S. households relocate yearly, and residential mobility rates are higher among low-income households, renters, and younger families. Neighborhoods vary in their levels of residential mobility as well, and housing units turn over more frequently in neighborhoods: (1) with low homeownership rates; (2) with larger shares of households without children or stable employment; and (3) undergoing changes in the built environment or local economy. While residential mobility is neither uniformly positive nor negative, the implementation and outcomes of community change initiatives are affected by the level and type of mobility in their target areas. As such, practitioners and policymakers need to make better use of available data and analytic methods to understand mobility in the communities they serve.

WHY WE NEED TO UNDERSTAND RESIDENTIAL MOBILITY

Community initiatives and organizations strive to benefit people and places, and data can measure the progress and effects of these efforts. However, the fact that residential mobility is one of the primary factors driving neighborhood change makes the interpretation of community indicators challenging. For example, a neighborhood may seem as if it is improving based on point-in-time indicators, but these "snapshots" of neighborhood measures cannot distinguish whether conditions are improving for current residents or whether change is being driven by an influx of newcomers who are better off than residents they are replacing. By digging deeper into the data, we can shed light on the questions of gentrification and displacement that often come up in community change initiatives.

An incomplete understanding of mobility can also lead to misinterpretation of data that indicate a lack of change in community conditions. Households, for example, may take advantage of neighborhood-based services and opportunities to improve their situation and then move, but the neighborhood socioeconomic profile may seem unchanged if these households are replaced by newcomers with similarly high levels of need. Relying only on point-in-time measures, one could incorrectly conclude that the assistance programs available in a neighborhood were not effective. A study of residential mobility and neighborhood change in 10 cities concluded that some neighborhoods that remained poor were really very dynamic, serving as launch pads for many residents who moved to better areas only to be replaced by poor newcomers.[1] Other neighborhoods that also appeared poor in consecutive snapshots were more like traps in which numerous poor residents were stuck in place for extended periods with few opportunities to move up, either residentially or economically.

Mobility also has implications for the success of community initiatives, since too many or too few moves can affect whether individuals are able to benefit from interventions intended to help them. Frequent residential moves resulting from stress or yielding no improvement in circumstances have negative consequences, particularly for children.[2] Community programs may create new housing or economic opportunities in a neighborhood, but if households are forced by circumstances to move frequently, they may not remain in the same area long enough to benefit from the programs. The goals of the community initiatives may also be thwarted if minority individuals have difficulty leveraging their new skills or assets to move to better neighborhoods because their freedom of movement is constrained by racial and economic segregation. By understanding the many ways that mobility can affect people

1 C. Coulton, B. Theodos, and M.A. Turner, "Residential Mobility and Neighborhood Change: Real Neighborhoods under the Microscope," *Cityscape: A Journal of Policy Development and Research* 14 (3) (2012): 55–89. http://www.huduser.org/portal/periodicals/cityscpe/vol14num3/Cityscape_Nov2012_res_mobility_neigh.pdf.

2 T. Jelleyman and N. Spencer, "Residential Mobility in Childhood and Health Outcomes: A Systematic Review," *Journal of Epidemiology and Community Health* 62 (7) (2008): 584–592.

and neighborhoods, practitioners can tailor programs to their particular context and knowledgably interpret indicators of neighborhood change.

PERSPECTIVES ON RESIDENTIAL MOBILITY

Gauging residential mobility as a positive or negative force, and then shaping interventions to suit, depends on understanding a number of factors such as the reasons for moving, the frequency and timing of moves, and the results of relocation for people and places. For individuals, moving to a new home can reflect positive changes in a family's circumstances, such as buying a home for the first time, moving to be close to a new job, or trading up to a better house or apartment. But mobility can also be a symptom of instability and insecurity, with low-income households making short-distance moves because of problems with landlords, creditors, or housing conditions. Similarly, staying in place can reflect a family's security and satisfaction with its home and neighborhood surroundings, whereas in other cases, it may reflect lack of resources to move to a better home or neighborhood. A study of disadvantaged neighborhoods in 10 cities found that only about one-third of movers left for better places, while two-thirds simply moved nearby to similarly distressed circumstances. Likewise, approximately two-thirds of those families who remained in place did so reluctantly, and only about one-third were satisfied with their situation.[3]

At the neighborhood level, residential mobility can be problematic but can also be a source of neighborhood vitality. As a negative force, excessive residential turnover can diminish neighborhood social ties, and weaken neighborhood institutions by disrupting neighbors' participation. High residential instability, combined with concentrated disadvantage, undermines the ability of neighbors to take collective action, and in turn limits the ability of residents to prevent crime and maintain safety and order in their neighborhoods.[4] On the positive side, increased housing turnover is key to maintaining housing market strength and preserving homeowner equity as areas attract newcomers.

---

3   Coulton et al., 2012.

4   J.D. Morenoff and R.J. Sampson, "Violent Crime and the Spatial Dynamics of Neighborhood Transition: Chicago, 1970–1990," *Social forces* 76 (1) (1997): 31–64. Also see R.J. Sampson, S.W. Raudenbush, and F. Earls, "Neighborhoods and Violent Crime: A Multilevel Study of Collective efficacy," *Science* 277 (5328) (1997): 918–924.

An optimal level of turnover can bring talent, vitality, and enrichment to the neighborhood. Moreover, mixed-income development, one important policy option for reducing persistent poverty and social exclusion, requires the replacement of at least some low-income households with middle-income households.

Finally, data on residential mobility must be interpreted in light of what is known about the structural influences shaping neighborhood selection. For low-income households, particularly those that are African American, the neighborhood selection process is fraught with roadblocks and constraints. A history of racial discrimination in housing markets and a lack of affordable housing make many neighborhoods simply out of reach. Studies of household residential mobility show African Americans are disadvantaged compared with whites regarding access to better neighborhoods.[5] This adverse neighborhood selection process tends to reinforce neighborhood inequality, often across generations, where families may be mobile but only within low performing neighborhoods that offer limited educational and economic opportunities. Because the cumulative effect of various neighborhood contexts affect individual well-being, structural barriers to residential mobility tend to reproduce social inequality over time.

MEASUREMENT ISSUES AND DATA SOURCES

Measuring residential mobility is not a simple matter, and a range of indicators is needed to capture different aspects of the process: residential mobility, residential instability, housing unit turnover, and neighborhood change. Researchers should carefully select data collection and analysis methods, paying attention to aspects of residential mobility that are of interest and practical to measure. For example, should the focus be on individuals, households, housing units, or neighborhoods? Should the measurement be based on a cross-sectional or longitudinal perspective? What is the definition of moving with respect to time and space? What data sources are available, such as individual or household surveys, administrative records, or interview data? The common approaches to measuring residential mobility differ

---

5 R.J. Sampson and P. Sharkey, "Neighborhood Selection and the Social Reproduction of Concentrated Racial Inequality," *Demography* 45 (1) (2008): 1–29.

regarding these questions, and these nuances must be taken into account in interpretation.

Cross-sectional measures of individual residential mobility

One of the most commonly used measures of residential mobility is from the U.S. Census Bureau's American Community Survey (ACS). The survey asks each individual in the sampled households whether he or she lived in the current housing unit for at least one year. If the answer is no, the survey asks for the respondent's previous location. The residential mobility rate for the neighborhood is calculated as the percentage of the population that was not in the sampled housing unit in the previous year. This ACS–based residential mobility measure is cross-sectional and can be interpreted as a one-year residential mobility rate for individuals. For small areas such as census tracts, the one-year individual residential mobility rates must be derived from the ACS five-year sample estimates. The summary measure reflects how many people surveyed each month during the five-year period had moved within the year. Although most residential moves are local, the ACS data also identifies the prior year's move as from outside the county, state, or country. Numerous studies of neighborhoods use this cross-sectional measure of residential mobility. It has played an important role in research on community social organization.

Household level measures of residential mobility

The measurement of residential mobility for households is a more complicated matter than for individuals because it is difficult to disentangle household moves from changes in household composition. Community initiatives are often interested in the latter because household turnover has different implications for their programming than does the movement of individuals. Households may be doubling up, for example, or children may be placed with relatives in new homes. The census measures do not distinguish between individuals who return to or become part of an established household, such as a child returning from college or the addition of a spouse to the family, and an entirely new household moving in. Capturing these distinctions requires survey data on the same households over time. The survey must contain information on the individuals who compose the household at each survey point, allowing analysts to compare household membership to determine whether individuals or the entire household moved.

Data collected in low-income neighborhoods in 10 cities for the Annie E Casey's Making Connections program provides an example of this kind of analysis.[6] By matching the individuals in the household rosters gathered during different waves of the survey, researchers were able to determine whether the entire household made a residential move, or whether specific individuals left or joined the household. Their analysis found that household compositional changes were much more frequent than residential moves that involved the entire household relocating.[7] This type of analysis was also able to characterize the household changes based on the ages and relationships of household members.

Frequency of mobility measures

Although most families move infrequently, community initiatives often want to estimate the level of recurrent mobility among residents since frequent movers face particular challenges. But cross-sectional mobility rates do not capture this information. Instead, frequent mobility can only be calculated using information on the number of residential locations in which individuals have lived during a specified period. For example, a longitudinal study of low-income families in Michigan asked mothers to provide their residential movement history at each wave of data collection. Using this fine grained information, researchers have been able to measure the frequency of moves for children at various ages to determine the patterns of movement that put children at risk at certain developmental periods.

Even longitudinal studies do not provide all of the answers. It is difficult to measure the extent of residential mobility at the community level because longitudinal surveys seldom have enough respondents to provide reliable indicators for neighborhoods. However, the advent

---

6   The Annie E. Casey Foundation's Making Connections initiative was a decade-long effort focused on target neighborhoods in 10 cities: Denver, Des Moines, Hartford, Indianapolis, Louisville, Milwaukee, Oakland, Providence, San Antonio, and White Center (outside Seattle). The target neighborhoods offer a unique and valuable window to the dynamics of low-income, mostly minority neighborhoods nationwide.

7   K. Bachtell, N. English, and C. Haggerty, "Tracking Mobility at the Household Level," *Cityscape: A Journal of Policy Development and Research* 14 (3) (2012): 91–114. http://www.huduser.org/portal/periodicals/cityscpe/vol14num3/Cityscape_Nov2012_tracking_mob.pdf.

of Integrated Data Systems is making this measurement of frequent mobility more feasible. These systems link administrative records from multiple agencies at the individual level. The data can cover states, counties, or cities, and increasing evidence suggests that they are cost effective data sources for longitudinal research and policy evaluation.[8] These systems can be a source for measuring frequent mobility if they capture address histories for individuals from the various administrative records. Such address history data can be used to estimate numbers and frequencies of moves for the population covered in the data system. With these types of measures, stakeholders can identify pockets of frequently mobile families or individuals and explore interventions, reduce mobility, or at least minimize the harmful consequences of frequent mobility.

Measuring housing unit turnover and neighborhood change

Housing unit turnover and the role that it plays in neighborhood change reveals another aspect of mobility. The housing stock of a neighborhood typically changes slowly, whether through construction, demolition, or rehabilitation. The dynamic movement of households into and out of housing units, though, is a continuous flow that can affect the neighborhood in many ways. Housing unit turnover can have positive or negative consequences for the community depending on its magnitude, velocity, and the characteristics of those moving in and out. Community initiatives have the potential to manage these shifting population dynamics so that neighborhoods thrive rather than crumble under the momentum, but only if they have information on the patterns of housing unit turnover and the resulting changes in the population.

Examining residential mobility through the lens of housing units enables an understanding of point-in-time neighborhood composition and the flow of households that shapes it. Investigating the stock and flow requires longitudinal data on housing units and their occupants, but such data sets are relatively uncommon. One exception is the American Housing Survey (AHS), which tracks a panel of housing units in selected cities. A limitation of the AHS for communities is that the sample of

---

8   The Actionable Intelligence for Social Policy program at the University of Pennsylvania provides support for this work and information on how to develop such systems (see http://www. aisp.upenn.edu/).

housing units is selected to be representative of metropolitan areas rather than neighborhoods, so the data cannot be used to describe small areas. Nevertheless, this data can be used to understand the dynamics of displacement and gentrification. One study using a national sample of housing units in high-poverty neighborhoods suggested that increases in average income of occupants were a combined result of richer households moving in, the exit of some poorer households, and income increases for low-income households that stayed in place.[9] Thus wholesale displacement of the poor was not the norm but, instead, the socioeconomic status of occupants gradually changed.

The Making Connections survey mentioned previously is an example of a data source that tracks a representative sample of housing units within specific neighborhoods. Therefore, it can also be used to look at the contributions of housing unit turnover to neighborhood change. An analysis of these data shows that residential mobility levels are related to housing unit and neighborhood conditions. For example, single-family rental homes are more likely to turn over to poorer residents, even though the rate of turnover is higher in multifamily buildings. This may be caused by the tendency of owners of single-family homes to defer maintenance when they convert the properties for rental occupancy. In addition, housing units tend to turn over to poorer occupants when the surrounding neighborhood has low levels of social cohesion and safety.[10]

Having data on housing unit transitions and how those shape the mix of households in neighborhoods can be useful to community planning and development. This type of information can help communities monitor issues of concern such as disinvestment, gentrification, displacement, and segregation. Knowledge of where these processes are occurring, both with respect to types of housing units and their locations, can help guide action and enable the evaluation of progress on these fronts.

9   I. Gould Ellen and K. M. O'Regan, "How Low Income Neighborhoods Change: Entry, Exit, and Enhancement," *Regional Science and Urban Economics* 41 (2) (2011): 89–97.

10 B. Theodos, C. Coulton, and R. Pitingolo, "Neighborhood Stability and Neighborhood Change: A Study of Housing Unit Turnover in Low Income Neighborhoods." Paper presented at Federal Reserve System Community Development Research Conference (Washington, DC, April 11, 2013). http://www.frbatlanta.org/documents/news/conferences/13resilience_rebuilding_theodos.pdf.

Qualitative measures related to residential mobility

The decision to move and the choice of where to move is the end result of a unique combination of household, housing unit, and neighborhood factors that are difficult to capture with quantitative data. Data gathered through in-depth interviews or focus groups with both movers and stayers shed light on how individuals take these factors into account when deciding where to live. Studies conducted with families that were offered the opportunity to move from extremely poor to low poverty neighborhoods as part of the Moving to Opportunity (MTO) experiment illustrate the value of qualitative data. Even though on average these families moved to lower-poverty areas, many MTO households were not able to move to significantly better, or more racially diverse, places.[11] In fact, their decisions were influenced by a number of considerations that would not have been easy to quantify, such as connections with family and friends, perceptions of whether the neighborhood and school were a comfortable fit for their children, and other qualities of the physical and social environment. In addition, movers often lacked information about housing options and neighborhood and school quality that could have been helpful in seeking the best locations for themselves and their children.[12] Combining qualitative and quantitative data allows communities to better understand the factors underlying residential mobility and to develop strategies that enable residents to make successful residential decisions.

CONCLUSIONS AND IMPLICATIONS

Community organizations with access to a variety of measures that can shed light on residential mobility processes will be best positioned to make strategic decisions about their work with people and places and accurately evaluate the effect of their efforts. Communities would be wise to look beyond census measures of residential mobility and demographic profiles to fully evaluate neighborhood change. Longitudinal surveys of households and housing units, although costly, can provide additional insight into characteristics of households that move, whether

---

11 X. de Souza Briggs et al., "Why Did the Moving to Opportunity Experiment Not Get Young People into Better Schools?" *Housing Policy Debate* 19 (1) (2008): 53–91.

12 S. DeLuca and E. Dayton, "Switching Social Contexts: The Effects of Housing Mobility and School Choice Programs on Youth Outcomes," *Annual Review of Sociology* 35 (1) (2009): 457–491.

or not they improve their circumstances, and how these individual deci-sions shape the trajectory of neighborhoods. The Making Connections survey is a good example of a useful community data collection tool.[13] Integrated Data Systems are also promising adjuncts to census surveys. Networks such as Actionable Intelligence for Social Policy share the lessons of what it takes to launch and sustain these systems and can help nonprofits advocate for these systems in their communities. Finally qualitative data gathered from in-depth interviews with residents moving in, moving out, or staying in place can provide additional insight into how residential choices are made. The field can do a better job of sharing procedures and protocols to help nonprofits conduct their own interviews or partner with other research organizations to do so.

Even with these data sources, measuring and understanding residential instability is a challenging task, particularly for nonprofits without in-house research capacity. Establishing partnerships with local researchers may be an effective method for more completely under-standing this important dynamic. Those conducting community initia-tives should do their best to map out the best strategies for data collec-tion given the resources and type of intervention, but the picture will be incomplete in many cases. Community stakeholders can also apply their on-the-ground knowledge and lessons from other studies in the field about how mobility affects low-income households and neighborhoods. Using this mosaic of sources, we can be smarter in designing programs that consider patterns of mobility in our neighborhoods, identifying how positive and negative mobility affects our progress along the way and in tracking and interpreting neighborhood change.

■ ■ ■

CLAUDIA J. COULTON *is the Lillian F. Harris Professor of Urban Social Research in the Jack, Joseph and Morton Mandel School of Applied Social Sciences at Case Western Reserve University. She is also codirector of the Center on Urban Poverty and Community Development. Dr. Coulton is a founding member of the Urban Institute's National Neighborhood Indicators Partnership and has been involved in the evaluation of numerous community initiatives. She is the author of many publications on urban neighborhoods, community research methods, and social welfare policy.*

---

13 For complete information about its use, visit http://mcstudy.norc.org/.

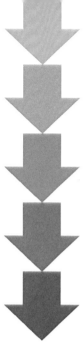

PUTTING DATA INTO ACTION FOR REGIONAL EQUITY IN CALIFORNIA'S SAN JOAQUIN VALLEY

Alex Karner
Arizona State University

Jonathan London
UC Davis Center for Regional Change

Dana Rowangould
Sustainable Systems Research, LLC

Catherine Garoupa White
UC Davis Center for Regional Change

In recent years, there has been a proliferation of new methods to identify, measure, and map issues of social and regional equity. Yet it is not always clear how best to use these methods to inform advocacy and policy change. The UC Davis Center for Regional Change (CRC) has taken up this challenge, combining innovative mapping tools, collaborative research, and technical assistance aligned with regional needs, to support policy change on a range of issues, from youth well-being to environmental justice and regional equity.

One area that the CRC has recently focused on is the implementation of California's Sustainable Communities and Climate Protection Act, Senate Bill 375. Passed in 2008, the bill requires metropolitan planning organizations (MPOs) to develop Sustainable Communities Strategies (SCSs).[1] The goal of each SCS is to reduce greenhouse gas emissions by coordinating land use and transportation planning, providing adequate affordable housing, and improving public transportation. Transportation planners at each MPO analyze the performance of their SCS using complex simulation models that provide estimates of future travel patterns and greenhouse gas emissions. To comply with the law, per-capita emissions from the plan must be less than a target set by the California Air Resources Board.

The bill's primary aim is to reduce driving; it contains no explicit requirement to analyze existing equity conditions or to ensure equitable conditions in the future. However, it does create a wider mandate for regional-scale planning aimed at reducing urban sprawl and redirecting growth and investment to dense locations well served by public transit. Sprawling patterns of development and overinvestment in highway infrastructure have led directly to current patterns of regional inequity. To the extent that SB 375 is intended to reverse these historical trends, it offers a chance to improve the health and well-being of the state's most disadvantaged communities.

Equitable outcomes are only possible if regional planners understand and embed specific elements into their SCSs. However, they often lack the policy mandate, data, and capacity to do so. California's San Joaquin Valley (SJV) is a case in point. Implementing SB 375 has been particularly challenging in this region. Despite the valley's substantial agricultural production and wealth, it is beset by acute social, political, and economic disparities. In particular, many of the region's poor and unincorporated communities lack strong political representation, are short on essential services, and are physically distant from urban job concentrations. These communities could greatly benefit from an equitable implementation of SB 375. However, most of the SJV's MPO planners have limited technical resources to develop SCSs with strong social equity components. Other challenges derive from the difficulties of coordinating the work of planners

---

1 MPOs are created by federal law to conduct transportation planning in urban areas with populations greater than 50,000. For more information on MPOs see: http://www.planning.dot.gov/mpo.asp.

and community advocates across all eight counties, when each county-scale MPO is developing a separate SCS.[2]

This is where the CRC has stepped in. Beginning in 2011, CRC faculty and staff have continuously engaged with diverse coalitions of social equity, environmental, and agricultural preservation advocates in the SJV. The goal has been to provide social equity planning tools and technical assistance to develop the area's SCSs to help meet the needs of the SJV's most disad-vantaged communities.

Specifically, the CRC has: a) conducted a Health Impact Assessment (HIA) of proposed SCSs in two counties; b) reviewed MPOs' environmental justice analyses in three counties; c) provided strategic advice to inform advo-cates' engagement in regional planning; and d) offered resources for MPO planners to integrate social equity considerations into their work. These efforts have helped achieve key victories. By calling attention to health disparities and transit access deficits in disadvantaged communities in Fresno and Kern counties, the HIA has led to new commitments from the Fresno MPO to study health and infrastructure needs and fund sustainable infrastructure and planning through a new grant program. In Kern County, CRC-developed environmental justice tools were incorporated by the MPO into part of their SCS.

The challenges and lessons learned from this work can be summarized in three points.

1 **Relationships Matter.** Integrating social equity into regional planning is not only a technical process. Its success also depends on the develop-ment of trusting and collaborative relationships between researchers, advocates, and planners.

To build such relationships, the CRC conducted a needs assessment with community advocates to identify the kinds of technical assistance that would best support their efforts. CRC staff participated in key advocacy gatherings, small workshops, and one-on-one consultations. Pre-existing relationships between the CRC team and the SJV's advocacy networks

---

2 Although most MPOs in the country span multiple counties, each of the eight counties in the SJV is also its own MPO. This fragmentation reflects the SJV's political culture that tends to emphasize local control of planning.

provided a strong platform for launching new collaborations. The CRC also worked with MPO staff to share social equity tools and data for SCS planning efforts. Staff at the Fresno and Kern MPOs later reciprocated by sharing data for use in the HIA.

2 **Capacity Matters.** The complexity of the data and tools used must be matched by the capacity of the intended users to engage in their development and application within the time available for planning and advocacy.

Following the initial needs assessment, the CRC team developed workshops and consultations with advocates and MPO planners to introduce tools and support their application. The novelty of the tools coupled with the urgent and shifting timelines of the policy process offered little time for advocates to fully absorb and "own" them. The short and simultaneous timeline of each MPO's SCS development also made it difficult for the CRC to assist advocates in evaluating SCSs while helping regional planners master new social equity tools. Effective future application of the social equity planning tools will require on-going capacity building activities aimed at both advocates and planners.

3 **Context Matters.** The successful implementation of social equity tools depends on the political climate and the attitudes of staff and decision-makers at regional agencies.

The SJV has a relatively conservative political culture that views issues related to social equity with some distrust. Engaging directly with planning staff was helpful for addressing these challenging politics. In Fresno County, CRC Director Jonathan London was invited to speak at the kickoff SCS planning event, introducing practical methods to put social equity and environmental justice "on the map." He also presented at a post-SCS Learning Exchange with the Fresno MPO to share lessons learned about integrating social equity into regional planning. In this and other communications with planners, the CRC framed social equity in ways that would align with local political values, emphasizing the relationship between regional equity, health, and economic prosperity.

Despite challenging political and social circumstances, the CRC and its community and agency partners have achieved notable success in shaping regional planning documents that reflect social equity values and that direct investments towards disadvantaged communities. The experience confirms that good data and analysis alone, while necessary, are not sufficient. Applied research and technical assistance must also be designed to account for the power of relationships, capacity, and context. This case study illustrates how diverse parties can work together to promote sustainable regional planning that guarantees healthy, prosperous and equitable outcomes.

Acknowledgment: The authors wish to recognize the generous funding of the Resources Legacy Fund, the many community and agency partners that made this work possible, and the editorial assistance of Dr. Krystyna von Henneberg.

■ ■ ■

The authors have extensive experience working across California and the U.S. to advance just, sustainable, prosperous, and equitable regions. The work documented in this essay was undertaken under the aegis of the UC Davis Center for Regional Change—a solutions-oriented research unit emphasizing community-based participatory methods, cutting-edge socio-spatial analysis, and a translational research orientation.

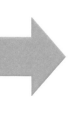

This essay examines the advantages and challenges of using shared measures in community development to evaluate the outcomes of complex revitalization programs, place-based strategies, or other initiatives. It explores how nonprofit organizations, intermediaries, and funders apply shared measurement within collective impact strategies and to evaluate similar programs implemented in different locations or for different populations in order to enhance learning about the myriad forces that drive community change. The essay concludes with questions and information that both organizations and funders can use to assess if shared measurement approaches would be a good fit for their community development evaluation needs.

SHARED MEASUREMENT: ADVANCING EVALUATION OF COMMUNITY DEVELOPMENT OUTCOMES

Maggie Grieve
Success Measures at NeighborWorks America

Community development involves long-term change in a complex environment, with many actors, strategies, and variables. Keeping track of all these components, let alone evaluating success, can be difficult. However, "shared measurement"—a method for assessing and understanding complex change—has captured the imagination of the community development and evaluation fields as nonprofit organizations, intermediaries, and funders seek more effective ways to understand the change that their programs and investments are making in communities.

Many organizations support or deliver similar programs that have the same intended outcomes. For example, financial capability programs delivered by multiple organizations throughout the country all aim to build financial skills and behaviors. Other community development efforts engage multiple organizations, each delivering its particular piece of a comprehensive strategy to accomplish a set of common outcomes. This approach is common in collaborative community revitalization efforts involving multiple organizations or multifaceted youth development programs. In both cases, evaluation using shared measures can be an effective and efficient way for organizations to learn whether they are achieving their intended outcomes.

This essay explores the benefits and challenges of using shared measures in community development. It also illustrates how shared measurement can be used for larger scale evaluation efforts that more fully engage organizations and their funders in defining how best to measure results of programs, collaborative efforts, or the field of practice. Finally, the essay examines how shared measurement efforts have built capacity and vocabulary for measuring outcomes among practitioners, while reducing the time and effort spent by an organization on evaluation after a start-up investment phase.

WHAT IS SHARED MEASUREMENT? WHY DOES IT MATTER?

Shared measurement approaches engage multiple organizations in using the same indicators or data collection tools to evaluate the performance or outcomes of their programs, place-based strategies or collaborative initiatives. Although applied across the community development field in several ways, organizations typically use common indicators and data collection tools to evaluate similar programs implemented in different locations or for different populations. For example, organizations draw on sets of shared measures to evaluate the outcomes of programs such as affordable housing development or community engagement in communities across the county. They may choose to share measures to better assess the most effective means of delivering similar programs. Alternatively, organizations may be primarily interested in under-standing the outcomes of their own programs, but want to enhance the validity of their own evaluation processes by drawing on tested measures used by other organizations in their fields. This use of shared measures can significantly streamline an organization's evaluation design process, saving both time and resources. Finally, a funder or intermediary may ask grantees or affiliates to use certain measures in common. In this case, the funder or other evaluation sponsor typically requests that organizations share data with them in order to look across the participating organizations to better understand the nature and scale of the outcomes achieved. Often, funders or sponsors may share their analysis to enhance learning and enable organizations to compare their own results within the context of the aggregated data set.

The most frequently cited application of shared measurement is within collective impact strategies. In these efforts, using shared measures enables a group of organizations working collaboratively to evaluate their progress toward a set of mutually defined common outcomes. For example, shared outcome measures may be used to assess outcomes of a comprehensive set of youth development programs including education, health care, employment, drug prevention, and mentoring. Rather than looking at the results of each program separately, organizations use a common set of measures across the programs to assess outcomes such as high school graduation rates, postsecondary education success or training goals, and the ability of youth to assume leadership roles. Using common measures in this way, organizations are likely to better align their program strategies, learn from the evaluation process collectively and use the results to strategize system-level enhancements that can significantly improve outcomes. In the most effective applications of shared measurement within collective impact strategies, the evaluation process itself strengthens the collaboration and can be a catalyst in enhancing program delivery to achieve intended program goals.

AN EVOLVING PRACTICE

Starting in the early 1990s, community development stakeholders began addressing the need for standard measures by developing common definitions for performance measures such as housing units developed or rehabilitated, jobs created or commercial properties developed. One of the earliest efforts was the Community Development Financial Institutions (CDFI) Fund's Common Data Project, notable for engaging a broad range of organizations within the emerging community development lending movement. Meanwhile, federal agencies were instituting performance measurement requirements, and national organizations, such as the International City/County Management Association, were developing a set of shared performance measures for local government services that covered response times for emergency services, provision of human services to youth and seniors, infrastructure improvements, and more.

As organizations began to master using common definitions to measure service provision and productivity, nonprofit organizations and funders wanted to better understand the broader change resulting from their work, including hard-to-measure changes such as quality of life and community resilience. Current shared measurement practice in U.S. community development emerged from this shift toward documenting outcomes rather than just units of service or other performance metrics.

Technology Fueled the Evolution

By the mid-1990s, advances in technology and greater availability of data led to the community indicator movement, another building block toward shared measurement.[1] The Urban Institute established the National Neighborhood Indicators Partnership (NNIP), which now includes 36 data intermediaries that support greater access to local and regional data on a range of community measures.

In the first decade of the 2000s, several sets of shared outcome measurement tools emerged. The earliest among these were the Aspen Institute's FIELD program's MicroTest for the microenterprise field; the U.S. Department of Health and Human Services' shared measures for Individual Development Accounts; and the comprehensive set of outcome measures for community development programs developed by Success Measures, an evaluation resource group at NeighborWorks America.

Technology played a pivotal role in the growth of shared measures. New tools provided accessible and secure ways to collect, access, manage, and analyze information to evaluate programs and place-based change. These included Efforts to Outcomes (ETO) by Social Solutions; the Success Measures Data System (SMDS) by NeighborWorks America Outcome Tracker by VistaShare; FamilyMetrics by Pangea Foundation; PolicyMap by The Reinvestment Fund; and the open-source Local Data application.

More recently, the impact investing movement developed sets of shared measures to monitor the financial, program, and social performance of a range of both domestic and international community development projects and social enterprises.[2] The Impact Reporting and Investment Standards (IRIS), an initiative of the Global Impact Investing Network (GIIN), is an example of a system designed to inform investors interested in tracking social return. The IRIS online catalog of generally accepted, shared performance metrics creates a common language for reporting social and environmental performance.

---

1   For more information on the community indicator movement, see Ben Warner's essay in this volume.

2   J. Freireich and K. Fulton, "An Industry Emerges." In *Investing for Social & Environmental Impact.* (San Francisco: Monitor Institute, 2009).

Today, the concept of sharing measures has become so widely accepted that, as a service to the field, online platforms such as PerformWell—a partnership of the Urban Institute, Child Trends, and Social Solutions—gather, categorize, and share data collection tools developed by other organizations throughout the country.

SHARED MEASUREMENT IN PRACTICE

The following examples illustrate how organizations are using shared measurement strategies to track short- and long-term outcomes in community development programs and investments.

Using Shared Measures to Evaluate Similar Programs or Strategies

Individual organizations interested in using shared measures to evaluate programs such as neighborhood revitalization, financial coaching, community engagement, or small business development can draw on available sets of shared measures or join with others to define and develop data collection instruments. These organizations may share a funder or intermediary interested in looking across a portfolio of similar efforts. They may be joined together in a network committed to a set of principles and practices or be completely independent yet interested in using measures established and vetted by others in the field. Typically, these organizations are motivated to use shared measures because they are primarily interested in examining their own outcomes or fulfilling funder accountability requirements. Having the ability to compare their findings with those of other nonprofit organizations using the same measures may not be important to them or be of secondary interest.

Shared Financial Coaching Measures: A recent example of funder-sponsored use of shared measures is the evaluation component of the Financial Capability Demonstration Project, a partnership between NeighborWorks America and the Citi Foundation. Thirty nonprofit organizations in 17 states used a common set of measures to document outcomes of financial coaching services. Drawing on a set of shared measures developed with input, review, and testing by experts and practitioners across the asset building and financial capability fields, these organizations used one common survey instrument to document their clients' household composition and measure changes in clients' financial status and saving, debt, and credit behaviors.[3]

With the support of technical assistance providers to plan and implement an evaluation, each organization selected at least one additional data collection tool to capture outcomes related to the specific focus of its coaching program, such as banking access, budget management, or college savings strategies. Over the course of the project, organizations also benefited from two convenings designed to provide training and peer exchange on key evaluation and data use strategies, as well as best practices. Using the Success Measures Data System, or its own client management systems, each organization collected at least two rounds of data on a sample of its financial coaching clients.[4] This structure provided each organization the data it needed to understand its own results and guide program improvements. It also allowed the funder to assess outcomes across the 30 organizations.

Results were aggregated for measures such as:

- Percentage of respondents who increased their credit score, as well as the mean increase.

- Percentage of respondents who started saving for the first time or increased savings.

- Percentage of respondents who decreased total unsecured debt and types of debt held, as well as the mean decrease in the amount owed.

- Change in number and type of bank, credit union, and long-term accounts.

- Changes in perceptions of ability to manage personal finances.

Shared Community Impact Measures: Another example of using shared measures for evaluation of similar programs is NeighborWorks America's Community Impact Measurement Project, which involves 23

---

3   NeighborWorks America, "Measuring Outcomes of Financial Capability Programs: Success Measure Tools for Practitioners." (Washington, DC: NeighborWorks America, 2011).

4   NeighborWorks America, "Scaling Financial Coaching: Critical Lessons and Effective Practices." (Washington, DC: NeighborWorks America, 2013). www.nw.org/FinCoaching13.

nonprofit members of the NeighborWorks Network.[5] These organizations are using the same measures to document change in communities across the country. The shared measures allow organizations to document the conditions of occupied and vacant residential and commercial properties, as well as levels of community engagement, resident satisfaction with neighborhood quality of life, and local economic impact.

In 2013, each organization identified an area of 500 to 1,200 households where it provides programs and received a data profile of the community's demographic, economic, and housing characteristics. Using a set of surveys and observation checklists, each organization systematically collected data, drawing on staff and community volunteers to complete the fieldwork needed. To ensure quality in this primary level data collection effort, experienced evaluators helped organizations draw appropriate respondent samples, train data collectors, plan survey implementation, and ensure high response rates. Participating organizations will collect this data again in future years for comparison. Economic impact is also analyzed based on performance data reported annually to NeighborWorks America by each organization.

The organizations are using their baseline data for a variety of purposes. For example, a number of them found that there were a greater share of longtime renters in their communities than they had assumed and that many were interested in remaining in the community to purchase a home. These organizations used this finding to direct some of their neighborhood marketing efforts toward current renters. In other communities, a detailed inventory of property conditions revealed patterns of roof, porch or other minor repair needs that led directly to new programs to address these problems. Other organizations focused on data they gathered on residents' confidence in their communities' futures and residents' willingness to become involved in working on community issues. In response, organizations are initiating or strengthening community outreach and engagement strategies.

Other noteworthy examples of this shared measurement model are Habitat for Humanity's Neighborhood Revitalization Initiative and the

---

5   NeighborWorks America supports the national NeighborWorks network of 245 independent community-based nonprofit organizations serving more than 4,600 communities nationwide.

Wells Fargo Regional Foundation's evaluation of its neighborhood plan ning and neighborhood implementation grant programs. Approximatel 100 of Habitat for Humanity's local affiliates throughout the country are using shared measures to evaluate the community impacts of their neighborhood revitalization programs. At the Wells Fargo Regional Foundation, based in Philadelphia, approximately 55 grantees working to revitalize communities in Delaware, New Jersey, and eastern Pennsylvania are assessing perceptions of community change using a common survey of residents' satisfaction with a variety of quality-of-life factors.

Benefits

In addition to the more general benefits of integrating systematic evaluation into their programs, organizations report several gains in learning and evaluation by drawing on shared measures. Organizations report that using shared measures:

- Helps streamline the evaluation design process.

- Gives organizations a shared language and experience that fosters peer learning to improve service delivery or development strategies.

- Allows organizations participating in citywide, regional, state, or national initiatives to contribute new understanding of program outcomes to the broader community development field.

The use of shared measures produced additional benefits for community development funders, researchers, and networks of nonprofits, including:

- A set of longitudinal, quantitative and qualitative primary level data on the effectiveness of various approaches to financial coaching or place-based revitalization; these data can inform policy, programs, and revenue streams.

- A shared evaluation vocabulary among funders and nonprofit organizations about outcomes.

- Greater capacity among hundreds of participating organizations to plan and implement evaluation.

- Standardized training and technical assistance processes that make it possible to implement an evaluation requirement across grantees or affiliates in ways that are perceived as fair and adequately supported.

- New organizational capacity to collect and use data at the community level; this capacity enables community-based organizations to become more effective partners with researchers addressing broad research questions.

Challenges

Community development organizations, intermediaries, and funders cite several challenges in implementing shared measurement evaluations.

Community Development Organizations

- Getting buy-in on the specific measures included in a common data tool. This is a particular challenge when programs target similar outcomes but employ different strategies, or when organizations are sharing data primarily with a funder or project sponsor but not with one another. This can be addressed by including in the common tool the core measures with broadest application and allowing organizations to add other data collection tools and questions to tailor their evaluation.

- Allocating the staff or volunteer time required for collecting primary-level data directly from clients and community residents. Organizations address this challenge by developing partnerships, recruiting additional volunteers, or in the case of client data, helping staff more seamlessly integrate data collection into program delivery.

- Addressing staff or leadership turnover and program or financial challenges. These organizational issues can easily derail a shared measurement effort regardless of an organization's initial commitment. Building in flexible technical assistance to bring new staff up to speed is essential for keeping the evaluation effort on track if there is turnover. Organizations facing program design or funding issues frequently need to set aside their evaluation efforts until those matters are resolved. Flexibility on the part of funders, partners or technical assistance providers can allow organizations to successfully resume their evaluation efforts at a later time.

- Ensuring data quality. This may be a particular challenge when an organization uses volunteers to collect data. A shared evaluation plan that clearly presents the data collection tools, data gathering process and method for checking data quality is essential. If also using a common technology tool for data collection and management, it is helpful to have a central source for accessible technical assistance to address issues organizations face along the way.

Intermediaries and Funders

- Setting realistic funder or project sponsor expectations about the scope of the results. In many cases, owing to the differing variables in the programs, the evaluation is not designed to compare results of different program models. Rather, the aggregate analysis demonstrate general trends in client or community results.

- Effectively directing technical assistance to support organizations in using shared measures. This is particularly challenging when many organizations are collecting data with the same measures. Online training, web-based materials, and remote phone and e-mail contact with a cadre of experienced evaluators on the topic have proven effective in addressing this issue.

Using Shared Measures to Evaluate Common Outcomes from Different Programs or Strategies

Shared measurement approaches are also used to evaluate collaboratively run initiatives striving toward collective impact. These efforts typically include a commitment among participating organizations to share data and, in some cases, jointly apply lessons learned. An example is the youthCONNECT initiative, a five-year partnership of Venture Philanthropy Partners and nonprofit organizations in the Washington, DC metropolitan area. YouthCONNECT is an effort to improve education, employment, and health behavior outcomes for low-income and at-risk youth, ages 14 to 24. Programs and services implemented by the six youthCONNECT network partners include college access; charter secondary education; youth development and services; HIV/AIDS prevention and treatment; and job and professional readiness through training, internships, and mentoring.[6]

When the youthCONNECT collaborative was created, the partner organizations committed to shared outcome measures to document progress. They defined the types of data each partner would collect and report. For example, organizations report which of their participants receiving youthCONNECT programming are enrolled in school and are on track to be promoted to the next grade level, which students graduate from high school, and which students enroll in and eventually complete postsecondary degrees. The partners also collect data on several other risk and protective factors, tracking data on youth who have positive adult relationships, avoid negative peer relationships, and avoid physical violence and substance use. Technical assistance provided by Child Trends played a key role in facilitating decisions about the evaluation design and is keeping the implementation of the shared measurement effort on track.

Benefits
The youthCONNECT partners identified key benefits of their shared measurement model. They found that it:

- **Reinforced partners' commitment to collaborative efforts.** Although the partners recognized that the toughest problems cannot be solved by any single funder, program, or agency, collective efforts were difficult to maintain. The shared outcome framework helped maintain accountability and participation by all engaged partners.

- **Enabled peer exchange and learning.** The use of common measures promoted teamwork when addressing data challenges, sharing training tips, and in peer-to-peer consulting.

---

6 The youthCONNECT partners include College Summit-National Capital Region, KIPP DC, Latin American Youth Center, Metro TeenAIDS, Urban Alliance, and Year Up-National Capital Region.

- Advanced project goals and created opportunities for the organizations to collectively reflect on their programs. Discussion about common measurement and evaluation procedures pushed the partner organizations to consider program refinements and to become more sophisticated in their thinking about key definitions and categories central to understanding their impacts.

Challenges

Key challenges identified by youthCONNECT partners include:

- Allocating the staff time and resources to the process. Developing and implementing a common outcome framework required significant time and commitment as well as a high level of critical thinking from each partner. This was managed by assigning one representative from each partner organization who could attend regular meetings, engage in organizational and community-level measurement discussions, and report to the respective organizations. However, the staff time still far exceeded initial estimates and, in response, the project funders provided supplemental funding to compensate for the additional resource needs.

- Agreeing on shared measures. Each partner organization needed to relinquish some degree of organizational autonomy for the project to succeed. To that end, organizations dealt with some of the practical challenges of collaboration by adopting common terminology, building relationships among the organizations' staff, accommodating program model diversity, and addressing differences in capacities to collect and use data.

LEARNING FROM PRACTICE: IS SHARED MEASUREMENT A GOOD FIT?

Shared measurement can be a useful, scalable approach that benefits individual organizations and advances practice on the whole. However, shared measurement takes time, resources, and sustained commitment. It also requires at least basic levels of data management and evaluation capacity within an organization and a willingness to balance individual organizational needs with the use of a standardized tool or framework. Funders and sponsors must have a realistic view of the cost to launch and sustain this effort. The time that nonprofit organizations and public-sector agencies must devote to a shared measurement effort must be adequately supported, particularly in the start-up phases. In addition, shared measurement cannot always be effectively aligned with proprietary program requirements in which each funder defines its own distinct outcomes, grant reporting requirements and technologies, and evaluation cycles.

How can organizations know whether shared measurement is appropriate?

Many factors must be considered, but the following questions can guide a range of stakeholders in determining whether using a shared measurement approach can advance their particular evaluation objectives.

For funders, intermediaries, public agencies, and other network or project sponsors:

- Are you interested in looking at outcomes across a grant portfolio, multisite initiative, or other major multi-organization effort?

- Is building the evaluation capacity of grantees, affiliates, or network members a priority?

- Does your organization have an interest in enabling peer learning among grantees or affiliates?

- Are you seeking tools to help organizations streamline outcome tracking and reporting?

- Will you need to scale an evaluation effort to a larger number of organizations or locations?

- Are you planning to sustain an evaluation effort in multiple sites through multiple rounds of analysis?

For local or regional nonprofit organizations:

- Are you involved in collaborative projects or part of a network interested in understanding your results according to common measures?

- Do you like the idea of having a head start in planning your evaluation process by drawing on sets of measures or data collection tools that others have developed for programs in your field?

- Are you interested in building your organization's ability to collect and analyze data rather than using an external evaluator?

- Is collecting qualitative data directly from program recipients or other local people or places essential to measuring your intended outcomes?

- Do you believe that shared measurement has the potential to advance learning in the field in a meaningful and consequential way?

If the answer is "yes" to several of these questions, shared measurement approaches can be a good fit. Organizations will also want to consider the range of practices, tools, and incentives that can make shared measurement more effective and useful. Ensuring adequate support and incentives can tip the scales to help sustain commitment to shared measurement by reducing the burden for nonprofits and funders. The following ideas drawn from applications of shared measurement provide a good starting place for organizations new to this approach.

Practices

- Providing training and technical assistance for practitioners is critical to ensure the collection of quality data and to troubleshoot organizational barriers to instituting shared measurement processes. Accessible, online training to build capacity is a scalable option, providing an affordable way to effectively reach a large number of organizations.

- Convening peer-learning opportunities, both virtual and in person, strengthens application of data to everyday organizational uses. Having a forum to share challenges and best practices can be valuable for practitioners and funders seeking to better understand the impacts for their investments in people and communities.

- Sharing successful examples of shared measurement models has the potential to advance community development and evaluation practice.

Tools

- Providing data collection tools that can be used in common is critical to successful shared measurement. To take full advantage of current and ever-evolving quality tools, investments must be made in menus and libraries of tested and relevant data collection instruments. Although the initial time and investment required can seem prohibitive, the resulting products form the backbone of a shared measurement process.

- Using technology to share measures and support data management, analysis, interpretation, and reporting is essential. Investment in technology can make a critical difference in the ability to consistently collect and aggregate quality data in shared measurement efforts.

Incentives

- Supporting a streamlined evaluation planning process through shared measurement offers a clear, practical way to determine what outcomes to measure and how to measure them. Organizations save time and planning effort because they do not need expertise in all aspects of evaluation to achieve quality evaluation design, tools, and analysis. Menus of common measures and data definitions that are easily accessible and understood by practitioners are a vital building block of an effective shared measurement process.

- Providing easy access to secondary data on communities, including key demographic, social, economic, education, housing market, human service, public safety, and other factors, is critical to shared measurement efforts in community development. Support for data intermediaries to assemble, analyze, and disseminate this data makes it possible for nonprofit organizations to cost-efficiently share data from secondary sources, streamline data access, and lower costs when primary data are not needed to address their evaluation questions.

- Adequately funding the evaluation activities to build and sustain shared measurement efforts is essential to recognize the value of an organization's time and to provide sufficient support for data collection, technology, analysis, peer engagement, or other specific needs. Clarity and commitment of funder support for shared measurement efforts are powerful incentives.

As this overview of shared measurement makes clear, application of the practices, tools, and incentives helps advance the field's understanding of the impacts of a range of community development programs and investments. As it continues to gain traction, this rigorous yet flexible method for capturing complex change is becoming an integral part of the community development tool kit, increasing the scale at which evaluation of people and place-based initiatives occur, as well as fostering stronger, more vibrant communities in the process.

DOCUMENTING HEALTH OUTCOMES OF HOUSING AND COMMUNITY DEVELOPMENT PROGRAMS

As more community development practitioners embrace the important linkages between community development and individual, family, and community health, the need for tools to measure these health-related outcomes has become increasingly clear. In response, Success Measures® based at NeighborWorks® America, is developing an evaluation framework and set of data collection tools for community development practitioners interested in documenting the health outcomes of a wide range of affordable housing, neighborhood revitalization, workforce development, supportive service, and community engagement programs. Drawing on social determinants of health research and using a health equity lens, the project is focused on the evaluation support needs of community development practitioners and complements efforts by leading funders, researchers, and others to identify core measurement issues at the intersection of health and community development.

Based on a literature review, stakeholder engagement, and the input of advisors drawn from the health care, public health, community development, and public policy fields, the final products of this effort will include an evaluation framework arraying the health outcomes along the spectrum of housing and community development programs, and a set of tested, validated data collection instruments to measure those outcomes. Similar to the data collection tools currently available through Success Measures and the Success Measures Data System (SMDS), these instruments will be developed for a range of community, cultural, and program settings, including translation into several languages, and will be applicable across populations from youth to seniors. Completion of the evaluation framework is anticipated in early 2015, with the data collection tools following later in the year. For periodic updates on this project, including information about opportunities to collaborate and participate in field tests, please see www.successmeasures.org.

■ ■ ■

MAGGIE GRIEVE *is vice president for Success Measures at NeighborWorks America where she directs a social enterprise offering evaluation consulting, technical assistance and technology services to national and community-based nonprofit organizations and funders. She previously served as director of research and evaluation at McAuley Institute where she co-directed the initial development of Success Measures as a shared measures approach to outcome-focused evaluation and managed the development of the Success Measures Data System, a web-based tool for data collection and evaluation support. She holds a BA in American Studies from the University of Minnesota and studied Urban Planning at the Graduate School of Fine Arts, University of Pennsylvania.*

This essay examines the ways that two recent Federal initiatives—Promise Neighborhoods and the Fair Housing Equity Assessment—encourage the use of data by local entities engaged in planning and implementing programs that aim to improve community-wide outcomes for children and policies that promote regional equity. It discusses how PolicyLink, acting as national technical assistance provider, has worked with other organizations to fill capacity gaps—both technological and non-technological—among grantees to foster strategic use of data for program targeting, improvement, and systematic change. This work is helping local educational partnerships to manage for better results, and enabling regional agencies to foster dialogue and action to promote greater access to opportunity.

NEW WAYS OF USING DATA IN FEDERAL PLACE-BASED INITIATIVES: OPPORTUNITIES TO CREATE A RESULTS FRAMEWORK AND TO RAISE THE VISIBILITY OF EQUITY ISSUES

Victor Rubin and Michael McAfee
PolicyLink

Federal place-based initiatives represent a great opportunity to motivate, encourage, incentivize or even require new ways of using data, measuring progress, and creating dialogue about findings and results at local and regional levels. If their planning and implementation includes a strong system for building the capacity of the grantee organizations and their partners, then truly significant change will be within reach. Several of the Obama administration's place-based programs have aspired to increase local capacity for collecting and interpreting data, though in very different circumstances and with different objectives. In this essay, we explore the experiences of two of these initiatives—Promise Neighborhoods and the Fair Housing Equity Assessment—and draw some early lessons about effective practices.

The two programs operate at vastly different scales. Promise Neighborhoods is focused on, and acts on behalf of, children and youth within locally defined urban, tribal, and rural communities. The Fair Housing Equity Assessment deals with long-range, multi-issue planning for metropolitan regions. The core idea of Promise Neighborhoods is to embed a "results framework" into the guidance, operations, and self-assessment of each grantee consortium. A results framework requires not only good data on processes and outcomes, but also a practical and insightful system to collect, analyze, display, and interpret the results. With this information and infrastructure, grantees can learn a great deal about whether, and how, children from the targeted low-income communities are progressing "from cradle to career," with the support of neighborhood factors as well as schools.

The Fair Housing Equity Assessment, a component of the Sustainable Communities Initiative, prompts grantees to use new spatial data and intensive public deliberations about that data to reorient local and regional policy toward creating "communities of opportunity." The process poses the question to regional leaders: What can we learn about the barriers to everyone in the region having not just equal legal and civil rights to housing, but also equitable access to the schools, services, jobs, and local environments that provide economic opportunity?

PolicyLink has had the privilege of working with the Promise Neighborhoods and Sustainable Communities programs on issues of data, mapping, and assessment, as well as advising the federal agencies that administer the programs and providing technical support to the grantees. We're now roughly two years into the first round of Promise projects and three into Sustainable Communities, and we can now take stock of our progress toward this ambitious goal of creating a society in which all are participating, prospering, and reaching their full potential.

THE PROMISE NEIGHBORHOODS OPPORTUNITY

Inspired by the Harlem Children's Zone (HCZ), the purpose of the federal Promise Neighborhoods Program is to significantly improve the educational and developmental outcomes of children and youth in the nation's most distressed neighborhoods. HCZ is a comprehensive set of wrap-around services for youth to help them succeed in school. HCZ principles are to:

- Serve an entire neighborhood comprehensively and at scale;

- Create a comprehensive pipeline of programs for children from birth through college graduation, and wrapping families in those programs;

- Build community among residents, institutions, and stakeholders who help to create the environment necessary for a child's healthy development;

- Evaluate program outcomes and create a data feedback loop to help management improve and refine program offerings; and

- Cultivate a culture of success rooted in passion, accountability, leadership, and teamwork.

Promise Neighborhoods is a manifestation of the Obama administration and U.S. Department of Education (DOE) efforts to listen to the voice, wisdom, and experience of local leaders. For years, these leaders have recommended that the federal government co-invest in place-based efforts with large, multiyear grants and flexible spending parameters. Promise Neighborhoods implementation grantees receive up to $30 million over five years to begin the projected 20-plus year journey of establishing cradle-to-career supports and improving outcomes for children and families.

The program is transforming neighborhoods by:

- Identifying and increasing the capacity of groups (nonprofits, institutions of higher education, or Indian tribes) that are focused on achieving results for children and youth throughout an entire neighborhood;

- Building a complete continuum of cradle-to-career solutions in both educational programs and family and community supports, with great schools at the center;

- Integrating programs and breaking down agency "silos" so that solutions are implemented effectively and efficiently across agencies;

- Developing the local infrastructure of systems and resources needed to sustain and scale up proven, effective solutions across the broader region beyond the initial neighborhood; and

- Learning about the overall effects of the Promise Neighborhoods program and about the relationship between particular strategies in

Promise Neighborhoods and student outcomes, including through a rigorous evaluation of the program.[1]

Promise Neighborhoods also represents an opportunity to demonstrate that HCZ operating principles can be successfully implemented in urban, rural, and tribal communities across America, and that the successes can be translated into smarter federal policies and programs.

As DOE's partner, the Promise Neighborhoods Institute at PolicyLink (PNI) provides local leaders with a system of support to help ensure their Promise Neighborhood is a success. This support entails technical assistance to: (1) accelerate local leaders' ability to achieve results, including results-based accountability training, supporting a community of practice,[2] and providing data infrastructure and leadership development; (2) build evidence of the effectiveness of cradle-to-career strategies through research, data analysis, evaluation, and communication outreach; (3) advocate for policies that support the expansion and sustainability of Promise Neighborhoods. PNI is a partnership of PolicyLink, HCZ, and the Center for the Study of Social Policy. It is funded solely by philanthropy, including support from the Annie E. Casey Foundation, Atlantic Philanthropies, California Endowment, Citi Foundation, Ford Foundation, George Kaiser Family Foundation, JP Morgan Chase Foundation, W.K. Kellogg Foundation, Open Society Foundation, Walmart Foundation and Robert Wood Johnson Foundation.

Data and Technology Infrastructure

Promise Neighborhoods has a strong results framework. The Department of Education requires Promise Neighborhoods implementation grantees to report on 10 results and 15 indicators, known as the Government Performance and Results Act (GPRA) indicators (see Figure 1 for two examples).[3]

---

1 U.S. Department of Education, "Promise Neighborhoods: Purpose" (Washington, DC: DOE, 2014), available at http://www2.ed.gov/programs/promiseneighborhoods/index.html.

2 As of 2014, the PNI community of practice included 61 communities—those that had won the federal planning or implementation grants, as well as those that submitted high-scoring applications.

3 For a full listing of the indicators and results, see J. Comey et al., *Measuring Performance: A Guidance Document for Promise Neighborhoods on Collecting Data and Reporting Results* http://www.urban.org/publications/412767.html (Washington, DC: U.S. Department of Education, 2013).

RESULT	INDICATORS
Children enter kindergarten ready to succeed in school.	Number and percentage of children age 0-5 who have a regular doctor or clinic, other than an emergency room, when they have health issues. Number and percentage of three-year-olds and children in kindergarten who demonstrate at the beginning of the program or school year age-appropriate functioning across multiple domains of early learning; these function are determined using developmentally appropriate early learning measures (as defined in the federal notice). Number and percentage of children, from age 0-5, participating in center-based or formal home-based early learning settings or programs, which may include Early Head Start, Head Start, child care, or preschool.
Students are healthy.	Number and percentage of children who participate in at least 60 minutes of moderate to vigorous physical activity daily. Number and percentage of children who consume five or more servings of fruits and vegetables daily.

Figure 1. Selected Promise Neighborhood Initiative Indicators

Establishing common measures like these increases the likelihood that local leaders will align their strategies to collectively make consistent progress turning the 15 indicator trend lines in the right direction. But common measures are not enough. Local leaders require guidance in developing the leadership, organizational, and programmatic capacity to effectively implement their cradle-to-career solutions so they can achieve population-level results.[4] They also require assistance designing and implementing accountability systems that empower them to use data for learning, continuous improvement, and shared accountability.

---

4   PNI defines population-level results as improving the quality of life in a place by implementing the appropriate mix of solutions that involve families, programs, policies, and systems. These solutions should improve the outcomes for at least 50% of children and families targeted.

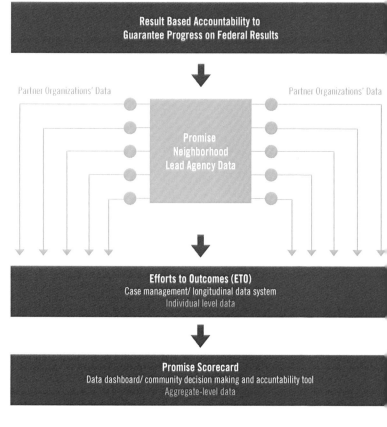

Figure 2. Data Platform Integration. The three data platforms are seamlessly integrated and designed to provide data in real time. The data can also be imported and exported across the platforms. When lead agencies and their partners enter program participant data into ETO, the results and indicators are transferred to the Promise Scorecard. Partners can then measure progress at both the individual and aggregate levels.

Planning grantees also need tools—tools that can help guide partners through a disciplined planning process, and, once they have moved on to implementation, tools that collect, store, and analyze data regarding progress. Community-based organizations, though, rarely have the in-house experience to evaluate the pros and cons of various tools. To speed up data collection and preserve valuable time that could be spent designing interventions, PNI partnered with members in its community of practice to develop data infrastructure that grantees could use to support the implementation of their Promise Neighborhoods program.

The data infrastructure includes both data platforms as well as guidance in using those platforms. PNI paid for the three data platforms—(1) results-based accountability tools, (2) a case management/longitudinal data system, (3) a data dashboard—to be integrated and makes the software licenses available at no cost. This allows leaders to seamlessly measure progress on the 10 results and 15 indicators. This national technology infrastructure can accelerate local leaders' ability to move from talk to action in a disciplined, results-based, and data-driven manner. PNI recognized that providing local leaders with national data infrastructure would help them focus on the hard work of organizing partners to implement their cradle-to-career continuum of solutions. Because PNI purchased the data licenses in bulk, staff calculate that providing a national data infrastructure is saving the community of practice members nearly $3 million annually compared to what it would have cost them to work with a vendor individually. This has also reduced the time that it takes to build and begin using a data system from approximately three years to six months, particularly for those program sites with previously limited data capacities.

Results based accountability (RBA): In 2011, PNI—in partnership with local leaders participating in its community of practice—chose Results-Based Accountability (RBA) as the preferred management tool for achieving the 10 specified results. RBA is a disciplined process in which local leaders articulate goals, craft strategies to achieve the goals, assess their progress, and regularly make necessary refinements to their strategies. RBA helps leaders answer seven questions that answer how much are we doing, how well are we doing it, and is anyone better off?[5]

---

5 Through RBA, local leaders move from talk to action by working through seven guiding questions: 1. *Who are our customers, clients, people we serve?* (e.g., children in a child care program); 2. *How can we measure if our customers/clients are better off?* 3. *How can we measure if we are delivering service well?* (e.g., client-staff ratio, unit cost, turnover rate); 4. *How are we doing on the most important of these measures? Where have we been; where are we headed?* (baseline data and the story behind the baselines); 5. *Who are the partners who have a potential role to play in doing better?* 6. *What works, what could work to do better than baseline?* (best practices, best hunches, including partners' contributions); and 7. *What do we propose to do?* (multi-year action plan and budget, including no-cost and low-cost items).

Longitudinal case management: PNI's case management/longitudinal data system is provided by Social Solutions' Efforts to Outcomes (ETO software.[6] By using the ETO software, the organizations implementing Promise Neighborhoods can enroll individuals in the system and collect data about them in a central location over time, whether initial descriptive information from case management interviews, program participation from service providers, or outcomes such as high school graduation. The system is tailored to allow partner organizations access to confidential or sensitive data based on their role. Program leaders can use the data in ETO to both measure the incremental progress of each program participant and produce aggregate outcome measures for the whole program. Staff can also use the resulting data to identify which efforts, staff, services, or programs are most effective in achieving desired results. More than one-half of the Promise Neighborhoods implementation grantees are using ETO software.

Data Dashboard: The Promise Scorecard, a data dashboard based on the Results Leadership Group's Results Scorecard, provides a way to visualize progress on the 15 indicators.[7] Local leaders use it to create a local culture of accountability, gain a shared understanding of the baseline conditions, and make data-driven decisions about what is working and where improvements must be made. In 2013, DOE purchased the Promise Scorecard licenses for the 12 grantees. PNI continues to make licenses available to planning grantees and high-scoring applicants in its community of practice.

Data Guidance: With the RBA management tool and the data platform in place, DOE recognized that local leaders would need formal guidance to ensure that Promise Neighborhoods grantees were using common data definitions, collection, and reporting protocols. The Urban Institute created "Measuring Performance: A Guidance Document for Promise Neighborhoods on Collecting Data and Reporting Results" to support grantees as they collected high-quality data. The document also

---

6   Social Solutions is the leading provider of performance management software for human services, connecting efforts to outcomes, people to social services, and service providers and communities to funders.

7   The scorecard is a product of the Results Leadership Group (RLG), which PNI rebranded as the Promise Scorecard. RLG consultants, educators, coaches, and facilitators develop the capacity of government and nonprofit organizations to produce measurable results for clients and communities.

supports the government's desire to collect as consistent data as possible across sites for program monitoring and future research. It is not only useful for the federal Promise Neighborhoods program but is applicable to any practitioner implementing a place-based effort. In addition, the document recommends data collection strategies, sources, and methods for leaders working to implement a Promise Neighborhood strategy, including the collection and tracking of demographic, family, and service delivery characteristics. These recommendations, while not formal requirements, are intended to guide local leaders on the best ways to collect information that they can use to improve the quality of their programs and services, evaluate the success of their initiatives, and most important, achieve better results. Together, the data guidance document, the use of RBA, and the integrated data platforms facilitate the development and implementation of common data standards and practices, thereby improving the ability to measure progress across Promise Neighborhoods.

PNI, DOE, and the Urban Institute are working to ensure that the data infrastructure is integrated and that all supports are well aligned. Senior staff at PNI and DOE meet monthly, and senior leaders from PNI, DOE, and the Urban Institute meet quarterly to hold each other accountable to the goals of the program.

This national data infrastructure enables high scoring applicants, planning and implementation grantees in its community of practice to learn and improve. To evaluate the effectiveness of PNI in the future, PNI, DOE, and the Urban Institute are combining individual- and program-level data files into a master file, and preparing a restricted-use data file that meets the congressionally mandated DOE National Center for Education Statistics' quality standards. In addition, PNI is partnering with Mathematica Policy Research to produce five case studies and to propose an evaluation framework for testing the efficacy of Promise Neighborhoods. The restricted-use data file, coupled with the proposed evaluation framework, will ensure that any evaluation is done with a credible and rigorous methodology and a context that acknowledges the family, program, community, policy, and systems complexity in a Promise Neighborhood.

Key Steps Underway in 2014

In 2014, the first cohort of sites were in their second year of implementation. The initial work of the PNI community of practice has shifted participants' mindset from that of applying for and receiving a federal grant to that of leading a multi-sector network of partners (e.g., school, health, housing, food, and public safety systems) committed to achieving collective impact, or in the RBA language, population-level results, through a cradle-to-career strategy.[8] In short, they are not simply running a program that expires in five years. To this end, the PNI community of practice has spent the past two years creating local cultures of accountability and building the infrastructure necessary for achieving population-level results.

Implementation sites have begun building out the programs in their cradle-to-career continuum by forming the appropriate partnerships and testing their solutions on a small scale. Expanding their efforts to a larger scale will take time. Partners will need to build organizational and leadership capacity, for example, as well as systems of accountability. The PNI community of practice is committed to achieving result at a scale and complexity rarely achieved by most place-based efforts. Every implementation grantee is using the RBA framework, and the Promise Scorecard data dashboard; and fifty-percent of the implementation grantees are using the case management system offered by PNI. They have also agreed to partner with the national technical assistance network to bring a disciplined approach to building an integrated strategy that will unfold over the next 20 years.

Three elements will be necessary to build these new systems:

1 Baseline data on the target community, including information on its schools and residents: Baseline data document the conditions at the outset and are necessary to measure progress. Baseline data also help local leaders determine areas of greatest need and opportunities to take action.

---

8 FSG defines collective impact as the commitment of a group of actors from different sectors to a common agenda for solving a specific social problem, using a structured form of collaboration.

2 Target or penetration rates: Measures of the extent to which the programs are reaching the intended populations within the Promise Neighborhood.

3 Performance measures: Measures of progress that also reflect the chosen strategy for effecting change. Local leaders should develop these performance measures in conjunction with partners to ensure that the partners can be held accountable for delivering programs or services and/or policies and system reforms. The leaders should also use data to manage program and project performance and report progress and outcomes to DOE, key partners, and community stakeholders.

Challenges Faced in Implementation

Leaders implementing a Promise Neighborhood cradle-to-career strategy have faced multiple challenges with using data for continuous improvement and shared accountability. In particular, they have struggled with: (1) conducting needs assessments and segmentation analyses, (2) designing longitudinal data systems, and (3) using the data collected to get results.

Conducting Needs Assessments and Segmentation Analyses: The Department of Education required grantees to conduct a needs assessment and segmentation analyses so they would have the information needed to tailor their interventions to the needs of neighborhood children. However, most nonprofits do not have the staff to conduct these types of analyses. In addition, leaders may not have yet developed the relationships or institutional capacity necessary to access administrative data from institutions such as a school district or health department. Consequently, when applying for funding that requires a needs assessment, the initial data collected is often insufficient for establishing baselines, targets, and performance measures. More important, the lack of access to administrative data makes it virtually impossible to fully understand the needs of children in the neighborhood and to appropriately customize interventions.

Designing a Case Management/Longitudinal Data System: The Department of Education believes that a case management/longitudinal data system is a piece of essential infrastructure to effectively target, track, and measure the results of interventions. It is also necessary to house data for future evaluations. Unfortunately, organizations rarely have systems that integrate multiple data sources with unique identifiers or connect with external data systems. It is also difficult, as noted, to access administrative data. Most local leaders have not yet developed a data agenda for how key pieces of missing data will be obtained. For example, school systems and service providers have a significant challenge tracking highly mobile students and families, who may move in and out of the target area or transfer between schools. Collectively agreeing on a multi-sector solution will save time and money and get local partners closer to crafting solutions that decrease mobility rates.

Developing the Capacity to Connect a Disciplined Approach to Achieving Results with the Use of Data: To get results, data must be connected to a disciplined approach to moving from talk to action and making progress on the 10 results and 15 indicators. Yet too often, the use of data is something done by one person and then simply reported out. In addition, the use of data is rarely linked to an evidenced-based approach to achieving population-level results. The challenge is to ensure that using data is not seen as another "add-on" to responsibilities. Rather, leaders must foster an organizational culture that views data as essential to getting results in every functional area of an organization, and by every person within the organization. Most important, partners must use data to guide decisions and manage the performance of those providing services. This is why the task of establishing baselines, targets, stakeholder solutions/strategies and performance measures is important.

The PNI system of supports is designed to focus leaders' attention to the following questions:

- What is the right mix of family, programmatic, policy and systems solutions that must be implemented to get results at a scale that will get a particular indicator moving in the right direction?

- What early results should be achieved by leading multi-sector stakeholders through the RBA process and obtaining their commitment to contributing to solutions?

- What does the process map for our cradle-to-career system look like?

- Who are the key partners at each developmental stage of our cradle-to-career continuum of solutions?

- What are each partner's results, indicators, targets, and performance measures?

- How does the use of data ensure that our cradle-to-career continuum of solutions has the appropriate mix of people, programs, policies and systems?

- How is the capital of multi-sector stakeholders being aligned to sustain our cradle-to-career solutions?

Without this disciplined execution and data work, it is difficult to create a culture of accountability and to achieve population-level results.

Early Examples of Impact

A culture of accountability and a disciplined approach to execution are clearly taking hold. Leaders from 61 communities have accelerated their work to establish baselines, targets, and stakeholder strategies linked to performance measures. In addition, local leaders are now developing data agendas and shared data agreements that are enabling them to break down data silos. Hayward, California, and Nashville, Tennessee, are leaders in this area.

Hayward Promise Neighborhood is establishing a successful data partnership with the local school district.[9] Its data agreement to acquire individual-level data from the Hayward Unified School District (HUSD) makes it one of the first Promise Neighborhoods in the nation to take action on this crucial step. Their shared data partnership demonstrates a deep commitment to getting results for children and families. Now that a community of partners has agreed that managing services and supports for children, families, and community members requires a powerful data management system, Hayward will be able to take a thorough approach to building a seamless cradle to career pipeline. In addition, this type of collaboration requires a level of trust among the

---

9 For more information see http://www.haywardpromise.org/.

partners to work through the difficult tasks needed to move the work forward. One of the next hurdles Hayward faces is how to collect the individual parental consent required before the district can share the data. Even with the remaining challenges, Hayward's commitment to the need for data-driven decision making and leadership by the school district position the Hayward Promise Neighborhood for transformativ work with children and families in the community.

Nashville Promise Neighborhood (NPN) is about to take their work to a new level.[10] The Promise Neighborhood team has announced the approval of its data-sharing partnership with Metro Nashville Schools to support common results around student achievement and family supports. Metro Nashville is one of the first school districts in the nation to establish a powerful data-sharing partnership with a Promise Neighborhood. As the *Tennessean* reported, the Metro Nashville Public Schools district "keeps a real-time, state-of-the-art data warehouse in order to track student progress and spot issues that could be interfering with performance."[11] Using the Efforts to Outcomes system to track the data, Nashville Promise Neighborhood is helping the city to comprehensively integrate school and community provider data into a single system. "We support collective impact models of transformation, and a key component of this is the sharing of information," Laura Hansen, Metro Schools Director of Information Management and Decision Support and co-chair of the Nashville Promise Neighborhood Data and Research Committee, told the *Tennessean*. Robin Veenstra-VanderWeele, director of the Nashville Promise Neighborhood, added, "The data partnership with the school district empowers the NPN to effectively link local schools and NPN Partner Organizations to change outcomes for students from kindergarten to college."

---

10 For more information see http://www.nashvillepromise.org/.

11 H. Hall. "Promise Neighborhood shares student data with nonprofits to improve help for kids." *The Tennessean*. (April 12, 2013). Retrieved from http://www.tennessean.com/.

THE FAIR HOUSING AND EQUITY ASSESSMENT: CREATING A REGIONAL BASELINE FOR IMPROVING ACCESS TO OPPORTUNITY

The second case of a new federal program that is changing the way data are used represents a new approach to a perennial issue: the documentation of, and response to, barriers to fair and opportunity-rich housing. In 2010 and 2011, the U.S. Department of Housing and Urban Development (HUD) awarded grants to 87 regions across the country to create and implement regional plans that would advance sustainability, equity, and economic resilience through the Sustainable Communities Initiative. These grants, which were a pilot program that emerged from the Partnership for Sustainable Communities, have brought together cities, counties, metropolitan planning organizations (MPOs), community organizations, equity advocates, foundations, universities and colleges, and economic development organizations. These new partnerships are using regional plans as a way to craft cohesive visions for future investment. This chance to support several agencies and organizations across a variety of issues and interests in creating "sustainable communities of opportunity" emerged at the same time that HUD was shifting its approach to fair housing enforcement and education. The new approach addresses not only literal discrimination but also structural issues of investment and disinvestment that have led to ongoing racial segregation and inequitable access to opportunity. The leadership of HUD asked the Sustainable Communities Regional Planning grantees to pilot this new regional and investment-focused approach to fair housing.

The grant program requires that recipients conduct a Fair Housing and Equity Assessment (FHEA) to quantitatively assess local and regional conditions relative to opportunity, broadly defined, and to propose policy solutions to diminish disparities. HUD provided the grantees with a set of indicators at the census-tract level on segregation, areas of concentrated poverty by race and ethnicity, and access to six aspects of neighborhood opportunity: housing affordability, transit, exposure to environmental hazards, exposure to poverty, economic opportunities, and school quality. Although grantees were familiar with some of the demographic and housing data, other indicators—such as access to opportunity and location of public investments relative to segregation trends – were new to most partners. Although HUD's assembly of consistent, nationally available data from a variety of sources in a single location was valuable in itself, the FHEA was not just an exercise in data analysis. Rather, grantees were encouraged to think of data collection and display as only a first phase. Deliberation about the data, and the ways that the data could inform regional and local decisions, were also key parts of the assessment process.

These assessments are currently underway or completed in 87 regions across the country, from the largest metropolitan areas to some of the smallest rural regions. PolicyLink and the Kirwan Institute for the Study of Race and Ethnicity at Ohio State University have been working with the consortia to strengthen their FHEA analyses, deliberations, and decision making and have published nine briefs to guide practitioners through all stages of the process.[12] This account is drawn from the briefs and the experiences of advising the consortia and reviewing their processes and reports.

Fair housing itself is a highly charged and sensitive subject, and addressing it adequately requires significant skill and capacity. But the breadth of the issues being addressed by the new FHEA presented unique challenges to regional grantees. The need to build new analytical capacities was only the starting point. More challenging were the needs to bring a wide range of partners to the table in considering the new issues and policy questions that the FHEA process brings to the fore, and to determine how to help those partners realign their activities toward regional equity.

The FHEA experience has required the regional partners to think about and organize their response to fair housing issues in more comprehensive ways. All partners, for example, needed to understand fair housing in HUD's new, broader framework of documenting and responding to disparities in access to opportunity. In particular, the regional teams needed to build staff and leadership capacity at MPOs to work within

---

12 Representative of this collection are "FHEA Resource: Emerging Practice in FHEA Development" and "The Fair Housing and Equity Assessment (FHEA) Deliberation Guide: Part 5–Using Data in Deliberation and Decision-Making," both published in 2013 by PolicyLink under a capacity-building contract with the U.S. Department of Housing and Urban Development.

a new paradigm that: 1) examined the interactions between sectors that are generally dealt with in silos; 2) built on civil rights and fair housing law that was unfamiliar to many; and 3) expected that planning, policy and investment decisions would be reshaped to remedy problems identified in the assessment.

The regional organizations also needed to act in new ways. Specifically, they needed to recruit and orient agencies and organizations that did not typically think about fair housing to see their work as critical to the effort. This could include local public health departments, whose perspectives and data on regional access to opportunity were critical, but who had not previously been involved in this area of planning. Or it could include many of the MPO's board representatives from suburban jurisdictions, usually elected officials for whom traditional fair housing issues or broader analyses of access to opportunity had not been significant. The consortia were also asked to engage equity-focused and community organizations in a substantive way that would inform both the analysis and the policy recommendations that followed. For many of these leaders, it was their first time working on a regional housing plan.

The assessments had different emphases depending on the local context, but the overarching policy challenge inherent in the new paradigm pushed beyond the typical responses to fair housing and the allocation of affordable housing resources. The efforts required partners to have conversations about how to balance calls to invest all future affordable housing resources in "high-opportunity suburbs" with the need to reinvest in low-income communities of color, even if those communities, mostly in the central city, had less access to opportunities, poorer quality schools, or were de facto racially segregated. This contrast between the goals of de-concentrating poverty and revitalizing urban neighborhoods was one of the central regional equity questions that these Sustainable Communities needed to address, so the FHEA helped to bring additional evidence and attention to bear on it.

Despite these capacity challenges, new players, and broader expectations for the process, some of the grantees are making significant progress:

- In the Seattle-Tacoma region, the Puget Sound Regional Council has used its FHEA analysis to inform how it allocates funding in their transportation improvement program. The complementary commitments and systemic policies to advance equity and social justice from planners and elected officials in the City of Seattle, King County and now the Puget Sound Regional Council enhance the prospects for the fair distribution of affordable housing within the major expansion of transit that is underway.

- The Chicago Metropolitan Agency for Planning has created a set of fair housing recommendations for local governments. The MPO has funded technical assistance to help local jurisdictions advance fair housing through new zoning, and general, comprehensive, and area plans. It has also helped to reframe a fair housing discussion in this heavily segregated region to focus on the benefits of economic inclusion across the spectrum from individual households, to municipalities, to competitive regions.

- In the Boston region, the Metropolitan Area Planning Council is creating a fair housing toolkit for local jurisdictions that helps cities and towns with higher-quality schools and service jobs but little affordable housing to set and meet new goals of zoning for and building of affordable homes.

- In Minneapolis-St. Paul, Minnesota, the Metropolitan Council is linking FHEA data to their Regional Transportation Plan and Comprehensive Economic Development Strategy to ensure that their regional housing, transportation, and economic development plans are all informed from the same baseline.

- The Lane County, Oregon, FHEA took the opportunity to amend and augment its national data with local survey data of all individuals who benefit from Section 8 rental vouchers or other affordable housing in Eugene, Springfield, and the surrounding county. Concerns identified in the survey included traffic safety related to sidewalks, speed, and crossing signals; and bus frequency, cost, and lack of night and weekend service. The recommendations for addressing safety and service have moved forward as action items for the Lane County Transit Authority.

- On the Pine Ridge Indian Reservation in South Dakota, data from their Equity and Opportunity Assessment identified the mismatch between jobs and residents on the reservation, and the need for more housing for working families. Local leaders are using the findings to leverage additional federal and philanthropic funding to develop more infrastructure and quality, energy-efficient affordable housing.

Although the policy changes as a result of FHEA are still in their early stages, the potential is significant for a long-term shift in the content and style of decision making. As more team members see their role in advancing fair housing, and see fair housing as critical to economic prosperity, we will hopefully see greater traction in reducing segregation and advancing opportunity for all. If more extensive and thoughtful use of data and mapping is embedded in the process of assessing regional opportunity structures and allocating public resources, then the pilot program will have been a success.

In June 2013, HUD released its draft "Affirmatively Furthering Fair Housing Rule." Many of the Sustainable Communities grantees that had conducted FHEAs weighed in with comments to the agency, supporting the rule and offering improvements based on their experience. Fair housing advocates, entitlement jurisdictions—and now regional planning consortia—all await the release of the final rule (expected late 2014/early 2015). The rule should help drive HUD investments and allied federal resources to the priorities flowing from data-driven assessments.

CONCLUSION

These two cases operate at different scales and in support of very different kinds of planning and implementation processes. One focuses all the resources of a community and outside sources toward a fixed but very ambitious set of goals for improving the life circumstances and educational outcomes of the community's children. The other case is casting a wider net across a region, bringing more issues, partners, and participants as well as a greater variety of data to bear. But whether they creating neighborhood or regional systems, Promise Neighborhoods and the Fair Housing Equity Assessment share the broad recognition that place matters—that the deficits in opportunity cannot be overcome without understanding the central role of neighborhoods, towns, cities, and regions in shaping people's lives. Place matters at the community level, where a child needs the supports provided by a Promise Neighborhood, and at the metropolitan level, where a family's access to good jobs, a clean environment, and excellent schools should not be a function of income or race.

Success in these place-based endeavors requires a strong system for data collection, analysis, and use. The system must also inspire multiple partners to improve the strategies they are using to reach these goals. HUD and DOE have not only recognized this, but they have encouraged and supported the growth of systems to help their local and regional consortia build their data management, research, planning, and implementation capacities. The federal departments have provided new information, set high standards, supported the proliferation of good management tools, and worked closely with a range of innovative intermediaries to assist the grantees and elevate the overall impact of the initiative. The early returns show that, when given this guidance and support, local leaders will make the most of it and seek to build strong, inclusive, results-driven partnerships. The federal agencies and all parties concerned with the success of place-based initiatives should continue to learn a great deal from their experiences.

Acknowledgement: The authors would like to thank Danielle Bergstrom and Kalima Rose for research and reflections on their experiences with the Fair Housing Equity Assessment.

■ ■ ■

VICTOR RUBIN, *PhD, is vice president for research at PolicyLink, a national research and action institute advancing social and economic equity. He has been an urban planning researcher, teacher, and consultant for more than 30 years. He has recently been leading consultations on equitable economic growth strategies in several cities and is co-author with Sarah Treuhaft of "Economic Inclusion: Advancing an Equity-Driven Growth Model," for the Big Ideas for Jobs project. Victor joined PolicyLink in 2000 after serving as director of the U.S. Department of Housing and Urban Development's Office of University Partnerships.*

■ ■ ■

MICHAEL MCAFEE, *EdD, senior director at PolicyLink and director of the Promise Neighborhoods Institute at PolicyLink, partners with leaders across America to improve the educational and developmental outcomes of children in our nation's most distressed communities. He oversees the institute's efforts to accelerate local leaders' ability to improve the well-being of children, build evidence that cradle-to-career strategies are working across the country, and scale and sustain the impact of Promise Neighborhoods so that millions of children are learning, growing and succeeding.*

The proliferation of data and new tools for data collection and analysis bring new relevance to an old question: Can community organizations prove they are making a difference? After 15 years climbing the data learning curve, LISC Chicago has concluded that effective use of data requires the same fundamentals as good community development work, such as paying attention to local context, local knowledge, and local capacity needs. This essay explores lessons learned about building data capacity through LISC's work supported by the MacArthur Foundation in Chicago.

EVERYTHING OLD IS NEW AGAIN: BUILDING NONPROFIT CAPACITY IN THE AGE OF BIG DATA

Susana Vasquez and Patrick Barry
LISC Chicago

Can local organizations make their neighborhoods stronger and healthier? If they can, how do they provide evidence that they are making a difference?

These are important questions, especially as millions of data points on neighborhoods become accessible via mobile apps, Web portals, and powerful databases. But these questions are not new. Former Federal Reserve chairman Ben Bernanke made the case for data-informed analysis of community work at the 2003 Community Development Policy Summit in Cleveland, suggesting that groups could raise funds and other types of support more effectively if they would "capture intangible social benefits, such as those that accrue to a neighborhood as residents become engaged in community planning activities, improve their financial literacy, and increase their access to employment opportunities through job training."[1]

Using data to demonstrate these types of effects has become a higher priority in recent years, as both foundations and government seek validation for the work they are supporting. But it's a tricky proposition, because first you have to show that something good has happened and then link those good results to a specific community improvement strategy, as opposed to a strategy or force from outside a specific organization's control.

---

[1] Ben Bernanke, Remarks at the 2003 Community Development Policy Summit, Federal Reserve Bank of Cleveland, Cleveland, Ohio, June 11, 2003. www.federalreserve.gov/boarddocs/speeches/2003/20030611/default.htm.

Just as important is the underlying framework for mounting the community improvements: the "logic model" or "theory of change." Jane Jacobs and Robert Moses went to war over these frameworks way back in the 1960s. Jacobs, Greenwich Village resident and author of *The Death and Life of Great American Cities*, argued that the complex networks of relationships in New York neighborhoods must be preserved and nurtured,[2] whereas Moses, New York City's construction czar, pushed for highways and urban renewal to bring economic benefits.[3] In his classic 1998 book, *Seeing Like a State*,[4] James C. Scott outlines numerous calamities caused by centralized planning that failed to incorporate local knowledge and marshal local capabilities. In addition to Soviet and Chinese failures, and the Brazilian folly of building its new capital on the country's distant central plateau, he recounted the data-driven efforts by 18th-century German forest scientists to create highly productive woodlots with a single species of trees, optimally spaced and free of competition from other trees. This experiment, like later efforts in the United States to build densely populated, isolated housing developments for poor people, sought to bring order to a complex reality, but led to failure.

After several decades of urban renewal in the United States, the weaknesses of centralized, top-down approaches became apparent, prompting new experiments to support "locally driven development." This framework departed from both top-down central planning and bottom-up community organizing. It moved nonprofit community groups into ownership and development of affordable housing and shopping centers, which required a business mindset and appealed to early supporters including the Ford Foundation and Senator Robert F. Kennedy. Nonprofit builders notched decades of successes, producing impressive outputs of housing units and commercial space, but eventually this too proved inadequate in the face of larger urban challenges. From that realization emerged the "comprehensive" framework, which

---

2 J. Jacobs, *The Death and Life of Great American Cities* (New York: Vintage Books, 1961).

3 R.Caro, *The Power Broker, Robert Moses and the Fall of New York* (New York: Vintage Books, 1975).

4 J. Scott, *Seeing Like a State: How Certain Schemes to Improve the Human Condition Have Failed* (New Haven, CT: Yale University Press, 1999).

folded education, health, safety, recreation, and other quality-of-life issues into the portfolios of community development corporations.

The comprehensive model has driven the work of Local Initiatives Support Corporation (LISC) Chicago and many other organizations for the past decade or longer, creating a rich dynamic that weaves central intermediaries such as LISC with community-based nonprofit organizations, social service agencies, local governments, foundations, corporate supporters, and subject-area experts on various issues.

This is complex and exciting work that *appears* to produce good results. But we still must ask, does comprehensive community development improve neighborhoods? And can we prove it?

DATA AND TECHNOLOGY

Rapid technology advancement and ubiquitous data create opportunities to begin answering those questions. But doing so will require strategies to address the same type of top-down, bottom-up tensions of earlier debates, as well as a clear understanding of the frameworks and theories to be tested. Perhaps most important, answering these questions demands a "data capacity" that is only beginning to be developed at the community level.

LISC Chicago has been nurturing this new capacity throughout its neighborhood work since the late 1990s, when it began emphasizing knowledge creation and journalism-style reporting around its comprehensive neighborhood initiatives. The early work was largely qualitative—more narrative than data portrait—but recently the data streams have been providing useful information about the reach and impact of LISC's work. Examples include the following:

- Data after the fact: Near a rough corner on Chicago's West Side, Breakthrough Urban Ministries has, since 2009, hosted Friday-night basketball tournaments that attract scores of youth and families. Whether it made a difference in crime was not clear until maps and charts—winnowed from millions of lines of police statistics on the City of Chicago Data Portal—showed that nearby crime had fallen for three consecutive years.

- Data for program tracking: Six weeks after the launch of the Affordable Care Act, LISC's partners in 24 neighborhoods had used the Web-based tool Wufoo to log contact with 4,314 people provided with health insurance information. (This number exceeded 14,086 by January 2014.) The shared, private database shows contact information, ages, language preferences, and locations, which helped insurance outreach workers track enrollment, flag individuals for follow-up, and develop program improvements. The ages alone offered important information, as the system needs enrollment of young adults to help balance the risk of older and less-healthy enrollees.

- Data for understanding: Surveys created by 10 community-based partners in the Little Village neighborhood provide detailed and, sometimes, disturbing portraits of at-risk youth, covering family life, academic attitudes, and stress related to violence at home or on the streets. In this low-income neighborhood composed primarily of Mexican immigrants, the information helps agencies better understand the youth they serve and provides a framework for more collaboration and coordination in youth programming.

What's remarkable about these data-informed snapshots is that they were generated by LISC-supported community groups working on the ground, not professional researchers. Until recently, regional think tank and "data shops" were the dominant purveyors of data because of their ability to access census tapes and other institutional data, which they filter and demystify for clients in city government, neighborhood organizations, or foundations. Today, trillions of data points can be accessed by just about anyone. New tools and technologies are invented nearly every day to collect, sort, and display the information. Responding to these opportunities, many nonprofit organizations in Chicago have caught the "data bug" and begun to recognize the importance of using data to improve programming and demonstrate impact.

But it's a steep learning curve to make sense of it all—and to do it right At the entry level, an organization must develop basic skills to interpret the data within a framework or theory of change. Such skills transcend simply manipulating Excel files. Rather, practitioners must learn at least one database, develop an ability to formulate query language, and know how to extract useful reports.

Next, the ever-evolving technical tools must be mastered. These tools include visualizations, "dashboards," and mobile apps for inputting or sharing data, all of which require technical and software skills. As organizations delve into the data, they discover the intricacies of survey methodology (particularly when tracking over time), the strict protocols for human-subject research and waiver requirements, and, in the health field or when dealing with schoolchildren, legal and privacy requirements that may hinder data collection and use.

This isn't something that can be done on the side or without commitment from an organization's senior leadership and the dedication of its staff. Although consultants may help, the work cannot be entirely outsourced. At least one person in the organization must have an innate curiosity about the data, and that person must be willing to experiment with data tools and demonstrate to colleagues the value of developing data-informed narratives.

BUILDING LOCAL KNOWLEDGE

For some nonprofit community organizations, a key driver for taking on these daunting challenges is economic survival. The prolonged recession caused many philanthropies to question whether their investments had any lasting impact—particularly if larger economic forces like the recent foreclosure crisis could undercut decades of incremental improvements at the community level. The recession also reduced endowments at foundations, cut government tax revenue, and trimmed corporate profits, leading to significant cuts to funding for nonprofit organizations. Faced with tougher decisions about which groups to support, funders demanded more evidence and data from organizations on not only "outputs," such as people served or dollars spent, but "outcomes," which require sophisticated logic models and the data to show what is happening.

Everyone, of course, wants to know if their work is having an impact. But the reality has been that most nonprofits simply have not had the expertise or capacity to capture data, sift the information, analyze and discuss the results, improve programming based on the numbers, and then prove effectiveness. More often, as foundations and government have demanded more metrics for the programs they fund, the harried nonprofit organizations have dutifully provided information, sometime devoting entire days to data input through multiple spreadsheets or databases. Unfortunately, these organizations rarely have had the time or inclination to find useful lessons in the data. Nor have they used data meaningfully at the front end of program development to inform strategy or monitor implementation.

LISC Chicago was one of these nonprofit organizations, more intereste in achieving results than proving a causal relationship. Even so, over many years of trial and error, LISC Chicago has gradually become mor involved with data and its various uses. The interest was driven by mor than a decade of learning from LISC's demonstration of comprehensive community development, the New Communities Program (NCP). The program used a relatively consistent methodology that has always included a respect for information flows, a bottom-up and top-down process, and strong support for knowledge building by NCP's primary funder, the John D. and Catherine T. MacArthur Foundation.

The New Communities Program began as a pilot in three neighbor-hoods in 1998 with nearly a year-long quality-of-life planning process that collected information from residents by using markers and newsprint sheets. The planning participants discussed and sorted these data into issue areas that could be addressed by interlocking strategies. A lead agency coordinated the neighborhood efforts, and in each plan, a chart showed the multiple neighborhood partners who had agreed to lead projects in their areas of expertise. As the plans were implemented coordinated sets of projects reached residents and produced concrete, visible improvements in the neighborhoods, like new employment centers, a community newspaper, youth-painted murals, and new retail development.

This was considered a sufficiently major accomplishment that, in 2003, the MacArthur Foundation supported a $17 million, five-year demonstration of the NCP method in 16 neighborhoods. Everything began with community engagement and planning, including some nicel bound data books that provided dense demographic and education tables, much of it from the U.S. Census, to help inform development of strategies. LISC contracted with urban planners to help guide the process, and hired former journalists—known as scribes—to document the discussions and create a coherent narrative about the neighborhood, its assets, and its challenges. The data books were ultimately not used extensively, but the plans incorporated a significant amount of local knowledge—what might today be called "little data." Those plans ultimately leveraged more than $500 million in new investments in the NCP neighborhoods and led to documented program-level outcomes in the areas of education, Internet use, and income- and credit-building.

When this work started, LISC and its partners were scouting the foothills of data. Navigation was mostly by instinct, as was program design and execution. LISC had partnered with a diverse set of community organizations from a range of low- and moderate-income neighborhoods. These groups could build partnerships with other neighborhood organizations and they had a stable commitment of operating and program funding from the MacArthur Foundation via LISC, so they were able to mount hundreds of small and larger projects in the first five years.

If someone had asked for proof that the MacArthur Foundation's initial investment was making a difference, LISC would have assembled a library of journalistic stories, thousands of professional photographs (another form of data), and a few charts showing where the money was spent. Local leaders routinely provided site visits at thriving new employment centers or rebuilt public spaces, and they used Web sites, fliers, maps, and reports to communicate that things were working and "producing impact."

But hard, organized data? The most important data collected early on were self-reported estimates of leverage, loosely defined as new investments in the neighborhood that were connected to specific strategies or projects in the quality-of-life plans. Some of these numbers were impressive, suggesting that the plans and their networks of partners had improved the "capital absorption capacity" of the neighborhoods.[5] But the data were unable to demonstrate causality—that the program

---

5 Capital absorption capacity represents "the ability of communities to make effective use of different forms of capital to provide needed goods and services to underserved communities," according to the Living Cities Integration Initiative, which identified gaps in such capacity as barriers to neighborhood improvement. See more at https://www.livingcities.org/work/capital-absorption.

caused a reduction in local crime or an improvement in graduation rates, for example—and were rarely consistent enough to support a theory of change.

A more subjective outcome, documented by the evaluation firm MDRC working for the MacArthur Foundation, was the creation by NCP of a platform of collaborative networks, financial resources, and technical assistance that produced significant positive activity in the NCP neighborhoods.[6] These networks had actually implemented the quality-of-life plans through discrete, concrete projects and programs, something that many previous comprehensive initiatives had been unable to do at scale. However, sufficient data did not exist to accurately track outcomes or correlate the projects with changes in traditional data sets being tracked by MDRC, such as mortgage originations or small-business loans.

CRUNCHING NUMBERS

These trends began to change during the second five-year commitment by the MacArthur Foundation. As the foundation's total investment grew to nearly $50 million over the ten-year period, LISC raised an additional $50 million from other funders. Some of those funds supported three multi-neighborhood programs that successfully integrated data use into the everyday rhythm. The number-crunching was tedious at first and required significant investment in database development, training, technical assistance, and supervision. Alongside the development of data expertise, LISC continued to emphasize storytelling and communications, deploying its own scribes to create meaning from the data. LISC also provided training and consultation to help neighborhood organizations develop these skills internally. Over time, as data were used to tell compelling stories, skeptics began turning into believers. The following are a few examples:

- Income- and credit-building: At 13 LISC-supported Centers for Working Families, participants are offered three core services: job placement and career development, one-on-one financial counseling, and enhanced access to income supports. Close tracking and incisive analysis found that those participants who used two or more services

---

6   D. Greenberg, et al., "Creating a Platform for Sustained Neighborhood Improvement," MDRC, February 2010.

are eight times more likely to increase net income than those who receive only one service. This result, confirmed for multiple years, has led to stronger integration of multiple services. Most recently, the centers added a fourth component, digital skills training, which is showing another layer of evidence in the form of improved job placement rates.

- School attendance: A multiyear commitment by the Atlantic Philanthropies allowed LISC partners in five neighborhoods to extend school days, add in-school health centers, and provide family supports at local middle schools. Close tracking of health data, including immunizations, showed that many students lacked the immunizations they needed to stay enrolled in school. Organizers identified these children and referred them to the health center for immunizations and health exams. Attendance rates, essential for academic gains, rose soon after, proving the positive impact. The neighborhood partner in Auburn Gresham was so impressed by the results that it analyzed immunization data at nearby elementary schools and rented buses to bring students to the health center. Again, attendance showed an upward trend. (This work required signed releases from parents of all students, which provided an important lesson on how much time and effort it takes to honor privacy and health information laws.)

- Digital skills: A federal stimulus grant to the City of Chicago funded intensive outreach and training that was coordinated by LISC Chicago in five "Smart Communities," where neighborhood "tech organizers" promoted and taught classes in basic computing, Internet use, and office skills. Baseline survey data found that people avoided the Internet because of lack of interest, high cost, and difficulty of use,[7] so the program was designed to provide free Internet access at neighborhood centers and hands-on training in basic tools such as e-mail, social media, and Microsoft Office. Early adopters became enthusiastic users and promoted the program to family and friends, leading to waiting lists and expanded offerings that produced 7,000 course completions and 17,000 visits per month to community Web portals.

---

7   K. Mossberger and C. Tolbert, "Digital Excellence in Chicago: A Citywide View of Technology Use," (City of Chicago Department of Innovation and Technology, July 2009). www.smartcommunitieschicago.org/uploads/smartchicago/documents/digital_excellence_mossberger_study.pdf.

Formal evaluation in 2012 showed a real impact: a 13-percentage-point gain in Internet use compared with similar neighborhoods nearby.[8] The City of Chicago is now promoting expansion of the model citywide.

In all of these cases, collecting and analyzing data served two distinct functions. First, they provided real-time information about program execution (the number of people served, in what capacities they were served, what types of services they received), which allowed program managers and their supervisors to identify strengths and weaknesses, to enforce accountability among local partners, and to implement program adjustments. Second, they created more meaningful data that allowed community-level program managers and professional evaluators to measure impacts. This documentation gives LISC Chicago confidence that its comprehensive, community-based efforts are making a quantifiable difference.

EXTENDING THE METHOD

The NCP method emphasizes the importance of local leaders having a voice and agency in decisions that affect their community. In today's world, this requires supporting local leaders' ability to interact with data systems and to apply the resulting information to the daily work of community development.

Capacity-building for data, from our point of view, doesn't start with data. It starts with the fundamentals of community engagement and planning, which of course are grounded in information about the neighborhoods. It starts with a methodology that brings in outside partners with data and tech expertise to add value to the community partners, who have their own local knowledge and program implementation expertise. It requires building sufficient trust so that local actors can safely unpack and question their own strongly held assumptions and theories about what works. It means having an entrepreneurial approach that allows innovative ideas to be tested and evaluated, to see if they work, and to be respectful if the answer is, "No, they don't."

---

8   C. Tolbert, K. Mossberger, and C. Anderson, "Measuring Change in Internet Use and Broadband Adoption: Comparing BTOP Smart Communities and Other Chicago Neighborhoods," (University of Iowa and University of Illinois at Chicago, 2012). http://www.brookings.edu/blogs/techtank/posts/2014/10/27-chicago-smart-neighborhoods.

And it recognizes that such capacity requires sustainable investment in an additional layer of information infrastructure that is beyond direct program costs. Unfortunately, building data capacity does not change the fundamental challenge of sustaining programs that rely on diverse streams of public and private funding.

After more than 10 years of extraordinary investment in and partnership with the New Communities Program, and only limited documentation of effective implementation in the official MDRC evaluation, the MacArthur Foundation asked LISC to further test its community development approach; to ramp multiple neighborhoods to a higher level of data use and evidence-based practices; to use that data to inform program design; and to track progress toward community-level change.

LISC responded by developing a knowledge-driven approach, called Testing the Model (TTM), which builds upon the NCP method and embeds data collection into focused strategies that neighborhood partners choose and tailor. Each plan includes a "theory of development," a series of related interventions, and datasets that help track activities and progress.

Knowing that it needed to build its own skills and those of its partners, LISC expanded its relationships with data-shop partners such as Chapin Hall at the University of Chicago and DePaul University's Institute for Housing Studies, which would offer guidance on data approaches, evidence-based practices, and research methodologies.

LISC worked intensively with a small cohort of its neighborhood lead agencies to develop data-informed community plans and the data capacity to effectively implement the plans and track the results. This involved significant amounts of time by program officers and scribes, who participated with the neighborhood groups and their data partners in a series of meetings that lasted for a year or longer. In each community, the budget covered support for a full-time program lead, a part-time data-entry specialist so that the data tasks would not distract from the core work, and seed funds to launch new strategies aligned with the plan.

The resulting collaborations provided learning experiences for all involved. The data and academic consultants had rarely worked so closely with community-level partners in the development and early implementation of programs, and they found these close relationships were more fruitful than the usual after-the-fact, arms-length observations. In the neighborhood, the initial reaction to the data partners was typically wary because community groups neither spoke the language nor had a background in data methods. Many early meetings included awkward moments and furrowed brows, including defensiveness among the neighborhood participants about being "pinned down" and made accountable for showing progress in particular ways. In time, however, as appropriate and meaningful data points were selected for tracking and new projects from the plan launched, neighborhood groups and their data partners became excited about what was being built.

SPREADING DATA SKILLS

While the TTM approach was being developed, LISC was building on its other data experiences with Centers for Working Families, the Atlantic Philanthropies middle-schools effort, and the Smart Communities demonstration. Sensing a desire for data expertise in its neighborhood network, LISC instituted a monthly series of informal gatherings called Data Fridays during which self-described data geeks explain their work to diverse and lively groups of 20 or more neighborhood development people. LISC also invested staff and consultant time to become familiar with powerful new tools such as the City of Chicago's data portal[9] and the various apps being created by the city's open data community.[10]

These continued investigations reinforced LISC's understanding that collecting data or digging into data sets was only the first step. Routine and useful application of data would require not only analysis but the artistic skills required to develop infographics and other visualizations, in addition to higher levels of technical knowledge to influence or design Web and mobile tools that facilitate data collection, retrieval, and presentation. A grant from Boeing helped LISC delve deeper in these

---

9   See https://data.cityofchicago.org.

10 Examples of work created by Chicago's data activists are at http://opencityapps.org/.

areas, most recently through a contractual engagement with a civic tech firm called DataMade, which specializes in creating vivid Web-based charts, maps, and tools related to crime, housing, and other civic data. This agreement is helping not only LISC but other neighborhood groups to become more involved with use of data.

After wading into the arcane world of civic hack-a-thons and "open government"—where discussions are laden with technical language about application programming interfaces (APIs), back-end databases, and URL query strings—LISC and neighborhood partners won support from the Knight Foundation for "Open Gov for the Rest of Us,"[11] which is helping a few of LISC's neighborhoods develop the technical language and data skills necessary to build bridges to Chicago's thriving tech and civic hacking scenes. The project provides funding and technical support to neighborhood partners who engage residents in trainings and discussions about local issues and how data might be used to address them.

BUILDING DATA CULTURE

Like many in the community development field, LISC and its partners are beginners in the use of data to inform and improve its programs. Over the years, we have learned a great deal about what it takes to build a data culture and how it can spread within and among organizations. Six lessons stand out:

- Community groups need to develop "data and information capacity." A June 2011 assessment by the Metro Chicago Information Center found that most of LISC's neighborhood partners (and LISC Chicago itself) had very limited capacity to collect and analyze data. Computer systems and databases were often inadequate, and many partners had limited or no in-house data expertise. LISC and many partners recognized the value of embracing data, however, and made commitments to build capacity through formal and informal methods. As LISC has directed financial, training, and technical resources into data capacity-building, many types of neighborhood partners have made significant progress on the data continuum. (This progression mirrors work performed five to seven years earlier when LISC and partners

---

11   Program description and video available at http://www.knightfoundation.org/grants/201346115/.

improved their digital communications skills including use of Web sites, social media, and video.)

- The right kinds of technical assistance are well received. Most organizations accepted the initial assessment without becoming defensive or feeling that data expectations were pushed on them by an outside force. Instead, they recognized the opportunity and many immediately made small changes such as improved computer networks or more attention to existing data collection. When LISC offered technical assistance from a variety of data support organizations, community groups responded favorably and shared their own lessons with peers. One neighborhood has even instituted its own "data geek squad," composed of senior staff members with strong data skills, a dedicated part-time data-entry specialist, and outside data consultants, to support other partner agencies.

- Peer-to-peer learning works. One of the least-threatening ways to spread data skills is through informal peer sharing, which can range from LISC's Data Friday gatherings to one-on-one encounters that demonstrate how a simple chart or visualization can bring data alive. LISC has found that community developers are hungry for this new knowledge and are excited about using it. Furthermore, LISC has learned that the best way to spread data culture is to create venues and programs that expose more people, at various levels, to data that are relevant to their work.

- Good enough is good enough, to start. Although early attempts to use data will likely be awkward and perhaps inconclusive, the only way to gain expertise is to experiment with the data. Many software developers use an "agile" approach that begins with a simplified working model that is then used, refined, used again, expanded with new features, and finally built into a fully tested product. The same approach has worked for development of the neighborhood data plans and the databases that support them. Unfortunately, philanthropic funding does not tend to follow this agile approach. Patient capital is needed if nonprofit organizations are to commit to learning and performing the data work.

- Data culture (or the wrong partner) cannot be forced on a group or individual. Although some groups and individuals are responsive to data, others may not be. LISC and its partners have experienced multiple instances of incompatibility or poor timing in which individuals have resisted or rejected data roles, and several organizations have had unsuccessful matchups with data partners. LISC used the initial capacity survey to gauge the readiness of partners, choosing the most "data-curious" for the first round of investments. The important test came when the work started and particular staff and partners had to collect and find meaning in the data. When that didn't work, in most cases, another attempt with different people and different partners—properly selected and supported—led to successful uptake of the data culture.

- The work still has to get done. To varying degrees, nonprofit partners with whom LISC has worked to integrate data into local programs have shifted their attitudes on the "burden" of data collection and analysis after having seen how it helps them discuss and learn from their programs. But for some groups it slowed the work to nearly a standstill as they struggled with partners over evidence-based models and data-sharing protocols. For others, a highly structured data-and-outcomes-driven plan did not align with the loosely structured, but highly productive local program design and staffing. The power of data to tell stories and prove impact only matters if the program gets implemented, residents benefit, and the work gets done. Along the data-capacity-building continuum, LISC recognizes "data-inspired" and "data-informed" as reasonable ground for community development practitioners to stand on.

HOW DATA ARE CHANGING LISC CHICAGO

LISC, with its partners, is learning how to use data to improve program design and implementation, to support the comprehensive development of neighborhoods, and to improve the quality of life of residents who live there. Although it is still not possible to prove that every program or approach is creating a particular measurable impact, staff members and partners are routinely asking the right questions, sharpening both the theoretical framework (e.g., "Why are we doing this? What do we hope to achieve?") and the daily routines of program implementation (e.g., "What is our baseline? Do we expect to see change?"). Despite the challenges, building data skills remains essential to improving the practice of community development and most importantly, the lives of the residents community development programs seek to impact.

Integrating a data mindset and skill set into LISC Chicago is analogous to realizing as a parent, on high school graduation day, that you should have photographed your child more often when she was entering kindergarten. It is challenging to attempt to build this capacity and retrofit the data models into a methodology that LISC has worked on for 15 years. Also, in the neighborhoods where LISC works, there are some things that data cannot help and data cannot do. Innovative practices will likely not have a baseline or evidence base, and serendipitous outcomes will not be captured by pre- and post-treatment surveys. Like parenting, community development is complex. Even as we try to capture the decisive moments, we must leave room for the unpredictable, the messy, and the surprise endings.

■ ■ ■

SUSANA VASQUEZ *is executive director of Local Initiatives Support Corporation Chicago (LISC Chicago), which connects neighborhoods to the resources they need to become stronger and healthier. She has more than 20 years' experience working with community organizing and community development organizations in Chicago.*

■ ■ ■

"Scribe" **PATRICK BARRY** *has been writing about neighborhoods and cities since the early 1980s, and for the last 14 years has documented the work of LISC Chicago and its partners. He has written for many civic organizations and a range of publications including the Chicago Sun-Times, Chicago Enterprise, Chicago Magazine, and U.S. News & World Report.*

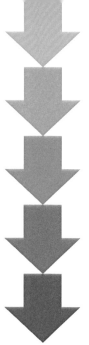

ENABLING AND DRIVING PERFORMANCE MANAGEMENT IN LOCAL GOVERNMENT

Cory Fleming and Randall Reid
International City/County Management Association

The International City/County Management Association (ICMA) was established in 1914 amid an atmosphere of broad-scale mistrust of city government. Its founding members sought to bring to municipal management a dedication to both ethics and professionalism to help restore public trust. Although the level of corruption in local government no longer compares to that of the early 1900s, several notable modern abuses of public trust—Bell, California; Detroit, and New Orleans—demonstrate that fraud and gross mismanagement still happen. During the first 100 years of ICMA's history, the organization has continued to see an accelerated demand for accountability and transparency locally as national media highlight mistrust and fiscal challenges.

The remarkable growth in the availability and usability of relevant data has both enabled and driven the expansion of local government performance management to respond to these challenges. The introduction of computers in the workplace in the 1980s enabled local agencies to automate their administrative records, making data much more reliable and easy to collect and analyze. For example, the ability to easily sort data and tabulate results allowed observers to understand whether agency performance was improving or declining and by how much. New data management systems for geo-spatial analysis and mapping, customer service, financial planning and assessment, and web use all provide the means to analyze and compare how effectively and efficiently local government is being managed.

In just the past few years, more timely and a greater variety of available data have enabled entirely new ways of conducting municipal business. From mobile devices placed in city vehicles to sensors on water meters, thermostats, and traffic signals, new forms of collection are allowing local governments to access unprecedented amounts of data in nearly real time. For example, the City of Rancho Cucamonga, California, has implemented a city sidewalk inspection program. A simple mobile app enables city staff to inspect sidewalks and document problems using nothing more than their smartphones. Even five years ago, such a program would have been technically impossible to institute.

But to improve performance, governments must create mechanisms to integrate the data into operational processes that improve the efficiency and effectiveness of government programs. Progress in this direction accelerated in the 1990s with the publication of *Reinventing Government,* which galvanized the practice of "results-oriented" management in the public sector.[1] The authors introduced the concept that government managers could use data to improve operations and meet citizens' expectations just as the private sector does.

In 1994, ICMA established the Center for Performance Measurement, now known as the Center for Performance Analytics, to advance these ideas. The center established the first national database of more than 5,000 measures used by local governments to gauge performance. One of the great advantages of this database is that it allows local officials to see how their own performance compares with similar local agencies elsewhere. This sort of comparative analysis, followed by reflection or studies of possible causes, can help establish useful benchmarks and a more nuanced understanding of the forces behind organization-wide performance.

By the late 1990s, a number of localities wanted to improve the effectiveness of their performance management efforts. The most prominent response was Baltimore's CitiStat program in 1999. The CitiStat program evaluates how efficiently city departments deliver services, and measures their performance in meeting mutually agreed-upon service delivery goals.

---

1 D. Osborne and T. Gaebler, *Reinventing Government: How the Entrepreneurial Spirit is Transforming the Public Sector* (Menlo Park, CA: Addison-Wesley, 1992).

Like most such efforts, this approach entailed a series of departmental meetings to review updates on a set of preselected performance measures. But CitiStat is distinguished by several features that motivated all participants to give it priority attention. Most important was the active, direct involvement of the mayor and other high-level officials. Department heads typically ran the meetings, and all staff members in attendance knew the mayor was regularly reviewing the results. Second, the meetings were held regularly and frequently. As a result, staff made extra efforts to generate better data to devise and track metrics that would be reliable and meaningful. They were also more careful in setting performance targets. As a result, city departments have significantly improved their performance and saved the city money in the process. The program, also known as "PerformanceStat," became a national model for using data to improve government performance. It has since spread to many other U.S. cities and some state agencies.

The initial CitiStat process had a reputation for taking a tough-minded approach when performance targets were not being met. As the model spread, it has evolved beyond its initial focus on poor performance to include a continuous improvement approach. In order to instead foster collaborative problem-solving, some local governments have adopted a "think tank" approach that enables executives and other leaders to analyze and propose new solutions when service problems are detected.[2] The focus is on using the data to learn about what is working, what is not, and why—in other words, using data to provide a sound basis for devising and adjusting strategies to truly improve results.

Increasingly, the practice of performance management is evolving beyond performance metrics. Mapping, in particular, generates potent new information. For example, Minneapolis 311 staff mapped service requests for nuisance complaints by supervisory districts and realized that the district with the most complaints had received twice as many as the district with the fewest.[3] Yet both district offices had the same number of support personnel. Likewise, the more complete data now available on the

2 C. Fleming, "Technology, Data and Institutional Change in Local Government," In *Strengthening Communities with Neighborhood Data*, edited by G. Thomas Kingsley, Claudia J. Coulton, and Kathryn L. S. Pettit (Washington, DC: Urban Institute Press, 2014).

3 C. Fleming, "Minneapolis 311 System," *Call 311: Connecting Citizens to Local Government Case Study Series* (Washington, DC: International City/County Management Association, 2008).

demographics of a neighborhood (for example, the proportion of children versus elderly) can be used to adjust the types of services provided in a neighborhood park or social service programming and thereby increase use rates and improve outcomes.

In an era of "big data," ICMA has recognized the need for greater analytic capability. Local governments require real-time data to proactively deliver services in communities. ICMA Insights, a new performance management software platform, automates data entry and introduces significant new tools for data-mining, analysis, and data visualization. More important, the new platform enhances the ability of local governments to respond to citizen demands for greater transparency. Daily, weekly, or monthly monitoring of performance metrics trends allows greater ability for managers to use predictive analytics to alter processes prior to failures or underachieving results.

The explosion of data available to local governments, along with increased pressure from the public for "open data" to assess government performance and program results, has already changed practice in dramatic ways. Going forward, local government employees will be much more likely to analyze rather than process data. Technological advances and software tools will continue to make data analysis easier. Better analytic tools, along with timely data, will help local governments re-engineer business processes and procedures, leading to improved service delivery, enhanced customer service, and greater transparency and accountability.

■ ■ ■

CORY FLEMING *oversees the International City/County Management Association (ICMA) 311–Customer Relations Management Technical Assistance Services and directed the ICMA National Study of 311 and Customer Service Technology from 2006 to 2011. Fleming has written in various capacities about the use of data for improved local government service delivery and performance measurement. She currently manages the #LocalGov Technology Alliance, an Esri-ICMA initiative to explore the world of big data, open data, apps, and what it all means for local governments. She served as editor of the GIS Guide for Local Government Officials and The GIS Guide for Elected Officials.*

■ ■ ■

RANDALL REID *serves as director of the ICMA Center for Performance Analytics and southeast regional director. As director for the Center for Performance Analytics, Randall sets the vision and strategic direction, provides leadership and operational management as well as identifies and develops partnership opportunities. As southeast regional director, Randall represents ICMA's professional development programs, services, and ethical values to communities to create excellence in local government by fostering professional management worldwide.*

5

ADOPTING MORE
STRATEGIC PRACTICES

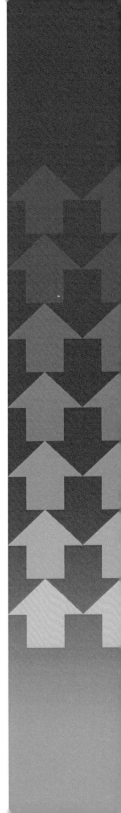

A consensus is emerging that policy would be more effective if evidence were more regularly brought to bear on key policy questions. However, the implementation of evidence-based policy is limited by several key issues. First, many have an overly narrow conception of what counts as evidence. More meta-analyses can help in this regard, as can the pursuit of more policy experiments in the field. But more importantly, evidence is often not coupled with a compelling narrative and presented to policymakers using an effective vehicle. After presenting examples of this problem, this essay argues that we should build institutional leadership for bringing together the disparate talents needed to meld evidence, narrative, and vehicle into effective policy strategies.

"NARRATIVE" AND "VEHICLE": USING EVIDENCE TO INFORM POLICY

Raphael W. Bostic
University of Southern California

"Wherever possible, we should design new initiatives to build rigorous data about what works and then act on evidence that emerges—expanding the approaches that work best, fine-tuning the ones that get mixed results, and shutting down those that are failing."
—*Peter Orszag, former director of the U.S. Office of Management and Budget*[1]

Any standard course in policy analysis will typically include a lengthy discourse about the importance of data and evidence. When policymakers or analysts face a problem, data can play at least four key roles in their decision-making process:

- Problem definition: Data can be used to focus attention on the precise problem policymakers are interested in solving;

- Option-building: Data can be used to identify the set of policy interventions that can have an impact on the problem;

- Prediction: Data can be used to predict how a particular policy intervention is likely to change conditions on the ground if implemented in a certain context;

- Evaluation: Data can be analyzed to establish whether a particular policy intervention has helped improve the situation.

These actions can generate a cache of evidence to help inform policy decisions to increase or reduce the scale and scope of a policy or

---

1 P. Orszag, "Building Rigorous Evidence to Drive Policy," Office of Management and Budget blog, June 8, 2009. www.whitehouse.gov/omb/blog/09/06/08/BuildingRigorousEvidencetoDrivePolicy.

program, modify a program's structure or incentives, eliminate a policy or program altogether, or introduce a new policy or program. This is classic policy analysis.

However, policymaking in the United States has not always followed this "textbook" approach, and consensus is emerging that policy would be more effective if evidence were more regularly brought to bear on key policy questions. This belief helped motivate the Obama Administration's multipronged efforts to promote evidence-based policy at the federal level.[2] The essays in this book focus on creating precondi tions so that: (1) the right data are available for policy analysts to conduct problem definition, option-building, prediction, and evaluation and (2) the right lessons are gleaned from these analyses. These are the building blocks of evidence-based policymaking.

However, the record of evidence translating cleanly into policy is not as stellar as it should be. For example, most scientists agree that the evidence is clear regarding the human role in contributing to climate change. A joint National Academy of Sciences and Royal Society report in 2014 summarizes the evidence and shows a direct correlation between the rise in planetary temperatures and more intensive human use of fossil fuels.[3] And yet this evidence has made limited inroads, at best, where new policy is concerned. A second example is in transporta tion planning. It is widely recognized that light rail projections used by transportation officials routinely overestimate ridership and under-estimate the cost of constructing light rail systems.[4] However, these projections are rarely adjusted and the erroneous projections still make the news, as if the variances were truly unexpected. In both examples, evidence has not translated into policy.

---

2   Orszag, 2009; Office of Management and Budget, "Circular Number A-11: Preparation, Submission and Execution of the Budget" (Washington, DC: Office of Management and Budget, 2012).

3   Royal Society and National Academy of Sciences, "Climate Change: Evidence and Causes" (Washington, DC: National Academy of Sciences, 2014).

4   C. Liu, "MTA Sees Success in Orange Line," Los Angeles Times, November 21, 2005, http://articles.latimes.com/2005/nov/21/local/me-orange21; A. Loukaitou-Sideris, D. Houston, and A. Bromberg, "Gold Line Corridor Study, Final Report." (Los Angeles, CA: UCLA Ralph and Goldy Lewis Center for Regional Policy Studies, 2007).

These cases reveal a simple truth: Developing evidence is not a sufficient condition for implementing evidence-based policy. More is needed. This discussion focuses first on the evidence that is useful for policymaking. Then it turns to the roles that "narrative" and "vehicle" can play in creating an environment in which evidence is recognized, understood, and incorporated into policy discussions and debates. A narrative is a simple, personal story that captures the relationship in a way the average person can understand. A vehicle is a conduit, such as a newspaper, through which the narrative is delivered. But even a strong narrative and vehicle cannot guarantee that evidence is incorporated into policy. Other elements, such as a focusing event that garners attention to a policy problem and an absence of gate-keepers committed to maintaining the status quo, are critical.[5] Unfortunately, researchers and others pay far less attention to creating a compelling narrative and vehicle than they do to ensuring that the latter factors are in place. The result is less use of evidence in policymaking.

WHAT COUNTS AS EVIDENCE?

A precondition for injecting evidence into the policy-making process is the existence of evidence that can potentially inform policy. There has been an ongoing debate about what constitutes actionable evidence. There is general consensus that the clearest evidence emerges from randomized, controlled trials (RCTs) in which people are randomly assigned to either a treatment or control group, and the study environment is closely managed or tracked to ensure that all other factors that could affect outcomes are controlled for. However, broad execution of RCTs within the social sciences is impractical because they are often difficult to design and expensive to run. Furthermore, RCTs raise ethical questions. How do you not offer a high-quality classroom experience, for example, to children in a control group? As such, few RCTs are undertaken in the social sciences.[6]

This leaves us in a world woefully short of "gold-standard" evidence in many policy areas. As a result, policymakers and analysts who insist

---

5   J.W. Kingdon. *Agendas, Alternatives, and Public Policies* (Boston: Little, Brown, 1984).

6   RCTs present other challenges in a policy context. In some instances, particularly those that have cross-sectional elements, some may question whether the design includes sufficient controls to identify and disentangle causal effects. Moreover, RCTs often do not yield results in a timely manner.

that the results of RCTs studies are the only valid form of evidence too often have nothing to use to support a position for changing policy, even when problems with particular policies are acknowledged. Strict adherence to an RCT–only view, therefore, can result in making decisions based on less information and evidence than is available, ultimately resulting in less evidence-based policy. This can also lead to a bias to preserve the status quo—no evidence equals no possibility of improvement.

But often other information can be brought to bear in policy areas lacking RCTs. There are many other types of high-quality studies that use valid data and sophisticated statistical methods that control for potentially confounding factors. I find these "imperfect" high-quality studies to be informative and useful as evidence, but I understand the reluctance of some in the research, policymaking, and research funding communities to embrace them. However, this hesitance need not result in policy stalemate, where one group says we have evidence and another says we do not. An underused statistical approach, known as meta-analysis, may be helpful in this regard. Meta-analysis synthesizes the findings of a set of research studies, which can be insightful, even when none of the studies is a randomized, controlled trial. It allows one to argue that "the preponderance of evidence suggests" using unbiased statistical techniques and thus can help build a policy consensus. While beyond the scope of this discussion, I would encourage more assessments of research on a given policy area using meta-analysis as a supplement to randomized, controlled studies, in addition to more support for those proposing such pursuits.

The use of meta-analysis would certainly have been helpful to the City of Fresno, CA. In 2012, city officials in Fresno embarked on an extended debate about whether to privatize their waste management services as part of a fiscal belt-tightening. The debate produced a divided city council, a 4–3 council vote to privatize the service, and then a citywide referendum reversing the privatization decision. The result: No change in service, hard feelings throughout the community, and tens of thousands of already-scarce dollars spent on the referendum vote rather than providing services to residents. The problem: The argument focused on the wrong issue, privatization. If the city had used results from an existing meta-analysis conducted by academic researchers, they could have clarified that the issue was not whether the service was provided by a public or private entity, but whether providers must compete for the franchise.[7] Competitive tendering leads to cost improvements regardless of whether the awardee is a private company or a public agency. This evidence would have made a big difference in Fresno, and left the community stronger.

But meta-analysis alone is not enough. We also need more policy experiments that generate information on observed effects from which we can glean insights into how programs and incentives work in practice. Two related examples from my former agency, the Department of Housing and Urban Development (HUD), highlight programs that represent such experiments at the federal and local levels. On the federal level, the Moving to Work (MTW) program allows local public housing authorities, with HUD approval, to modify some operating guidelines in rental assistance programs to lower costs and promote self-sufficiency among residents. There are now more than 35 MTW housing authorities, and they have instituted dozens of new program policies. Sadly, the follow-through on evaluating these changes has not been as robust as one would like. But there remains an opportunity to learn much.

The way the Denver, CO, Public Housing Authority (PHA) manages its portfolio exemplifies a policy experiment by local governments. The PHA maintains a public housing portfolio that has two distinct configurations. One portion of the portfolio consists of large block of units located at a single site—the quintessential image of public housing. A second portion consists of individual or small sets of units scattered throughout the PHA service area. Denver's policy for new recipients was to randomly assign them to either the concentrated block of units or scattered site housing. This distribution offers a natural experiment that allows for the policymaker to assess the effects of concentrating rental assistance units, with potential implications for how best to maintain and adjust public housing portfolios to increase residents' quality of life and improve outcomes for program participants. This experiment

---

7   G. Bel, X.Fageda, and M.E. Warner (2010), "Is private production of public services cheaper than public production? A meta-regression analysis of solid waste and water services," *Journal of Policy Analysis and Management*, 29(3), pp. 553–577.

differs from the large-scale demonstrations, such as HUD's 20-year Moving to Opportunity demonstration, that include a purposeful decision to implement a research design. Here the Denver PHA simply implemented their program to mimic a research design, which provides high-quality insights. I believe there are many more such natural experiments in the field.

USING EVIDENCE EFFECTIVELY: NARRATIVE AND VEHICLE

Although evidence is the precondition in evidence-based policymaking, two other tools are required: a narrative and a vehicle. Too often, evidence is presented and made available in lengthy academic documents that appeal to only researchers and academics. Policymakers rarely have the training or the time to sift through such documents to fully digest the results. What they need is a narrative, a concise short story that presents the evidence in a way that is memorable and intuitive. The narrative serves as a shorthand distillation and translation of the compiled evidence and becomes the embodiment of the lessons learned and actions to be taken. The most effective narratives will include clear explanations of directly-supporting evidence. But the story leads with the narrative, not the data and evidence.

An appropriate vehicle for delivering the narrative is also essential for the effective implementation of evidence-based policy. We all have read a good book or short story and wondered why it didn't gain traction. One possibility might be that the author or publisher didn't promote the work in the most powerful way. The same challenge can arise for evidence and a narrative. It is not enough to publish significant results of studies in academic journals or publications. When the vehicle for the narrative is not on policymakers' radar, it is hard to inject evidence into policy.

What represents the ideal combination of narrative and vehicle? It depends on the audience. A different approach is needed if the intended audience is composed of key lawmakers, leaders, and staff who have an ability to shape legislation and policy or if the target audience is the general public or the social circles of the key lawmakers, leaders, and staff.

To target key players, the vehicle should be a short document (one to two pages) with main conclusions from the evidence laid out clearly and concisely. The document may be slightly longer if it is generated "on the inside," as a principal is likely to have a longer attention span if a trusted staff person has produced the document. Simple bullets with bolded key sentences or phrases make central points stand out. Finally, the piece should incorporate a straightforward narrative drawn from experiences in the field. A document that is too data-oriented runs the risk of becoming abstract and distant. A document designed to achieve these many different goals requires considerable effort and time, but the payoff is substantial.

To reach the general public, researchers and others must leverage the media via television, newspapers, or magazines. Because these pieces will be lengthier than the one- to two-page document for the targeted lawmaker, a narrative may be developed more completely to personalize the issue. Moreover, skilled writers or producers can use visuals to relay the key ideas quickly and memorably.

Today's social media and online publishing options offer additional avenues. Increasing numbers of people, including policy experts, are now using Facebook, Twitter, and other social media applications to exchange information. However, our understanding of how social media can be used to promote policy change continues to evolve. For example, relatively little is known about what makes evidence go viral. A second challenge with these vehicles is credibility; virtually anybody can post information without regard to accuracy. That said, we are increasingly seeing information outlets in this space. For example, the Office of Policy Development and Research at HUD has an app that allows people to read accessible summaries of research and innovative practices in the field. Figuring out how to navigate these waters is a current frontier, and many learning opportunities are ahead.

For both the targeted and public strategy approaches, authors must take care to ensure that a narrative is not viewed as a one-shot exposé with limited generality or a thin advocacy piece. It must be clear that the evidence used to draw the conclusions is credible, definitive, and weighty. Sometimes, though rarely, a single study can accomplish this.

However, a definitive conclusion regarding a particular policy issue typically arises through the cumulative effect of multiple studies conducted
in varied contexts that produce a body of mutually reinforcing evidence.

The next section presents two case studies that demonstrate the power
of narrative and vehicle for injecting evidence into policymaking. The
first example describes a successful strategy that targeted the public. The
second example shows the harm that can arise when an effective vehicle
is absent. It also demonstrates how the subsequent introduction of an
effective vehicle can change the tenor of the policy discussion. In both
case studies, having a body of evidence that generated clear implications
for policy was essential but not sufficient.

EVIDENCE, NARRATIVE, AND VEHICLE WORKING TOGETHER

Homelessness in Reno, Nevada: While working at HUD, I had a pair
of "aha" moments during the budget-wrangling with Congress during
President Obama's first term. These moments revealed the importance
of a narrative and a vehicle. During the 2010 and 2011 budget deliberations, Congress was in a serious belt-tightening mode. Line items were
being pitted against each other to try to bring budgets in line with
the reduced total spending that Congress authorized. At HUD, this
meant difficult decisions regarding whether vouchers, public housing,
block grants, or Secretarial initiatives should bear the bulk of the
austerity burdens.

Homelessness was noticeably absent from the conversation about
trade-offs. Almost nobody talked about reducing funding for the suite
of programs designed to reduce the incidence and severity of homelessness in the United States. Why? Because everyone in Washington—from
policy experts, to staffers on the Hill, to elected officials—shared the
same understanding about the large returns to up-front investments
targeted at treating and preventing homelessness.

The question, of course, is: How did such a consensus emerge? A key
part of the answer can be found in an article by Malcolm Gladwell that
appeared in *The New Yorker* in 2006, titled "Million-Dollar Murray."
The article tells the story of Murray Barr, a chronically homeless man
in Reno, Nevada, and the police officers who were regularly called to

pick up Murray and deliver him to the hospital or county jail. Gladwell reports that local police estimated that Murray had racked up at least $100,000 in hospital bills in only six months. But he'd been repeating the same pattern during his 10 years on the streets, meaning that he'd likely cost public services more than $1 million—far more than what it would have cost to provide him housing or supportive services.

Although the story would have been quite useful for informing homelessness policy in Reno, Gladwell went further. He chronicled the work of many researchers—including Dennis Culhane, now widely recognized as a leading researcher on homelessness—to highlight consistent evidence supporting the notion that there are Murray Barrs in every U.S. city. The key takeaway from Gladwell's piece is that most of the costs associated with homelessness owe to the troubles of a small number of people who are chronically homeless. If we focus treatment on these people, he argues, we can see both short- and long-term savings.

While Gladwell provided the narrative (and it is good reading!), success occurred in part because *The New Yorker* was an ideal vehicle. Its readership is broad and it is popular among the better-educated urban people who would know of homelessness but not necessarily understand it. It gave this group, which undoubtedly included some policymakers and aides, a new way of thinking about the problem and its potential solutions. The vehicle helped the story quickly make its way through a broad set of circles and its takeaways became generally known. Hence, a common understanding emerged, and the funding for homelessness prevention policy was resilient in the face of intense budget stress. Evidence coupled with a narrative and a high-quality vehicle translated into the effective use of evidence to inform policy.

Housing Counseling: A second example is housing counseling. During budget tightening, unlike the case for homeless services, housing counseling became a target of congressional appropriators, and its line item was ultimately zeroed in the House's budget prescription. Many assumed this was an impossibility. By 2011, everyone was aware of the housing crisis and its devastating effects on families across the country. It was widely understood that many people got into trouble due to a lack of understanding of the risks associated with some mortgage instruments and homeownership more generally. Moreover, stories abounded of how a specific housing counselor had saved the day for a desperate homeowner. So how could counseling be stripped of funding There were two issues here. First, somewhat surprisingly, policymakers did not know about the quantified benefits of housing counseling. After the House action, HUD convened the major housing counseling agencies and advocates to determine a response. During these discussions, it became clear that little effort had gone into building the case for the return on investment (ROI) for housing counseling. Counseling was at a disadvantage compared with other policy areas that had such cost/benefit figures because it was difficult to demonstrate that counseling was more cost-effective than another policy. Second, the lack of a vehicle was a problem. Appropriations staffers were unaware of the narratives regarding the benefits of counseling and did not hear about them during the budget process. Clearly, the narratives were not effectively deployed. These factors doomed the program.

However, the story ended on a somewhat happier note. The loss of funding galvanized the counseling industry to correct both of these problems. A coalition of key players, including service providers, advocates, and government staff, worked together to assemble data on the costs and benefits of counseling. Their analysis showed that housing counseling resulted in almost $400 in benefits for every $1 spent.[8] Second, a bevy of counseling providers and housing policy advocates descended upon the Hill with a coordinated information campaign to make sure that the cost-effectiveness and efficiency arguments were too loud to ignore. Ultimately, some funding for counseling was restored.

ADVANCING THE USE OF EVIDENCE TO INFORM POLICY

Producing the narrative and finding the right vehicle consistently and effectively require drawing from the knowledge and expertise of people with varied backgrounds. Researchers and analysts are necessary to distill a body of research into its essential messages. Practitioners and advocates often are aware of the experiences that can put a personal face on the messages and provide the basis for a compelling narrative.

---

8 This estimate was generated from internal modeling and projections by the Office of Policy Development and Research at HUD.

Public affairs and media professionals are skilled in crafting pieces that have maximum impact. Purposeful collaboration among these groups will increase the likelihood of success. Yet few organizations set bringing together teams of people with these diverse skills as a key goal or mission. More need to. Governments can be effective in this regard, but changes in administrations bring changes in goals and priorities, so there can be an ebb and flow in government's participation. Perhaps philanthropy, which can be more stable in its objectives, can play a catalyzing role in this regard.

A more fundamental issue is exemplified by the counseling example. The translation from anecdote to general lesson depends on the presence of indisputable evidence and consensus on what the evidence means. Success would be enhanced if there were monitoring to ensure that these preconditions exist and, if they do not, to determine what needs to be done to get the field to that position. In the case of counseling, the budget crisis would have been less likely to occur if there had been an organization that was mission-driven to ensure that there was a strong evidence base and that the lessons from existing evidence were easily available to key decision-makers.

This process would run something like this. Ask the question: Has anyone summarized what is known about a given policy? If so, the next issue is to wrestle with whether clear lessons or implications emerge from the existing evidence. It is likely that the author of any summary will make declarations about key takeaways. But independent scrutiny is important to preserve the credibility and validity of subsequent efforts. Furthermore, if no summary has been done, take the time to do it and craft the lessons to be drawn from what was found.

I am unaware of organizations that view this as their role. My unit at HUD embarked on a two-year Research Roadmap process to determine what questions in a number of policy directions still needed attention. The effort was difficult, precisely because few institutions and experts ask these questions in the course of their everyday work. This is a gap that requires filling, though there are some encouraging examples of this kind of work. The multi-institution What Works Collaborative, established at the start of the Obama administration, had as its goal identifying promising policy implications from existing research and supporting other research that had promise to answer key questions. Similarly, the recent collaboration between the Federal Reserve Bank of San Francisco and the Low Income Investment Fund that resulted in *Investing in What Works for America's Communities* yielded a produc that purposefully incorporates the varied expertise of multiple groups.

Along similar lines, we would benefit by having some institutions that viewed it as their charge to maintain a real-time, current record of wha we know about a particular policy arena. Given the continuous flow o studies and reports issued by universities, think tanks, advocacy group and others on various issues, it can be a significant challenge to maintain pace with policy changes, and individual researchers often do not provide straightforward syntheses of their work that place the results i a useful policy context. Support to assign some individuals or organiza tions with this role would be quite helpful.

Finally, timing is a key barrier to the effective use of evidence in policymaking. Too often, evidence is not available when policymakers are looking for it. An ongoing, real-time summary of what is known would mean that answers to policy questions, such as we have them, will be readily available when the policymakers want the knowledge, rather than the present reality in which requests for knowledge are often met with a reply that study results will be ready in 18 months.

CONCLUSION

More evidence-based policymaking will require attention to all of the elements of the undertaking. We will need to compile the right data and conduct the highest-quality analyses and evaluations. As the housing counseling example demonstrates, assuming the appropriate evidence exists is problematic, even in mature policy areas. Housing counseling had been offered for decades, and yet the evidence was not there. We cannot advance effective policy if we do not know what works, or if we—at a minimum—can't clearly demonstrate that certain policies work. Lacking an evidence base will almost always be fatal in this pursuit. We need to address evidence gaps, which will require an assessment of existing data and data systems to identify barriers and find solutions for overcoming them.

But we should also consider other parts of the equation, because the existence of evidence is insufficient to guarantee its use by policymakers. Is there a narrative that captures the essence of what we know in a way that is personal and memorable? We must find stories as compelling and straightforward as the Murray Barr story for all of our policy areas. We must then deploy resources and skills to ensure the story is told to maximize its effects. Do we have a vehicle that can spread this narrative broadly and to the right audiences, so that our knowledge becomes common knowledge, particularly among those involved in making policy? Too often, knowledge in academia never becomes general knowledge, or if it does, it happens several years after the initial point is established. The end results of slowly disseminated knowledge are more societal costs and fewer societal benefits than should be realized. Purposeful attention to identifying and leveraging the right vehicle to gain the broadest possible understanding of the evidence and its implications can significantly improve the likelihood that better policies are adopted and implemented.

Both these dimensions need to be someone's responsibility. Ideally, an organization would take on this role so that institutional memory about the evolution of policy and evidence could be broadly shared. Without a "ring leader," the use of evidence to inform policy will happen, at best, on an ad hoc or somewhat random manner. We can do better and should not leave such matters to dumb luck. Success here will mean having a robust strategy for effective use of evidence in policymaking, resulting in better policies that are adopted more quickly. Failure will risk having this conversation again, and again, and again. I, for one, would like the cycle to end here and now.

■ ■ ■

DR. RAPHAEL BOSTIC *is the Judith and John Bedrosian Chair in Governance and the Public Enterprise at the Sol Price School of Public Policy at the University of Southern California. He served for 3 years in the Obama administration as the Assistant Secretary for Policy Development and Research at the U.S. Department of Housing and Urban Development. His work spans many fields including home ownership, housing finance, neighborhood change, and the role of institutions in shaping policy effectiveness.*

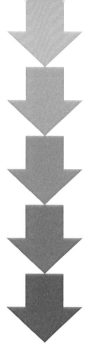

SUSTAINING DATA CULTURE WITHIN LOCAL GOVERNMENT

Erika Poethig
Urban Institute

I joined the City of Chicago's Department of Housing in 1999, just after Julia Stasch, then Commissioner of the Department of Housing (now Interim President of the John D. and Catherine T. MacArthur Foundation), had put the final touches on the City's second five-year plan for affordable housing. Largely due to Julia's leadership, this iteration of the City's plan was produced in collaboration with affordable housing advocates and the development community. This collaborative approach stood in contrast to the contentious process that produced Chicago's affordable housing plan six years earlier.

The "Affordable Housing and Community Jobs" ordinance of 1993, which required the City of Chicago to produce an affordable housing plan, was the result of considerable work led by Alderman Toni Preckwinkle (now President of the Cook County Board of Commissioners) and the Chicago Rehab Network, a network of community development organizations and nonprofit affordable housing developers. With support from local foundations, the Chicago Rehab Network mobilized a campaign over several year that pressed the City to make long-term commitments of resources—federal, state, and local—to the development and preservation of affordab housing for Chicago's neediest residents.

Armed with "The Chicago Affordable Housing Fact Book: Visions for Change," community organizers were positioned in neighborhoods across the city to mobilize support. With data from a variety of local and federal sources, including the newly released 1990 census, the Fact Book served as the evidence and guidebook for policy change. One of its features was a housing misery index. The index ranked the 77 community areas on indicators such as "communities with less than $5 million invested by conventional lenders," "communities that lost 10 percent or more of their total units between 1980 and 1990," and "communities where at least 10 percent of children under age 5 suffer from lead poisoning."[1] These indicators were also broken down for all 50 aldermanic wards. Two of the Fact Book's most impressive charts compared Chicago's spending on affordable housing with that in other U.S. cities. In 1989, Chicago spent $0.66 per capita for low-cost housing compared with $101.89 per capita in New York City.

This huge gap between Chicago and New York motivated a campaign that used data to demand increased local resources for affordable housing. The resulting ordinance required the city to create five-year estimates for affordable housing commitments and submit quarterly progress reports with accompanying testimony to the City Council's Housing and Real Estate committee. A sample for these reports was even attached to the ordinance. In the end, the City Council approved a five-year commitment of more than $500 million that was estimated to produce and preserve just over 36,000 units of affordable housing.

In my role as Assistant Commissioner for Program, Policy and Resource Development, I was charged with creating the quarterly reports for the second five-year plan. Notwithstanding the collaborative process that led to the plan, assembling these reports felt like a great imposition. At the time, the reports served only to fulfill a regulatory requirement. Each quarter I cajoled colleagues to provide data. If I was lucky, they submitted the data in an Excel spreadsheet, but there were still a few program managers who tracked every small loan or grant using paper and pencil. My staff and I would pull all these disparate pieces together into one unified report that tracked the funding sources (CDBG, HOME, GO Bonds, LIHTC, etc.), project type (rental housing, improvements, affordable mortgages, etc.), who was served (income and ethnicity), and the location. The resource was painstaking to produce, but even worse, it was woefully underused.

Soon after I arrived at the department, Julia moved over to become Mayor Daley's Chief of Staff, and Jack Markowski replaced her as commissioner

1   Chicago Rehab Network, "The Chicago Affordable Housing Fact Book: Visions for Change."(Chicago Rehab Network, 1993), pp., 12–13.

in 1999. A seasoned public servant, Jack transformed the data-rich quarterly reports from a regulatory requirement into a management tool. He held monthly "stat" meetings to hold program managers accountable. As a result, the data started to improve and so did the outcomes. These stat meetings marked the advent of data-driven policymaking and program management for affordable housing investments in the City of Chicago. In fact, the City recently completed its fifth five-year housing plan.

At the same time, the Chicago Rehab Network continues to push from the outside. Although the network and the City have collaborated over the years, they are not always on the same page about the City's progress toward meeting its goals, even though they use the same data. The network continues to produce its own review of the quarterly reports and to testify before City Council.

The lesson I take from this experience is that although data can be powerful in fortifying the "outside game," that is, the pressure from advocates or other community stakeholders necessary to spur major policy change, it is not sufficient to sustain that change. An "inside game," driven by those within government who know how to leverage bureaucratic processes, is also needed to ensure that data are used effectively and systematically to hold the public sector accountable.

The challenge is that the quality, utility, and use of data depend on its currency with leadership and managers. Investing in local government capacity to create, manage, and analyze its own data may well be a necessary condition to significantly improve housing and community development policy. But to get the most out of data, changes to organizational culture are also needed. Strong internal leadership that helps staff at all levels recognize the value of data for decision making will help ensure that programs and policies remain data-driven over the long term. It is also important that mayors, city councils, and federal and state funding agencies reward public officials who use data and information to advance the public good.

Acknowledgment: The author would like to thank Kevin Jackson, Rachel Johnston, Jack Markowski, and Stacie Young for providing important source materials and background on the Affordable Housing and Community Job Campaign and Ordinance and the subsequent five-year plans.

■ ■ ■

ERIKA POETHIG *is an Institute fellow and director of urban policy initiatives at the Urban Institute. She recently served as acting assistant secretary for policy development and research at the U.S. Department of Housing and Urban Development, and was also a leading architect of the White House Council for Strong Cities and Strong Communities.. At the John D. and Catherine T. MacArthur Foundation, she was associate director of housing. She also served as assistant commissioner for policy, resource and program development at the City of Chicago's Department of Housing.*

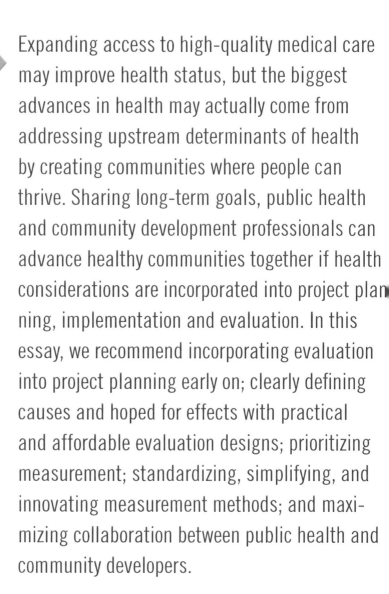

Expanding access to high-quality medical care may improve health status, but the biggest advances in health may actually come from addressing upstream determinants of health by creating communities where people can thrive. Sharing long-term goals, public health and community development professionals can advance healthy communities together if health considerations are incorporated into project planning, implementation and evaluation. In this essay, we recommend incorporating evaluation into project planning early on; clearly defining causes and hoped for effects with practical and affordable evaluation designs; prioritizing measurement; standardizing, simplifying, and innovating measurement methods; and maximizing collaboration between public health and community developers.

EVALUATING SOCIAL DETERMINANTS OF HEALTH IN COMMUNITY DEVELOPMENT PROJECTS

David Fleming, Hilary N. Karasz, and Kirsten Wysen
Public Health-Seattle & King County

We know the all-too-familiar statistics—despite the United States spending almost twice as much as other developed countries on health care, we rank 33rd in life expectancy. Although expanding access to high-quality health care is important, improvements in medical care delivery can be expected to reduce preventable deaths by only about 10 percent.[1] To make bigger improvements in health, we need to look outside the walls of the clinic to the places where we live, learn, work, and play. Individual health is based in large part on the health of the communities in which one lives, homes free of toxins, accessible parks and community centers, convenient and safe transit, biking and walking trails, and access to good food, child care, and jobs. These "social" or "upstream" community determinants of health can influence as much as 60 percent of preventable mortality.[2]

Almost without exception, the goals of community development projects include improving one or more of these upstream determinants of health. In theory, then, a logical outcome of successful community development should be improved community health, although this is neither a necessary nor intentional outcome. Also, in theory, evaluations quantifying the health improvements resulting from well-designed community development projects should be plentiful and broadly disseminated. Unfortunately, practice has not caught up with theory,

---

1 S. Schroeder, "We Can Do Better Improving the Health of the American People," *New England Journal of Medicine*, 357 (September 2007): 1221–1228.

2 Ibid.

and our evaluation cupboards are mostly bare. In part, this may be the result of not prioritizing evaluations, but in truth there are significant obstacles to successfully measuring the effects of community development projects on health.

One early example of this kind of upstream intervention was recent multi-sector work in King County, Washington, to improve school nutrition and student physical activity and reduce obesity in some of the poorest school districts in the county. This work, led by the public health department of Seattle and King County, involved the collaboration of K-12 education, the food system, urban planning, small business and other sectors to make concentrated investments in specific location

At the end of the two-year initiative, results showed that for children living in the project area, obesity prevalence dropped by a highly significant 17 percent, whereas obesity remained unchanged in other parts of the county.[3] Hidden behind this one-sentence result are lessons in front-line complexities of conducting this type of evaluation. Drawin in part from this experience, the essay outlines some of the steps that should be considered in community development projects that aim to improve the health of residents, among other goals.

INCORPORATE EVALUATION INTO PROJECT PLANNING EARL'

Evaluation should be part of project planning at the earliest conceptualization phase. Too often, evaluation is an add-on after the bulk of planning has been done, when time and budget are short and it is too late to make significant changes to the project.

The King County project had a strong evaluation component from the start. Evaluators played an important role in project design and were active participants during the start-up phase of the project, when adjus ments were made to the project design based on early results. Almost 10 percent of the total project cost was dedicated to data collection an evaluation, a signal of the importance of evaluation to the project.

---

3 E. Kern, N.L. Chan, D.W. Fleming, J.W. Krieger "Declines in Student Obesity Prevalence Associate with a Prevention Initiative—King County, Washington, 2012." *Morbidity and Mortality Weekly Report*, February 21, 2014 / 63(07); 155–157.

Incorporating evaluation early is not only more efficient than doing evaluation post-hoc, it also may allow for more deliberate incorporation of health interventions. If health is a desired goal of a housing development project, planners can think through in advance how to incorporate opportunities for residents to be physically active. They can install sidewalks and bike paths, provide green spaces and walking destinations such as shopping, and take into account transit routes so people can walk to and from buses and trains. This explicit planning simplifies evaluation. If walking paths are being incorporated into a project to increase exercise, it becomes clearer that a primary goal of an evaluation will be to determine whether these paths are being used.

Thinking about evaluation early may also create opportunities for more elegant evaluation through smart project implementation. For example, a larger scale renovation project may allow for testing of the impact of design elements by sequencing the construction and comparing results in renovated versus not yet renovated areas (newer buildings, for example, may prioritize the placement of the stairway to encourage using the stairs instead of elevators, unlike older buildings).

CLEARLY DEFINE CAUSES AND HOPED-FOR EFFECTS. THEN PICK A PRACTICAL AND AFFORDABLE EVALUATION DESIGN FOR MEASURING THEM

One of the most difficult evaluation barriers to overcome is the overpowering conventional wisdom that the best (and in some minds the only) way to scientifically conduct a valid evaluation is through a "gold standard" randomized, double blinded, placebo-controlled trial (RCT). RCTs eliminate many sources of bias and are a great design for identifying whether a new drug or vaccine works—but usually not for whether a community development project is improving health. Using RCTs to evaluate the effects of upstream determinants of health is plagued by problems, including the impracticality of random assignment of subjects, the difficulty in limiting exposure of the intervention to just the experimental group, the impossibility of blinding people or researchers to whether they have received the intervention, and the costs.

There are many alternative, more practical and less expensive approaches to evaluation, and community developers have an importa co-conspirator here: the public health scientist who spends his or her life in the same "real world" trying to evaluate the same kinds of interventions. Examples of interventions with strong evidence bases from a variety of study designs can be found in the Centers for Disease Control and Prevention's (CDC) "Community Guide." This online resource is an important collection of evidence-based practices, which continues to expand.[4]

The bottom line is that an evaluation should help determine whether what was done did what it was hoped it would. At its core, evaluation usually involve measuring what was done, what happened, and, in son way, what would have happened if nothing had been done (the reason for the placebo arm of an RCT). As a consequence, one of the most important features of any evaluation design is a comparison group tha did not receive the benefit of the intervention. The use of a comparison group dramatically strengthens the power of the evaluation but most often entails additional data collection costs.

Different types of comparison groups are possible. Quasi-experimental elements such as the 1811 Eastlake study of medical care costs for homeless people with alcoholism, for example, used such a design to compare 95 housed participants (with drinking permitted) with 39 wait-list control participants.[5] The results showed impressive health improvements and cost savings, and this type of Housing First approac is being adopted throughout the country after years of little agreement on how to reduce chronic homelessness. Other designs are simpler still Examples include sequential implementation, in which a comparison group receives the intervention after a group that receives the intervention in the first round. Another example is a pre/post design, in which group serves as its own comparison by measuring changes in the grou

---

4 The Cochrane Review and the Coalition for Evidence-based Policy also have public access compendiums of a small but growing number of proven practices along with indications of the strength of evidence about community interventions.

5 M.E. Larimer et al., "Health Care and Public Service Use and Costs Before and After Provision of Housing for Chronically Homeless Persons with Severe Alcohol Problems," *JAMA*, 301(13) (2009):1349–57.

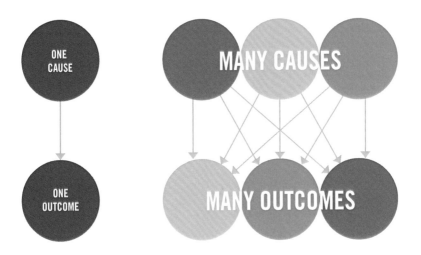

Figure 1. Potential pathways from causes to effects.

before and after the intervention (yet another reason to incorporate evaluation early).

The problem with a comparison group that has not been randomly drawn from an initial set of eligible participants is that it may not be comparable and observed differences between the groups may be for reasons other than the intervention. Comparing drug treatment outcomes between individuals who voluntarily enter treatment with those who decline, for example, may reflect differences in motivation to quit rather than effectiveness of treatment. Statistical and study design elements can minimize these problems. For example, regression analysis can separate the effects of the chosen intervention from other known influences and can limit the chance of faulty conclusions owing to confounding factors extraneous to the intervention (a type of analysis where evaluators can really earn their pay).

In the King County obesity reduction project, project evaluators used existing data sources to compare obesity data in the intervention districts with similar data in the other 12 King County districts that did not participate. The two groups were somewhat dissimilar in that the intervention districts were lower income and more poorly resourced, while the nonintervention districts were much higher income. The risk

INTERVENTION	RATIONALE	SHORT TERM OUTCOME	MEDIUM TERM OUTCOME	LONG TERM OUTCOME
Bike paths accessible within 300 feet of all homes	Easy access facilitates bike use, which increases overall physical activity level	X% of residents use bikes compared to people without access to bike paths	Increased physical activity improves cardiovascular health	Less heart disease, stroke

Figure 2. Sample logic model describing the relationship between bike paths and health.

was that natural improvements in the wealthier districts could have obscured intervention group improvement.

Community development evaluations must overcome the challenge assessing cause and effect in which interventions (such as housing or preschool education) commonly act through more than one pathway to improve health and also may influence more than one health outcome (Figure 1).

Logic models—visual depictions of the relationships between inputs and outputs—can help overcome this difficulty by providing a way to see and agree on the interventions, outcomes, and the intervening pathways. For example, Figure 2 shows a simple logic model describing the relationship between bike paths and health.

Actual logic models likely will be more detailed, particularly if there are multiple interventions and outcomes. In community development projects that address health risk factors, logic models can be integrated into the original project design and evaluation plan. Developing a logic model allows project managers to talk through assumptions about how design decisions will impact health and set expectations about short term, medium term, and long term impact.

PRIORITIZE MEASURING WHAT COMES FIRST

Sometimes, in evaluating interventions to improve health, it is easy to fall prey to a "tyranny of outcomes" mindset that prioritizes measuring important health outcomes above all else. This desire may be intensified by a belief that potential funders will be most receptive to a promise of "hard proof" that their money has improved health. Like the conventional wisdom that the randomized control trial is the gold standard of evaluation design, this "tyranny of outcomes" mindset is often incorrect and can lead to inefficient, ineffective approaches.

By their nature, community development projects are most likely to be targeted at upstream determinants of health (bike paths as in the logic model example above, increased social connectedness, better access to healthy food, etc.). Generally, evaluations should prioritize identifying and measuring the earliest expected outcomes. One advantage in using a well-planned logic model to guide evaluation is that it should indicate what these first outcomes are. Measuring the most important earliest signs of success will show whether the project is on the pathway to better health. If it is not, the program managers may want to revise the intervention or modify the expected outcomes.

For example, an evaluation of a housing project with nutrition and physical activity attributes designed to reduce the rates of diabetes should not focus first on measuring changes in diabetes rates. Instead, evaluation should first monitor whether the planned health assets were implemented on time and as designed (good project management). In this housing project example, the first step may be to ensure that the exercise facility for the housing project was completed and opened. Subsequently, evaluators can measure how frequently it is being used. If time and resources allow, the next step would be to think about short-term indicators of health in residents using it. Finally, for well-funded projects, longer-term follow-up could more clearly establish the evidence base that these short-term outcomes do lead to longer-term health improvements.

Optimally, evaluations should prioritize measuring intermediate outcomes that have been shown by prior research to be connected to longer-term outcomes. For example, antismoking interventions routinely measure changes in tobacco use rather than waiting 30 years to measure reduction in lung cancer mortality. Similarly, an intervention to increase physical activity by installing bike paths probably should not target its evaluation dollars to measuring reduction in heart disease, but rather look farther upstream in the logic model, to links between exercise and obesity reduction and less hypertension. The most important measure is probably one of bike use. The downstream health outcomes such as causes of death can be left for another day, assuming the interim outcome measures along the way (and the budget) are adequate.

The King County obesity prevention project's intent was to improve health in the targeted school districts through policy, systems, and environmental change. Its logic models showed that the first significant outcome to measure was the number and type of policies that changed, such as adoption of physical education curriculum or lunchroom cafeteria food purchase standards. Had no policies changed, then measuring health outcomes would have been a wasted effort. The intermediate outcome in this case was obesity prevalence, and the long term outcome, something that would not be measurable for a decade or more, was heart and other chronic disease where obesity is a risk factor.

Greater use of intermediate outcomes, process measures, and rapid-cycle surveys can speed the process of obtaining information measures sufficient to take action and make mid-course corrections by rolling with interim results rather than waiting for the results of lengthy trials. Micro-trials are becoming more common in medical research, and in these early days of community development/public health collaboration it makes sense to measure as many project approaches as possible to rapidly determine what works and to eliminate approaches that do not. New research methods, such as rapid online survey data collection and text responses, can provide nearly real-time feedback.

STANDARDIZE, SIMPLIFY, AND BE INNOVATIVE ABOUT MEASUREMENT METHODS AND APPROACHES

In addition to building a database of what works, the pathway to more effective and efficient evaluations will be aided by both more standardization in and greater use of emerging, smarter approaches to evaluation.

Our collective knowledge will increase faster if the results from different sites and studies can be compared. Unfortunately, if results and health outcome measures from different studies are not defined in the same way (standardized), their outcomes often cannot be compared—a significant problem unless you really like apples and oranges. For example, "prevented hospital emergency room visits" is a compelling outcome measure for housing and social services, but when there isn't agreement on what health outcomes are preventable in the first place, it makes it difficult to determine the relative cost-effectiveness of different approaches. This lack of standardization is a significant problem in public health, community-based interventions, and the Community Guide, which we mentioned earlier, has struggled to identify the cost-effectiveness of different community-level preventive approaches because of the differences in how outcomes have been measured across studies.

Another benefit of standardization is that results can be aggregated across many evaluations when a standard definition and data collection protocols for outcomes and interventions are used. The federally funded Community Transformation Grant Program, which King County also particpated in, required sites across the country to report activities and results using the same online data collection template. This uniformity provides evaluators with a much stronger ability to understand the effects of different approaches and allows findings to be analyzed much more robustly than if each of the more than 100 sites could only be compared against itself. New partnerships, such as the Build Healthy Places Network, offer promising efforts to standardize this new field as well.

Just as important as standardization is overcoming barriers to effective data collection. It is usually much less expensive to use information that someone else has already paid to collect. Examples include ongoing data collection efforts involving state health care claims data and public health disease-specific registries. An important obstacle, however, is the general lack of data on health at the *neighborhood* level. In general, community development work touches the lives of hundreds or perhaps thousands of people in specific neighborhoods. Existing health surveys often do not have an adequate sample sizes to offer meaningful or stable estimates in small areas. Instead, state or perhaps county or city estimates are typically as low as you can go. For example, one of the best measurement systems, the Behavioral Risk Factor Surveillance System (BRFSS) survey, a telephone survey that is the basis of most communities' knowledge of risk factors such as diet, physical activity, and tobacco use, was designed to report state-level results. The BRFSS requires additional local funding to produce local results for counties or cities, and additional funding still would be needed to measure outcomes from community development projects in a single neighborhood.

In King County, evaluators used standard methods and data across project activities. For example, data were used from BRFSS survey as well as the Healthy Youth Survey. In some cases, project funds were used to oversample in targeted geographic areas to ensure adequate sample size to detect a difference.

Careful thinking about the best measures to use, and in particular selecting outcomes that are common, can help avoid part of this problem. A neighborhood intervention to improve pregnancy outcome might be hard pressed from a statistical standpoint to identify a decrea in infant mortality (with a base rate of a few deaths for every 10,000 births), but reductions in low birth weight (among every 100 births) might be feasible. Additional solutions to this problem of sample size limited by small geography may come from new information technolo-gies. Geographic Information Systems (GIS) capability and ease of use are rapidly improving. Websites such as County Health Rankings and Community Commons[6] allow users to trace the ZIP code and census tract distribution of social determinants of health and health outcomes in ways that were not possible in the past. New requirement on nonprofit hospitals to assess and report on the health profiles of the communities they serve has led to progress in the capacity to map and track changes in social determinants in smaller geographic areas through resources such as CHNA.org. In addition, analytic techniques such as data smoothing, which uses information from nearby census tracts, and the use of multiple-year rolling averages, can help build stable small area estimates for health and social determinants measures In the future, as health outcomes become available through electronic health records, registries of specific health conditions and mapping

6 See www.countyhealthrankings.org and www.communitycommons.org.

will become more useful in understanding the complex pathways from community conditions to disease and disability (while ensuring the privacy of individual health information).

Minneapolis/St Paul's "Hennepin Health" is an example of a health system that has invested in social determinants because they have access to timely and actionable data. Hennepin Health is a county health plan for 10,000 of the highest need residents. The project spent considerable time and expense to create a near-to-real-time data warehouse for all the health services used by enrollees. When the Hennepin Health physicians could see a complete picture of all recent services, they observed multiple emergency room, physician, and pharmacy visits that did not contribute to optimal health nor efficient use of services. Using the data warehouse information, they were able to coordinate care and use the resulting shared savings to invest in social determinants like supportive housing and a sobering center.

There are also new tools to help think about and see data, such as network mapping and data visualization. Network maps that illustrate the connections between many organizations and the clients they serve can identify where duplication, fragmentation, and gaps in the system occur and how the entire system could benefit from specific policy changes. New data visualization tools allow policymakers to see at a glance complex relations in large data sets. For example, the Institute for Health Metrics and Evaluation's Global Burden of Disease project (www.healthdata.org) has interactive online resources that use shape, size, and color to instantly and clearly show relationships of risk factors such as diet, sedentary lifestyle, tobacco use, and mental health to leading causes of death and disability over time and by location. As data visualization advances to show effects at a smaller scale, local policymakers will have a more data driven basis for decision making.

MAXIMIZE INNOVATION THROUGH COLLABORATION

Community development and public health are natural partners because both are focused on practical ways to improve the lives of people in their communities. Both are also interested in simple, inexpensive evaluation strategies. That said, the cross-disciplinary approach to evaluating how community development projects affect social determinants of health is in its infancy. More tools are needed to aid collaboration. For example, a national clearinghouse that provides timely access to best practices and evaluation findings would allow those of us working on community development and public health to advance more quickly than separate efforts working in isolation on similar problems. We should be working collectively to develop logic models and establish causal connections between social determinants of health and health outcomes so these links can be explored and replicated, and evidence can be established in this new territory. We also should create mechanisms to standardize definitions and measures, particularly for community- as opposed to individual-level health determinants, such a availability of healthy food, open space, access to child-care, and other

The King County project brought together experts across many sectors to develop and implement evidence-based projects to improve the community's policies, systems, and the environment that affect health. Each sector has its own research and language; it took much work to just begin to be able to talk and share best practices with one another. Had we not had experts in so many fields, it would have been impossible to break into other disciplines to locate best practices. For example, few public health professionals are deeply engaged in the business of school siting, yet we know that schools within walkable distances of homes will encourage physical activity. A national clearing house of best practices would have been useful to streamline this work

Knowing what works also takes investment, and evaluation needs resources. For example, the CDC recommends that 10 percent of tobacco prevention grant program budgets should be allocated to eval ation activities—this for a health issue with a relatively well-establishe evidence base.[7] Community development is a $100 billion effort annually. The Department of Housing and Urban Development's (HUD budget of $45 billion includes 0.3 percent for research, evaluation, and demonstration projects.[8] In short, the needed financing for measuring

---

7 Centers for Disease Control and Prevention. Best Practices for Comprehensive Tobacco Control Programs—2014.Atlanta: U.S. Department of Health and Human Services, Centers for Disease Control and Prevention, National Center for Chronic Disease Prevention and Health Promotion, Office on Smoking and Health, 2014, page 61.

8 U.S. Department of Housing and Urban Development, "FY 2013 Budget: Housing and Communiti Built to Last" (Washington, DC: HUD, n.d.).

the social determinants of health is not yet available, and we need a strategy to develop it.

The field also needs more cross-sector agreement on the concept of "return on investment" (ROI) as it relates to health measurements. In the strictest sense, of course, ROI is a monetary return for dollars invested. Some health interventions, particularly some prevention interventions (immunizations, asthma management, and tobacco cessation), do yield a financial return to the health care system. Another type of health intervention (for example, nurse home visiting for high-risk infants) has a monetary ROI, although the investor (public health) is different from the party reaping the economic benefit (criminal justice and economic sectors). Health improvements resulting from community development activities would most likely fall into this second category— improving multiple health outcomes, but with the return not necessarily to the original community development investors. Evaluations should be constructed to capture this second set of returns as well.

The public health world has taken this concept of ROI one step further, recognizing that health itself has a monetary value. As a consequence, often the ROI on health investments is not reported as dollars, but as health benefit for dollars invested. Increasingly, this metric is being standardized as a "healthy year lived" or "disability adjusted life year" (DALY), a measure that combines benefits from both reduced mortality and reduced morbidity. For example, childhood immunizations cost $7 per added healthy year lived, while heart surgery costs $37,000 per additional healthy year lived.[9] Optimally, the cost per healthy year lived or DALY gained by investments in community development will be calculated and compared to costs from medical interventions. Being able to quantify health returns in this fashion may bring more investors to the table to make community improvements.

SUMMARY

Monitoring the effects of upstream determinants on health seems at first blush a straightforward task. But there are significant challenges that

---

9   *Disease Control Priorities in Developing Countries. 2nd edition.* D.T. Jamison, J.G. Breman, A.R. Measham, et al., editors. (Washington, DC: World Bank, 2006).

must be overcome. We have suggested five approaches to lessen these challenges, as summarized below.

Incorporate evaluation into project planning early on. Incorporating evaluation early on increases the likelihood of a useful evaluation, ma allow for more deliberate incorporation of health interventions, and could create opportunities for more elegant evaluation through smart project implementation.

Clearly define causes and hoped for effects. Then pick a practical and affordable evaluation design for measuring them. Clearly defining the intervention, hoped for effects, and if possible, a comparison group are key first steps. Randomized control trials are not the only option. Community developers have a co-conspirator in public health scientist who routinely conduct and evaluate similar kinds of interventions.

Prioritize measuring what comes first rather than focusing on long-ter outcomes. Logic models are excellent tools for identifying the paths from inputs and activities to short-, medium-, and long-term outcome. A logic model will help focus evaluation on measuring the first expect results so that program managers can know early whether they are on the right track. These "first results" with evidence-based links to longer-term health outcomes are among the most relevant to commun development projects.

Standardize, simplify, and innovate measurement methods and approaches. Using simple and standard measurement methods will accelerate progress for both the community development and health fields and will allow for more accurate comparison across projects. Using existing health data is one strategy, but it is hampered by limite information at the neighborhood level. Selecting common outcomes, more effective use of GIS and analytic methods that identify health outcomes at smaller geographic areas, and the potential use of electro health care records are all positive steps.

Maximize innovation through collaboration. The field is early in the process of figuring out how to effectively measure the social determinants of health, and inventing wheels is easier when you collaborate. A national clearinghouse of evidence would speed good intervention design and evaluations and assemble known links in logic models. Given the size of the investment this country is making in community development, identifying resources for sound evaluation must be a priority. Work is also needed to develop shared understanding of the concept of return on investment, including reporting on this return in not only dollars but also in health gains.

We are at the beginning of an interdisciplinary collaboration that has the potential to increase the effectiveness of both the community development and the health fields. Working together in smart ways will move us forward quickly, and signs of early successes could create momentum for greater investment in neighborhood-level improvements from new sources, such as health care payers, insurers, and hospital community benefit programs. As evidence (and our sophistication in obtaining it) grows, it should enable the goal of using measures of community features (such as grocery stores, bike paths and health clinics) to accurately predict and improve both health and economic outcomes.

■ ■ ■

DAVID FLEMING, *MD is health officer of Public Health—Seattle & King County, a large Metropolitan Health Department that serves 2 million residents. Dr. Fleming has also served as the director of global health strategies for the Bill and Melinda Gates Foundation, the deputy director of the Centers for Disease Control and Prevention, and the state epidemiologist for the Oregon Health Division. He has participated in multiple national and international boards and advisory committees, has published on a wide range of public health topics, and has faculty appointments at the University of Washington and the Oregon Health and Science University.*

■ ■ ■

HILARY KARASZ, *PhD has been with Public Health—Seattle & King County since 2001. She is currently a public information officer, where she works with the media, staff, community members and others to provide high quality health information to King County residents. She is also the director of a six-year CDC funded research project that examines the potential for mobile health applications such as text messaging to be used at the local public health department level. Hilary received a BA in History from the University of California and a doctorate in Communication from the University of Washington.*

■ ■ ■

KIRSTEN WYSEN, *MHSA, has worked at Public Health—Seattle & King County since 200.*
She is the initiative director of communities of opportunity, an early strategy of the
King County Health & Human Services Transformation Plan. Before that, she analyzed
Medicaid programs at the National Academy for State Health Policy in Portland, Maine.
In the 1990s, Kirsten served as the Deputy Program Manager for the Washington Basic
Health Plan and as a Policy Analyst at the state Health Services Commission and the
Medicare Payment Assessment Commission in Washington, DC. She graduated from
Brown University and the University of Michigan School of Public Health.

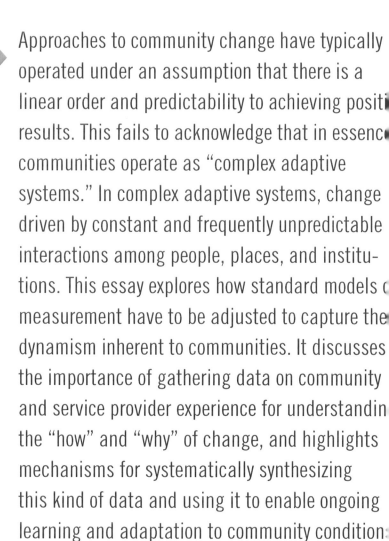

Approaches to community change have typically operated under an assumption that there is a linear order and predictability to achieving positive results. This fails to acknowledge that in essence communities operate as "complex adaptive systems." In complex adaptive systems, change driven by constant and frequently unpredictable interactions among people, places, and institutions. This essay explores how standard models of measurement have to be adjusted to capture the dynamism inherent to communities. It discusses the importance of gathering data on community and service provider experience for understanding the "how" and "why" of change, and highlights mechanisms for systematically synthesizing this kind of data and using it to enable ongoing learning and adaptation to community conditions.

USING DATA TO DRIVE CHANGE IN COMPLEX COMMUNITY SYSTEMS

Patricia Bowie and Moira Inkelas
University of California, Los Angeles

Many cross-sector and multidisciplinary efforts are underway, all aimed at achieving better outcomes for residents within a community, neighborhood, or other designated area. Whether known as collective impact, "Promise" or "Choice" neighborhoods, neighborhood revitalization, cradle to career, place-based, or comprehensive community initiatives, these efforts seek to improve outcomes not only for a specific group of individuals or families, but for the full population across the life course. Although this is a time of optimism for the newest attempts in this arena, it is also an important time for reflection. What works, what doesn't, and why?

A major challenge in answering these questions is that measuring change and impact is exceedingly difficult in cross-sector, geographic-focused initiatives. In large part, this is because we have not adjusted our practices to fully acknowledge that communities operate as "complex adaptive systems." In complex adaptive systems, linear relationships between cause and effect do not apply. Instead, change is driven by constant and, frequently, unpredictable interactions among all elements of the system. In communities, this plays out as intentional, or unintentional, interactions among a range of community stakeholders, including residents, those providing services and supports, and others who shape community resources from both inside and outside the community. The dynamism inherent to the interactions among all these players renders standard models of organizational practice and leadership, and in particular, measurement, incomplete.

Through our long-term involvement with the Magnolia Community Initiative, and more recently with other community initiatives striving to improve population outcomes, we have had the opportunity to rethink the approach to measuring change under conditions of complexity. In this essay, we illustrate a set of measurement principles and approaches that have helped service providers and community residents better understand and respond to the complexity inherent in community change.

BACKGROUND

The Magnolia Community Initiative is a voluntary network of 70 organizations and resident groups working in a five-square mile area near downtown Los Angeles. The network's vision is to help the 35,000 children within the 500-block area break all records of success in their education, health, and the quality of nurturing care and economic stability they receive from their families and community. Partners include multiple departments operated by the Los Angeles County Chief Executive Office, including social services, child support, and child protection. They also include regional organizations responsible for populations of children such as the Los Angeles County Unified School District; the Women, Infants, and Children (WIC) nutrition program; and child care resource and referral services. In addition are the private and nonprofit community-based organizations providing health care, early care and education including Head Start and Early Head Start, family support, and banking and economic development services and supports.

The Magnolia Community Initiative aims to connect these diverse groups, programs, and providers in a system of shared accountability, emphasizing sustainable and scalable data-driven practices. This involves creating a systemic approach to community change based in problem solving, learning, and discovery. Data are employed to help vast numbers of individuals—including residents, providers, and leaders—identify ways to change their behavior to collectively improve conditions and outcomes for a local population of children and families

CHANGE IN A COMPLEX SYSTEM

Approaches to community change have typically operated under an assumption that there is a linear order and predictability to achieving positive results. Standard strategic planning starts with defining the problem, deciding on a strategy or action plan, establishing a timeline with benchmarks to mark progress, implementing the interventions, and then confirming through measurement and evaluation that the intended results are achieved. The result is a blueprint of success that others can follow.

However, if we begin by acknowledging communities are complex adaptive systems, it is easy to see that the constant interplay of actors and actions produces outcomes that are impossible to fully predict, and that "success" may look different from what we imagined. In systems, change is constant, and there are too many moving parts to plan for every circumstance. As complex systems, communities are never permanently "fixed." Although programs can be planned and implemented, it is impossible to plan and specify all of the detailed actions necessary to produce a better community-wide or population outcome. As such, improving outcomes for a community goes beyond the "right" service strategy, resource, or planning process. Similarly, measuring progress and evaluating success in these endeavors must go beyond tracking the "right" set of high-level benchmarks or indicators.

Complexity expert Brenda Zimmerman offers a grounded way of thinking about the unique approaches required under conditions of complexity.[1] She uses the examples of baking a cake, sending a rocket to the moon, and raising a child to distinguish between simple, complicated, and complex conditions, respectively. For the first two, one can be reasonably assured that with the right level of knowledge and expertise, the results will be similar each time. However, with complex problems, like raising a child, having expertise or experience offers no certainty of success. Any parent knows that strategies used to raise one child may not apply to a second child. In complex tasks, we must continually seek information that helps gauge whether the theory

---

1 S. Glouberman and B. Zimmerman, "Complicated and Complex Systems: What would successful reform of Medicare look like?" Discussion paper No. 8. (*Commission on the Future of Health Care in Canada*, 2002).

undergirding actions is relevant to real-life conditions. If not, we must adapt our actions and seek alternative solutions.

DATA CAN PROVIDE A MORE COMPLETE PICTURE OF CHANGE

Gathering data on multiple levels across the system is critical for generating a more complete picture of what is happening and how the system is performing. To understand baseline conditions, the Magnolia Community Initiative developed a system map, which allowed the network partners to examine how the various actions of service providers, residents, and others were linked in affecting community results. In looking across the system and coming to a shared understanding of the interdependencies across players and chain-reactions among their actions, network partners could begin to see avenues for changing patterns in the system that would produce better results.

The Magnolia Initiative partners then instituted techniques to gather and display timely data and information about multiple components of the system. Our aim was to learn how the system was functioning in (nearly) real time to refine and continually improve actions. Timely data are critical to this approach and allow us to fine-tune changes at a much faster pace than what is typically possible from program evaluations or research.

Breadth and depth of data are no less important. Agencies typically collect and report on only their actions or outputs, for instance, counts of clients served. Yet, this level of data does not reflect what families or individual staff experience when receiving or providing services, and it sheds little light on why or how those services result in change (or do not result in change, as the case may be). Data that capture the experience of program users or participants can give providers a better sense of the true results of their efforts. This means getting more granular than looking at counts of services delivered at the front end and then tracking high level "outcomes" such as rates of obesity or high school graduation. It means instead that outcome data should be coupled with information about individual experience as well as family and community context, all of which affect how well the system can function to achieve better results.

Clients Asked About Family Stressors

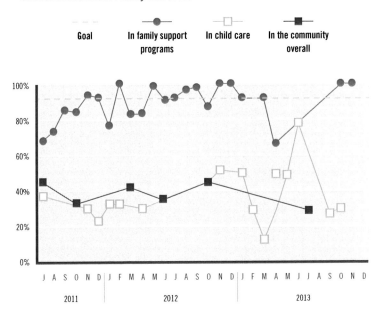

Figure 1a. The Dashboard monitors resident experiences and trends in the community overall and in particular Magnolia Initiative partner settings. This chart shows a sample of a Care Process measure, which assesses the extent to which organizations are carrying out the work that the Initiative partners believe will improve outcomes. Goals (dotted green line) are set at ambitious levels that are considered achievable. Data are self-report measures from monthly client surveys collected by organizations. The Dashboard also includes charts that monitor Health Routines, such as "Percent of Parents Reading Daily with their Child."

The Initiative uses a data dashboard to synthesize and make these multiple levels of data accessible for partners and others. The dashboard displays a range of items from day-to-day actions (e.g., rates of daily reading to children) to care processes (e.g., how frequently service providers ask clients about family stressors) to the family conditions that ultimately drive outcomes (e.g., family stability, food security, access to needed care and supports).The dashboard serves as the data visualization for our theory of change and functions as a tool to coordinate efforts and foster shared learning and joint accountability for results. It displays the various measures chosen by the partners to reflect their agreed upon actions and the intended short-term impacts (see Figures 1a and 1b). Short-term impacts serve as indicators for the longer-term changes, and ultimately these long-term changes are positi indicators that the efforts are leading to community-wide change.

The Magnolia dashboard differs from many others by having real-time and regular measurement, much the same way that the dashboard of a vehicle displays both current speed, indicating how the driver is doing at the moment, as well as miles accrued, indicating cumulative progres We find the dashboard holds promise as a tool to align leaders and organizations around collective action and long-term results.

DATA CAN PROMOTE LEARNING AND CHANGE

In determining the scope of information needed to support community change, the Magnolia Initiative partners began by adopting a set of measures that tells the story as they imagined it would unfold based o the network's theory of change. That theory holds that the outcomes for a population of children and families depend on the day-to-day actions of individuals and organizations supporting families and other neighborhood residents. Progressive changes in these actions contribut to shifts in family and neighborhood conditions as well as changes in individual health and parenting behaviors. Taken together, all of these small shifts build toward the longer-term improved outcomes for children. As such, the partners have constructed a measurement system th aims to concurrently capture information about each of these elements The measures are clustered in the following categories, indicating whic aspect of the system they shed light on:

- Actions of individuals or organizations to support positive behavior change. Examples of these types of measures include whether providers or staff asked residents about their well-being, concerns about their family, and whether they were guided to local resources to address their concerns. Another measure asks whether service providers and staff were able to respond to needs expressed by residents or clients using their own resources or by linking to other local organizations.

Parents of Children 0–5 With Protective Factors

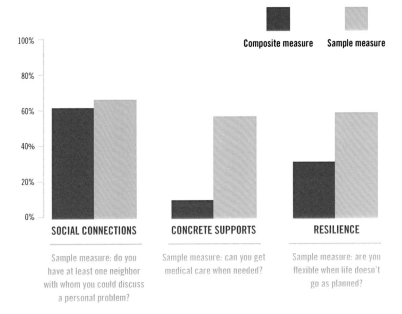

Figure 1b. The Dashboard also displays results of a biannual survey of community residents that assesses protective factors: social connections, concrete supports in times of need, and individual resilience. The chart shows composite measures in blue, representing the percent of respondents affirming all measures in a given category. The light green represents the percent of respondents affirming the noted sample measure from each category.

- Conditions of families and neighborhoods that enable people to sustain health-promoting behaviors. Examples include residents reporting that they have social connections with other residents or social support for personal needs or problems, sufficient food, feelings of safety in the neighborhood, safe places for children to play, enough money to prevent frequent moves, and positive role models for parenting.

- Individual behaviors that contribute to positive health and economic outcomes. This includes asking residents about behaviors that promote health, such as physical exercise and healthy eating, in addition to daily habits such reading books to young children and other parenting routines that are associated with children's learning and development. Residents are also asked about the extent to which they have regular contact with family and friends and know their neighbors.

- Outcomes or results the system is producing. Examples of these measures include the social and emotional well-being of children as they start school, the percentage of local children who are proficient in reading in third grade, the percentage of children in middle school reporting that they have positive relationships with peers and adults the rates of children graduating from high school, and rates of child abuse or neglect.

The Initiative partners have also included other measures such as "reach" to understand the extent to which the target population is linked into the network or system, and therefore experiencing the improvements. For example, if several health clinics improve their services, but together serve only 20 percent of the local population, that helps explain why changes might only be seen for a subset of the community.

Data that only helps to identify a problem is not adequate. The data must also help fill in the details of the possible pathways for addressing the problem. Without the latter, organizations find it difficult to use the data when designing system-level improvements. For example, test scores can show that students are not reading at grade level. Although group might have additional information about the extent to which th children are receiving tutoring and test-day breakfasts at school, other influences—such as study habits, family stability, and parent interest in their child's academic success—can be even more important to both the near-term (test results) and long-term (high school graduation) outcomes. Without data on those facets of student life, it's impossible gauge opportunities for improvement. If, in drawing boundaries arou our problem set, we fail to consider the potential causes of a situation and lack information that allows us to test our assumptions, we can miss critical intervention opportunities.

DATA NEEDS VARY ACROSS THE SYSTEM

We've learned through our experiences that the different data needs of different types of actors in a system must all be taken into account in designing a measurement approach. Leaders in a system require a set of measures that indicate whether and how the day-to-day operations are achieving a larger impact—e.g., headline statistics such as third grade reading scores or rates of low birth weight births. But doctors, social workers, classroom teachers, and parents need other kinds of data to guide actions within their sphere of influence. They need the data that help them achieve the specific day-to-day actions for which they are responsible, and that contribute to these long-term results along with the actions of many others. By providing the various stakeholders information that is relevant to their particular roles, everyone receives the information they need to take actions within their realm of responsibility or influence. Putting the measures together in a dashboard allows everyone to see if everyone's collective actions are resulting in meaningful change. Consider the different data needs for the following stakeholders:

- Policymakers, system leaders, and public agency leaders have the responsibility for systemwide outcome measures and results. This refers to numeric targets (e.g., 90 percent of children enter kindergarten ready to learn) for what success would look like. Beyond policymakers and system leaders, community members and stakeholders can also use these outcome measures as motivation for their own actions. This may involve advocating for improved neighborhood and larger community conditions.

- Organization and program leaders focus on operations and strategy for their particular organization, and need information about whether actions and practices among staff are contributing to the intended goals and aims of the organization. For example, a strategy might call for empowering clients to take charge of their health. Survey questions that ask clients if service providers paid close attention to what they were saying and let them tell their story without interruption help identify whether service providers are providing care in a manner that helps clients have a voice in the process. If not, it is the responsibility of managers or program directors to design training or coaching strategies for staff so that the system is delivering on actions that are consistent with an overall strategy.

- **Frontline providers** (such as doctors, social workers, teachers, and intake workers) need access to regular and timely data that offer feedback about the care they provide. They often need this information daily, weekly, monthly, or soon after the service date so they can easily see if their actions are leading to an improvement. The data that are gathered monthly and quarterly inform day-to-day actions that support improvements in practice. Frontline staff gather and receive timely and consistent feedback through surveys that ask clients about their experiences with the care received. For example, one of the goals of Magnolia is to routinely identify and respond to family stressors. Clients are asked during all encounters with providers and staff if anyone asked them about any changes or stressors in their home, and whether they received information about other programs that could be helpful. Reports are then shared with providers and staff to show that, when repeated, these measures can detect whether intentional changes in practice are producing the desired result. If not, the data can point to areas ripe for adjustments that might produce a better result, such as staff using a checklist as a reminder or prompt to take certain actions. Although this type of report and data display has rarely been available to frontline providers or managers, we have found that it is a powerful motivator to improve practice. Although the social sector has just begun to use these types of methods, there are numerous examples in the business and health sectors of employing real-time data to improve practice. Ironically, frontline providers often spend considerable time gathering and entering data, and yet they often do not receive it back in a meaningful time frame, or at all.

HOW COMMUNITY MEMBERS CAN USE DATA

Community members use data differently depending on their focus. Measures may be relevant to them in their capacities as neighborhood residents; as participants in services; as clients working in partnership with organizations; as parents striving to create safe, nurturing and development-promoting home environments for their child; or all of these.

In their capacities as neighborhood residents, community members have found it helpful to know the actual counts of children in their neighborhood who are "on track" in health, development, and learning. Knowing this generates engagement and concern among residents. However, to identify which steps to take to change conditions, residents also need information about the factors that shape children's developmental progress. The Magnolia Community Initiative uses a holistic measure of child health and well-being—the Early Development Instrument (EDI). The EDI is a measure of children's development at age 5 based on a checklist completed by kindergarten teachers. The EDI consists of more than 100 questions measuring the following five developmental areas: (1) physical health and well-being, (2) social competence, (3) emotional maturity, (4) language and cognitive skills, (5) and communication skills and general knowledge. These areas correlate closely with nationally accepted measures of school readiness.

EDI results and other measures of family well-being in neighborhoods are geocoded and mapped to the local neighborhoods using boundaries defined by local residents. Examples of these measures fall in the realm of social cohesion (e.g., are people willing to help their neighbors?) and informal social control (e.g., would neighbors do something if children are hanging out on the street? Do the parents on a neighborhood block know one other?).

Mapping and publicizing these measures help galvanize direct actions that can alter family and neighborhood life because the data can help neighborhood residents organize around broadly shared concerns and perceptions. The information also allows residents to see how their neighborhood compares with others in terms of the well-being of children and adults. Some have used the information to advocate for changes or new resources in their neighborhoods. For instance, community members have used information to inspire others to participate in Neighborhood Watch. Others have been inspired by data to change their personal behavior, such as exercising more or reading together with their child. It is important to support community members with the right information tailored to their purpose. The type of information that motivates one to advocate for resources or safety should not be assumed to be the same type that is needed to help parents change their personal behaviors at home. Motivation to advocate can come from neighborhood-level measures of well-being, whereas motivation to change one's own personal actions requires measures of individual daily activities and their impact.

In their capacities as parents striving to create positive home environments for their children, parents have benefited directly from information on whether they are meeting their own specific goals. For example, child care providers and others can track how often parents are able to read books with their young child, and then can help parents with goal setting and tracking progress. This is a similar process that organizations follow in trying to effect a change. While the measurement process and the display of data can be tailored to the specific user, the concept of individuals having regular information about their goals and progress toward those goals is as relevant to a parent as it is to an organization.

ACHIEVING SCALE AND SUSTAINABILITY

This kind of a data system can only work when it is *scalable* and *sustainable*, such that all network partners who need to be involved to achieve a system-level, community-wide change can actually adopt measurement as part of their routine practice. This means ensuring that the data system is affordable, contains measures that are relevant across organizations and sectors, and is not burdensome in the time and resources required for regular data collection. In addition, the number of measures being tracked must be limited so as not to overwhelm use.

There are well-recognized features that can serve as guiding principles for selecting useful measures to drive change for programs and systems as well as for community systems that are striving for a population impact. Valid measures represent the intended concept. Reliable measures dependably gauge the intended concept over time. Measures should be sensitive to change so it is possible to know whether actions taken to improve a process or experience are producing better results.

In deciding which measures to collect, we have also found that it is important to consider what measures will motivate people to focus on collective action. Individuals and organizations need to see how their contributions contribute to the shared goal. This helps move from an individual or client perspective to a collective responsibility for population outcomes.

It is also essential to consider *scale* when the intention is to have an impact on a geographic population of children and families. Working at scale means that the data collection needs to be feasible for all involved organizations, under all conditions. Some data collection systems that track information about children and families are proprietary and costly to organizations. Data systems that are costly to maintain, or difficult for organizations to use, are unlikely to be adopted by the number of organizations required to achieve a population change. Also, data systems adopted for a specific, time-limited project or a specific sector that are not designed with other goals and sectors in mind are unlikely to meet the needs of long-term, community-wide change processes.

The key is to have measurement become a routine part of practice and regularly reviewed to inform decision making, assess progress, and support improvement over time. To that end, the measurement system must be designed for the long term. It is important to sustain the measurement long enough to see the learning, testing, and implementation take effect.

Measurement that takes too much time to collect and that is not built into the regular process of caring for clients or one's daily routine, or is simply overwhelming for leaders and practitioners to track, is unlikely to be sustained as a permanent part of a community system. At the end of the day, all measures come at a real cost, so it is essential to choose measures carefully. Although almost counterintuitive in today's era of "big data," selecting a modest, balanced number of measures (10–15) is much more effective than larger sets.[2]

CORE PRINCIPLES FOR USING DATA IN COMPLEX SYSTEMS

By introducing a disciplined approach to learning, organizations can move quickly from an idea for change to testing and implementing that change. In this way, the network "acts" rather than "plans" its way

---

2 G. Langley et al., *The Improvement Guide: A Practical Approach to Enhancing Organizational Performance* (San Francisco, CA: Jossey-Bass, 2009).

into a new system.[3] A systemic approach to learning equips partners to adopt new practice and policy as it emerges. It enables organizations t translate cutting-edge ideas into care processes that work across many people and organizations, even those in the most challenged settings. A critical part of this process involves attending to human reaction to change. Introducing measurement without attending to personal aspec of what helps people change their actions and behavior is enough to limit the impact of even the most robust theories and approaches. It's a old saying that while everyone wants progress, nobody likes change! A such, we have found that more meaningful and lasting change can occ when path-breaking ideas are introduced in conjunction with coaching on ways to take action.

The purpose of measurement is understanding and reflection, plus change. To that end:

- Select a set of measures that reflect your theory of change from actic to results, being mindful not to overwhelm those you hope will participate by adopting too many measures.

- Design a measurement system for scale so that all the community members, community-based organizations, and decision makers who are important for the outcomes will receive the information they need to take the appropriate actions at their level. This also means attending to cost considerations to develop, maintain, and partici- pate in a data collection system, as well as considering open versus proprietary information systems.

- Design for sustainability so that the data support an enduring change process. Designing measurement support for a two-to three- year process may inform some change, but it is unlikely to deliver community-wide change or provide families with a supportive environment for a long enough time to improve their conditions, actions, and well-being.

---

3   A.S. Bryk, L.M. Gomez, and A. Grunow, "Getting Ideas into Action: Building Networked Improvement Communities in Education." *In Frontiers in Sociology of Education*, edited by M. Hallinan (New York: Springer, 2011).

- Consider all the different roles that community members play when providing or helping gather and use information. They are a critical voice in showing how a system is performing and in creating the demand for change. Recognize that information for one purpose may not be helpful for other purposes, with the understanding that not all community members will play all possible roles.

- Avoid giving people (actors, stakeholders) measures without a change process that helps them to take actions in their sphere of influence. It is also essential to shift to providing timely, monthly progress on process of care measures overall and by service sector to provide diverse programs and providers both shared accountability and a common change process. Understanding variation within an organization, or across a system, is a cornerstone of effective improvement.

- Offer coaching and other support to make a change. Remember that having information alone is insufficient to drive change in professional practice, in resident actions, or in personal behaviors.

- Be ready to change both measures and strategies if they appear not to be as informative, effective, or change-inducing as predicted.

OPPORTUNITIES GOING FORWARD

A key design imperative is to collect data in a way that meets the needs of the user, which in a change effort is the entity or actor responsible for the targeted change. We know from our experience in supporting population change efforts, such as the Magnolia Community Initiative, that program directors, evaluators, and leaders of community change efforts are better able to support change when they use methods of data collection, display, and analysis that are designed for dynamic systems. Fortunately, the cost and ability to gather data are shifting enormously, creating opportunities to use data and measurement in new ways.

We have seen a growing appreciation that small data samples repeated more often are not only more feasible than conventional evaluation methods but also more powerful for real-time learning and knowledge. As the value of process improvement becomes more evident to stakeholders, comfort with using time series and real-time data to support frontline providers will increase. A greater appreciation of the value c these methods can provide an important opportunity to equip all actc with data they need for action and for gauging change over time.

There is also great value in collecting and sharing resident and client voice in a productive way, for reflection and action at all levels of the system. For residents and practitioners in community serving organiza tions, measures of neighborhood conditions can be much more moti vating and useful than regional, city, or countywide measures, so ther is a need to help residents and others secure these data. For neighbor hood change, it is imperative to help residents identify and use measu and data collection processes that align with their needs and that are affordable and sustainable for the period of time they will need them.

Lastly, while it is often stated that "what gets measured gets done," it also common knowledge that "you can't fatten a cow by weighing it." Data alone are insufficient for driving significant change, particularly in complex community systems. Rather, more attention needs to be placed on creating learning environments. This means that in additio to support for data collection, there must also be support for efforts to make meaning of the data, make a prediction, and learn our way forward. Many fields offer examples of collaborative and iterative learning methods that can accelerate innovation and improvement.[4] What these efforts have in common is a successful transition from usi data for generating information to using data for reflection and chang

■ ■ ■

PATRICIA BOWIE *has over 20 years of experience developing community based initiati aimed at improving the well-being of children. She is currently working with the UCLA Center for Healthier Children, Families and Communities as part of the Transforming Early Childhood Comprehensive Systems (TECCS) team. One of her long term endeavor has been contributing to the design and implementation of the Los Angeles-based Magnolia Community Initiative. Also in partnership with UCLA, Ms. Bowie coordinates a national cross-site learning community supported by The Doris Duke Charitable*

---

4   Ibid. Also see C.M. Lannon and L.E Peterson. "Pediatric Collaborative Networks for Quality Improvement and Research," *Academic Pediatrics* 13(6 Suppl)(2013):S69-74; A. Billett et al. "Exemplar Pediatric Collaborative Improvement Networks: Achieving Results." *Pediatrics* 131(Su 4)(2013):S196-203.

Foundation. This community of learners—which includes the Magnolia Community Initiative and groups in Binghamton and Brooklyn NY, Boston MA, Hartford CT, Milwaukee WI, San Antonio TX, Sarasota FL, and Tulsa OK—is dedicated to improving population outcomes within a specific geography.

■ ■ ■

MOIRA INKELAS, *PhD, MPH is associate professor in the Department of Health Policy and Management, UCLA Fielding School of Public Health, and assistant director of the UCLA Center for Healthier Children, Families and Communities. Her research and policy studies examine how systems of care influence quality and performance of children's health services and supports. She has directed innovation and improvement collaboratives with networks of health care providers to improve child and family outcomes. She has also designed measurement and change processes to support cross-sector efforts involving health, education, child care, social services and others to achieve population health goals for children and families.*

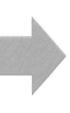

Impact investors use targeted investments to create market-based positive social and environmental change. Investing is a blunt instrument, however, and regularly creates both positive and negative impact. Getting impact investing right requires access to comprehensive impact metrics like Impact Reporting and Investment Standards (IRIS) and sophisticated ratings and analytical tools like the Global Impact Investing Ratings System (GIIRS), B Impact Assessments, B Analytics, and B Corporation certification. This essay explores these data-driven tools and speculates on how they may evolve to support a new class of impact investments known as Pay for Success.

THE ROLE OF DATA AND MEASUREMENT IN IMPACT INVESTING: HOW DO YOU KNOW IF YOU'RE MAKING A DIFFERENCE?

Ian Galloway
Federal Reserve Bank of San Francisco[1]

At best, data help us predict the future and understand the past. At worst, they mislead us and obscure the truth. Investors—in the business of predicting the future—know this better than most. Data are the coin of the investing realm: economic data; industry data; company performance data; and now, increasingly, social and environmental data—information that some investors use to gauge the impact of their investments. These "impact investors" are using these data to invest "into companies, organizations, and funds with the intention to generate measurable social and environmental impact alongside a financial return," according to the industry trade organization Global Impact Investing Network (GIIN).[2] These investors may target a particular sector like Fair Trade agriculture, for example, or companies with explicit social or environmental missions such as those committed to sustainable supply chains (Ben & Jerry's), hire disadvantaged employees (Goodwill Industries), or dedicate business revenue to a social cause

---

1 The views expressed in this essay belong to the author and do not necessarily represent the views of the Federal Reserve Bank of San Francisco or the Federal Reserve System.

2 Global Impact Investing Network. Impact Investing Resources: What is Impact Investing? Available at http://www.thegiin.org/cgi-bin/iowa/resources/about/index.html.

(Ethos Water).[3] These investments all have an expected financial return (or at least an expected return of principal) and, crucially, measurable impact.[4]

CHALLENGE: INVESTING IS A BLUNT INSTRUMENT

At root, impact investors are motivated by the belief that the market can be both a source of economic growth and a force for good. The challenge they face, however, is that this pathway to impact is indirect; investing in companies (or funds, which invest in companies) is uncertain to lead to impact, much as investing in a promising company is uncertain to lead to profit. In truth, an impact investment may not create the desired impact given any number of changing or conflicting business and market conditions beyond an investor's control.

Consider an investment in Walmart. The largest retailer in the world, Walmart may seem like an unlikely place to look for impact. But the data tell a different story. According to the Solar Energy Industries Association, Walmart is a global leader in solar energy production. For years, the company has been installing solar panels on store roofs generating two times more renewable energy than its closest commercial solar power competitor, Kohl's. To put this in context, Walmart's solar power generation is more than 35 states and the District of Columbia *combined*. And Walmart is just getting started: the company plans to double its solar panel installations by 2020.[5] On this basis, an investment in Walmart would seem to be spectacularly impactful.

But this underscores the difficulty of using impact investments to affect social or environmental change. It quickly becomes messy. An

---

3 Ben & Jerry's current social mission statement, which includes a commitment to sustainable supply chain management, is available at http://www.benjerry.com/values. Goodwill Industries is committed to "addressing poverty and unemployment for people with disabilities and other challenges to finding jobs." More information about Goodwill's social mission is available at http://www.goodwill.org/global/. Ethos Water, now owned by Starbucks, was created to help raise awareness about water scarcity and increase access to clean water. Every bottle of Ethos Water that is sold contributes $0. to the Ethos Water Fund, totaling more than $7.38 million. More information on Ethos Water is available at http://www.starbucks.com/responsibility/community/ethos-water-fund.

4 Global Impact Investing Network. Impact Investing Resources: What is Impact Investing? Available at http://www.thegiin.org/cgi-bin/iowa/resources/about/index.html.

5 Solar Energies Industries Association. "Solar Means Business 2014: Top US Commercial Solar Users," available at http://www.seia.org/sites/default/files/resources/17ay15uqAzSMB2014_1.pdf.

investment in Walmart, for example, creates two extreme impacts: a decrease in carbon emissions and, potentially, an increase in low-wage jobs (a negative impact many investors with social impact preferences would have a hard time accepting).[6] And Walmart is by no means alone. Many companies create both good and bad impact, even those committed to sustainability and corporate social responsibility.[7]

IMPACT DATA AND ANALYTICS ARE KEY

The complexity and unpredictability of the market require investors to arm themselves with sophisticated impact data and analytical tools to help guide their decision-making and maximize the chances that positive impact will flow from a targeted impact investment. While there are a number of public and proprietary systems that measure impact, the gold standard in impact metrics is IRIS.[8] Conceived by a group of impact investors convened by the Rockefeller Foundation in 2008 and now maintained by GIIN, IRIS was created to serve as a free centralized repository of generally accepted impact metrics.[9]

IRIS also serves as a cross-sector glossary of common impact terms and definitions to encourage the standardization of language across the impact investing field so that investors, companies, fund managers, grantmakers, government, and nonprofits can better communicate their activities and impact preferences.[10] The U.S. Small Business Administration (SBA), for example, recently announced that all fund managers applying to the SBA's Small Business Investment Company

---

6   C. Fishman. *The Wal-Mart Effect: How an Out-of-Town Superstore Became a Superpower.* (Penguin Press: 2006).

7   Clara Barby and Mads Pedersen. "Allocating for Impact: Subject Paper of the Asset Allocation Working Group." Social Impact Investment Taskforce: September 2014, available at http://www.socialimpactinvestment.org/reports/Asset%20Allocation%20WG%20paper%20FINAL.pdf.

8   Impact Reporting and Investment Standards (IRIS).

9   IRIS: History, available at http://iris.thegiin.org/about/history.

10 These metrics span: 1) financial performance; 2) operational performance; 3) product performance; 4) sector performance; 5) and social and environmental objective performance. More information on IRIS metrics is available at http://iris.thegiin.org/guides/getting-started-guide.

(SBIC) Impact Investment Fund "must commit to measure their social environmental or economic impact" using IRIS-compatible metrics.[11]

IRIS is also designed to feed a number of impact investor tools. The Global Impact Investing Ratings System (GIIRS), for example, turns company and fund-specific positive social and environmental information into impact ratings for investors. These ratings are intended to make the process—usually very labor-intensive—of identifying and comparing investments based on their impact potential, easier.[12]

Another investor tool, B Analytics, is a customizable platform used by impact investors to measure, benchmark, and report on their impact. The platform, maintained by the nonprofit B Lab, includes searchable impact information on over 1,600 companies and 90 investment fund Investors use B Analytics to evaluate their investments against a custo ized set of IRIS metrics and metrics of their own choosing.[13]

A third tool, the B Impact Assessment, evaluates the social and environmental impact of small- and medium-sized businesses. It includes 60-200 IRIS-compatible questions on company leadership, employees, consumers, community, and the environment.[14] Companies that score minimum of 80 out of 200 possible points on the B Impact Assessmen are eligible to become certified B Corporations.[15] Like a GIIRS rating, B Corporation certification acts as an industry stamp of approval signaling to the company's investors, customers, and stakeholders that it is committed to positive social and environmental impact. Over 5,00 companies have completed the B Impact Assessment and 900 of them have become B Corporations. Impact data from B Impact Assessments and B Corporations are compiled for investors on the B Analytics

---

11 U.S. Small Business Administration. "SBIC Program's Impact Investment Fund Policy Update." September 25, 2014, available at http://www.sba.gov/sites/default/files/articles/SBA%20Impact%2 Investment%20Fund%20Policy%20-%20September%202014_1.pdf.

12 About GIIRS: How GIIRS Works. Available at http://giirs.org/about-giirs/how-giirs-works.

13 B Analytics: About Us. Available at http://b-analytics.net/about-us.

14 The Foundation Center. Tools and Resources for Assessing Social Impact: The B Impact Rating System. Available at http://trasi.foundationcenter.org/record.php?SN=29.

15 Ibid.

platform to allow for industry-wide impact benchmarking and market trend spotting.[16]

CASE STUDY OF AN INVESTOR: KL FELICITAS FOUNDATION

The KL Felicitas Foundation was created in 2000 to support global social entrepreneurship, particularly in rural areas. The foundation invests a significant percentage of its corpus in impact investments—55 percent in 2009, well beyond the 5 percent grant or program-related investment minimum required to maintain their nonprofit tax status. Historically, the foundation measured its impact largely by counting the number of people served by its investments. This proved inadequate to the foundation's founders—Charly and Lisa Kleissner, however, who asked for a baseline against which to compare the foundation's impact.

To that end, the foundation adopted five IRIS metrics in 2009—two social, three financial—as common core impact indicators to measure the impact of its impact investment portfolio. In 2011, the foundation added five more sector-specific IRIS metrics related to health, energy, water, land conservation, and restoration. These ten metrics were further enhanced by six proprietary qualitative metrics developed by the foundation to capture anecdotal data related to company innovativeness and scalability.

Combined, these sixteen impact metrics are used to evaluate and compare the impact performance of the foundation's impact investments and to "deepen the foundation's understanding of whether, how, and why its investments helped social enterprises gain scale and increase their respective social impact." The foundation intends to integrate the metrics into its traditional due diligence process to ensure that in the future, 100 percent of the foundation's corpus aligns with its mission.[17]

---

16 B Impact Assessment: Case Studies. Available at http://bimpactassessment.net/case-studies; and B Analytics: Follow Market Trends. Available at http://b-analytics.net/products/market-trends.

17 Global Impact Investing Network. KL Felicitas Foundation: Case Study. IRIS Case Study Series. April 18, 2011, available at http://www.thegiin.org/binary-data/RESOURCE/download_file/000/000/226-1.pdf.

CASE STUDY OF AN INVESTEE: ETSY

Etsy is the largest online handmade craft marketplace in the world wit over 40 million members and $1.35 billion in total sales.[18] In an effort to more fully integrate impact in the company's core mission, Etsy completed a B Impact Assessment to become a certified B Corporation Initially, the company scored just above the minimum certification level. The process, however, was a worthwhile one, revealing several impact areas in which the company excelled—such as composting and community engagement—and several opportunities for it to increase i potential impact in the future.[19]

Committed to boosting its initial score, the company organized a "Hack Day" for employees to brainstorm ways to improve its impact on the community and the environment. Several ideas from the brainstorm session became official company policy, including "an updated volunteer leave policy and program, carbon footprint tracking, Etsy School (admin-taught internal school), IdeaCraft (an internal speaker series), living plant walls, and female-driven learning and development workshops."[20] These ideas and others implemented by Etsy increased the company's B Impact Assessment score by over 2. percent in one year.[21]

Etsy considers these efforts to be consistent with its core social and environmental values. They also make the company more attractive to impact investors. Etsy's B Corporation certification allows investors to more easily evaluate the company's impact potential and the additiona impact data now regularly collected by Etsy as a result of its B Impact Assessment make it easier for investors to monitor Etsy's impact on an on-going basis.

IRIS metrics and the analytical tools they support are state of the art. Many social enterprises, such as Etsy, depend on them to track and

---

18 Certified B Corporations: Etsy Case Study. Available at http://www.bcorporation.net/community/et

19 Interview with Jennifer McKaig, Social Impact Lead at Etsy. B Impact Assessment Case Study: Etsy Available at http://bimpactassessment.net/case-studies/jennifer-mckaig.

20 Ibid.

21 B Impact Assessment. Etsy Improvement Report. Available at http://bimpactassessment.net/ etsy-improvement-report.

communicate their impact to investors and other stakeholders. That said, companies don't operate in a vacuum; they are subject to global forces outside of their control. Even a data-driven impact investment may not be sufficient to keep a company on track for impact. This is the downside to harnessing the market to affect change: it can be difficult to predict the outcome. But what if impact investors could be more surgical in their search for impact? What if, instead of gently nudging the market towards sustainability with targeted investments, investors could invest directly in impact itself? That is the tantalizing promise of a new class of impact investments called "Pay for Success."

A NEW WAY TO INVEST IN IMPACT: PAY FOR SUCCESS

Pay for Success (PFS), also known as Social Impact Bonds, allows investors to invest in organizations that directly "manufacture" impact.[22] These organizations can be nonprofits, social enterprises, or for-profits but their distinguishing characteristic is that they produce a defined impact and are able to sell it into the PFS marketplace (usually to government but potentially to any organization that is willing to buy it). Like any other company that produces and sells a product, these organizations are able to borrow money based on how much of their product—impact, in this case—they are likely to sell and at what price. That is the investable opportunity created by PFS.

Consider the Salt Lake County PFS project, for example. In an effort to increase school readiness among low-income kindergarteners, Salt Lake County and the United Way of Salt Lake offered to pay $2,470 plus 5 percent annual interest, per student, for every year of remedial special education avoided through sixth grade as a result of high-quality

---

22 There are currently five PFS projects underway in the United States: in New York City, Salt Lake County, New York State, Massachusetts, and Chicago. Each of these projects is designed to produce a predetermined impact ranging from reduced prison recidivism to improved kindergarten readiness for low-income students. Each raised upfront investment from impact investors to pay for a program designed to create the pre-negotiated impact. Depending on how effective a given program proves to be, its investors will receive, in most cases, mid-single digit returns with an opportunity for higher returns for higher levels of impact. More information on the current state of the PFS market is available at http://www.payforsuccess.org.

preschool.[23] On the basis of this future payment commitment (and a three-year study demonstrating an 85 percent track record of success) the Granite School District high-quality preschool program was able to raise $1.1 million in impact investment from Goldman Sachs Bank and the philanthropist J.B. Pritzker to provide 600 low-income three- and four-year olds high-quality preschool.[24] The investment will earn a return based on how effectively the Granite School District preschool program can increase school readiness among a subset of those students that were highly likely to need special education as a result of a skills deficit beginning before kindergarten.

But no investment is without risk, of course. If the Granite School District high-quality preschool program fails to increase school readiness as promised, Salt Lake County and the United Way of Salt Lake will not be obligated to "pay for success" and, as a result, there will be no revenue with which to repay Goldman Sachs and J.B. Pritzker. Impact, in this case, is the entirety of the investment and not just an ancillary benefit to be measured alongside financial returns.

In another PFS example, the state of Massachusetts is attempting to reduce recidivism among at-risk young men aging out of the juvenile justice system. To do this, the state procured the nonprofit Roca to provide a range of behavioral and employment services to young men recently released from prison and on probation.[25] The state, with the help of an $11.7 million grant from the U.S. Department of Labor, agreed to pay investors in Roca up to $27 million if Roca succeeds

---

23 This payment rate drops to $1,040 per student, per year, once the investors have recouped their principal investment. More information on the Salt Lake County PFS project is available at http:// www.goldmansachs.com/what-we-do/investing-and-lending/urban-investments/case-studies/impact-bond-slc-multimedia/fact-sheet-pdf.pdf; and John Williams. "Letting Investors Take a Shot at Cure Social Ills." *Wall Street Journal.* Opinion Section. September 24, 2014.

24 Low-income students in Salt Lake County without access to high-quality preschool require special education 33 percent of the time. When exposed to Granite School District's high-quality preschool that rate dropped to five percent. "In our opinion: Social impact bonds offer a way to get measurable results for social service investments." Deseret News Editorial. May 19, 2014, available at http:// www.deseretnews.com/article/865603339/Social-impact-bonds-offer-a-way-to-get-measurable-results-for-social-service-investments.html?pg=all.

25 Young at-risk men in Massachusetts typically reoffend 55 percent of the time within three years.

in measurably reducing recidivism and unemployment among a target population of at-risk young men.[26]

Roca, whose tagline is "Less Jail, More Future," has successfully served more than 20,000 high-risk 17-24 year olds since 1988. This year, 92 percent of Roca's program participants have avoided arrest and 80 percent have retained employment for at least 90 days.[27] Most important to Roca's investors, however, was a study by the Harvard Kennedy School Social Impact Bond Technical Assistance Lab (Harvard SIB Lab), which demonstrated a 33 percent reduction in recidivism rates among Roca program participants compared to the state average.[28] That rigorous evaluation, combined with Roca's historical impact data, was sufficient to convince Goldman Sachs, Kresge Foundation, and Living Cities to invest a total of $12 million in Roca, allowing it to serve 929 at-risk young men over a seven year period.[29]

But the Massachusetts and Salt Lake County PFS projects are unusual in a crucial way: the relative availability of robust project-specific impact data. Today, there are very few evidence-based interventions on par with Roca and the Granite School District preschool program or rigorous program evaluations like that administered by the Harvard SIB Lab. This may soon change, however, as impact investors' interest in PFS grows. Over time, metrics systems like IRIS may be more readily adapted for PFS use and certification tools like GIIRS and B Corporation may evolve to extend investor "stamps of approval" to organizations like the Granite School District and Roca.

LOOKING AHEAD

There are admittedly many potential data related challenges with PFS. For one, narrow definitions of impact can create potentially perverse incentives. If an investor can achieve impact by denying access to critical services—special education for eligible children, for example—in order to

---

26 The Massachusetts Juvenile Justice Pay for Success Initiative Fact Sheet, available at http://www.thirdsectorcap.org/wp-content/uploads/2014/01/MA-JJ-PFS-Frequently-Asked-Questions.pdf.

27 Roca. What We Do: Proven Outcomes. Available at http://rocainc.org/what-we-do/proven-outcomes/.

28 Massachusetts Fact Sheet.

29 Several foundations also contributed grants to support the Massachusetts PFS project and both Roca and the project intermediary, Third Sector Capital Partners, agreed to defer a portion of their fees conditional on impact.

increase their return on investment, it could do great harm to already vulnerable populations. For another, tying financial returns directly to impact raises the stakes for efforts to calculate and validate it. If PFS investments are going to enter the mainstream, the impact data collection and analysis process will need to be unimpeachable, which difficult even for trained evaluators.

But these challenges also illustrate the great opportunity created by P investing: accurately measuring impact is at its core. If impact is not created, the investment is lost. This elevates impact to a central role i the impact investment, not simply a side benefit, as can be the case w impact and financial returns are calculated separately. PFS projects al require a very high level of statistical rigor: experimental evaluation designs, such as Randomized Control Trials, are used often to prove impact, for example. And promisingly, as more PFS deals are done th impact-investing field will have access to increasingly high-quality da and analytics on social interventions.

PFS is by no means a panacea, nor should it represent the entirety of impact investing market.[30] Nevertheless, it allows for a direct approac to impact investing that will eventually serve as a useful complement to existing investor efforts to harness market forces for good. It will also create more demand for data and help foster a robust data infra-structure (as we now have in the traditional capital markets) that wil contribute greatly to our knowledge of what counts.

■ ■ ■

IAN GALLOWAY *is a senior community development research associate at the Federal Reserve Bank of San Francisco. Ian was a contributing editor of the 2012 book, Invest in What Works for America's Communities, and his article "Using Pay for Success to Increase Investment in the Nonmedical Determinants of Health" was published in the November 2014 issue of the health policy journal Health Affairs. Previously, Ian devel a social enterprise (virginiawoof.com) for the Portland, Oregon homeless youth agenc Outside In. He holds a master's degree in public policy from the University of Chicago a bachelor's degree in political science and philosophy from Colgate University.*

---

30 Daniel Stid. "Pay for Success is Not a Panacea." *Community Development Investment Review.* Volume 9, Issue 1 (2013), available at http://www.frbsf.org/community-development/files/pay-for-success-not-panacea.pdf.

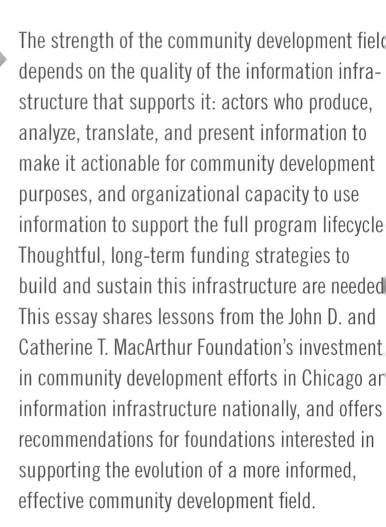

The strength of the community development field depends on the quality of the information infrastructure that supports it: actors who produce, analyze, translate, and present information to make it actionable for community development purposes, and organizational capacity to use information to support the full program lifecycle. Thoughtful, long-term funding strategies to build and sustain this infrastructure are needed. This essay shares lessons from the John D. and Catherine T. MacArthur Foundation's investment in community development efforts in Chicago and information infrastructure nationally, and offers recommendations for foundations interested in supporting the evolution of a more informed, effective community development field.

STRENGTHENING COMMUNITY DEVELOPMENT: A CALL FOR INVESTMENT IN INFORMATION INFRASTRUCTURE

Alaina J. Harkness[1]

John D. and Catherine T. MacArthur Foundation

In January 2014, the 50th anniversary of the War on Poverty sparked a round of animated debate about the impact of efforts to meet the basic needs of Americans and to support economic mobility.[2] As is often the case, the numbers support multiple, complicated narratives: The official poverty rate has decreased slightly, from 19 percent to 15 percent, but more than 46.5 million Americans were poor in 2012, more than any point in history.[3] Despite trillions of public and privately funded investments to combat poverty and all of its effects, it persists in the United States at levels that many consider intolerable for a country with such wealth and stature.

For everyone concerned with conditions in and around the metropolitan areas where the vast majority of poor people live, the stubborn correlations between place, race, and poverty are even more unsettling.[4] We want urban neighborhoods to be both anchor and springboard for their

---

1 While this article is informed by my experience working at the John D. and Catherine T. MacArthur Foundation, the views expressed are mine alone and do not represent the views of the institution, its Board or its grantees.

2 Zachary Karabell, "What America Won in the 'War on Poverty'," *The Atlantic*, January 12, 2014. http://www.theatlantic.com/business/archive/2014/01/what-america-won-in-the-war-on-poverty/283006/; "Does the U.S. Need Another War on Poverty?" *New York Times*, January 5, 2014. http://www.nytimes.com/roomfordebate/2014/01/05/does-the-us-need-another-war-on-poverty.

3 Urban Institute - http://www.urban.org/poverty/.

4 Patrick Sharkey, *Stuck in Place: Urban Neighborhoods and the End of Progress towards Racial Equality* (Chicago, Illinois, University of Chicago Press 2013); Richard Florida, "The Persistent Geography of Disadvantage," Citylab, July 25, 2013. http://www.theatlanticcities.com/neighborhoods/2013/07/persistent-geography-disadvantage/6231.

residents, but research has shown that chances of advancement, and even survival, are greatly diminished for residents of low-income place With more than five decades of community development policy and practice behind us, it is unsurprising that the field should be so preoc- cupied with the question of what works. For nonprofit organizations, foundations and other funders responding to the mounting evidence that poverty and place are connected, but under pressure to demonstr results from investments in periods even shorter than 50 years, finding better ways to measure progress at neighborhood scale is essential.

While the big-picture goal of community development—to build place that help their residents thrive—has remained remarkably stable over time, the strategies and tactics have evolved. Information has always been an essential factor of production in the community develop- ment field, as valuable a resource as money, time, and human capital. Information matters now more than ever, and it is increasingly likely t be the determining factor in the success of both people and organiza- tions. For individuals, access to information is a baseline need for successful participation in society, influencing every aspect of quality of life, from healthcare and housing to employment and education.[6] For organizations, access to information and the ability to use it determin their ability to craft and execute effective solutions, track progress, and advocate for support. To take advantage of the (ever increasing) abundance of information resources, organizations need to become more flexible, agile, and aware.

Understanding what is working in community development—and importantly, how it is working—requires a zoom lens: looking beyond headlines, statistics, and longitudinal studies to the organizations and individuals working in neighborhoods to address specific conditions on the ground. Long-term, large-scale research projects are important for helping us understand the big picture of community change, but

---

5   The Equality of Opportunity Project

6   Karen Mossberger's seminal research on digital connectivity—access, skills, and meaningful use—a connections to community development objectives has informed and grounded the MacArthur Foundation's ongoing investments in this arena. See for example: http://cpi.asu.edu/project/smart-communities John Horrigan has also helpfully pushed the connection between "digital readiness" economic participation. http://jbhorrigan.weebly.com/uploads/3/0/8/0/30809311/digital_readiness horrigan.june2014.pdf.

only fine-grained, closer-to-real-time information about context and program operations make it possible to adapt to changing conditions on the ground and make the corresponding adjustments to program design and strategy. The complexity of community development efforts creates special challenges for measurement and tracking progress, as has been noted elsewhere in this volume. However, this complexity only increases the importance of having reliable information to help set priorities, refine program strategies, and evaluate what works. There is ample room for improvement.

Many excellent resources address performance management and how to become a learning organization, so I won't cover that ground here. What I want to emphasize in this essay are two kinds of investments that are undervalued (and hence, with a few notable exceptions, underfunded) in the community development field:

1 Information infrastructure: the ecosystem of local, state, and national organizations and individuals who produce, analyze, translate, and present information to make it useful and actionable for specific community development purposes; and

2 Organizational capacity to use information to support the full program lifecycle, from planning and design through implementation and evaluation.

The call for more and better investments in organizations' capacity to access and use information is certainly not new, but it is one worth repeating and refining until all of us in the social sector absorb it fully into our theories of change and funding strategies. The sector-wide under-investment in data collection and performance management has been documented for at least a decade, but organizations still say it is nearly impossible to find funding to support these critical systems and functions.[7] Why? The reasons may have more to do with a failure of framing than a failure of the concept itself. As recently stated in an excellent compendium of writings on the use of information in the social sector from Markets for

---

7 Two seminal articles that discuss the importance of building capacity to use information in nonprofit work are (1) Ann Goggins Gregory and Don Howard, "The Nonprofit Starvation Cycle," *Stanford Social Innovation Review*, Fall 2009, http://www.ssireview.org/articles/entry/the_nonprofit_starvation_cycle and (2) John Kania and Mark Kramer, "Collective Impact," *Stanford Social Innovation Review*, Winter 2011, http://www.ssireview.org/articles/entry/collective_impact.

Good, the term *information infrastructure* doesn't exactly roll off the tongue.[8] This infrastructure is often invisible. There's no ribbon cutting or grin-and-grab when it's successfully built, and its failures aren't spectacular like a bridge collapse, or even a mundane annoyance, like potholed road. Donors don't aspire to have their names on databases. Yet the vitality of the social sector—in an age when data talks as much as money does—depends on significant, sustained, conscious investments in information infrastructure if we are to take advantage of the benefits that the explosion of information resources offers to advance the public good.

A simple call for more funding is insufficient. The community development field needs thoughtful, long-term funding strategies that pay attention to the whole universe of available (and unavailable) data to inform program strategies and the evolving array of options available to those seeking to build or buy capacity to use information more effectively. For too long, funders (public and philanthropic alike) have focused on trying to understand the measurable impact of their grant making without making commensurate investments in their grantees' own capacity to measure. In the turn to focus on outcomes, funders became too narrowly interested in the value of information to demonstrate what happened at the end of an investment. More attention should be paid to how organizations are using information to plan for and advance their work, and to the long-term challenge of building, maintaining, and evolving the tools and capacities that make information actionable.

The imperative for organizations to keep pace with these changes is clear: access to better information at lower cost, the ability to add new information about conditions on the ground to higher-level planning processes (the "little data" Susana Vasquez and Patrick Barry describe in their essay in this volume), and the potential to deploy other scarce resources more effectively to increase benefits to people and their communities. But the roadmap to becoming a more informed community development partner is not clear. It is a crowdsourced map, one that all of us in the field are building as we go.

---

8 Markets for Good is an initiative of the Bill & Melinda Gates Foundation and the financial firm Liquidnet to "improve the system for generating, sharing, and acting upon data and information in the social sector." http://www.marketsforgood.org/making-sense-of-data-and-information-in-the-social-sector/.

This remainder of this essay aims to contribute to the map-building project by sharing lessons from the John D. and Catherine T. MacArthur Foundation's investments in community development efforts in Chicago and in information infrastructure nationally. Then the discussion turns to observations about what foundations can do to support the evolution of a more informed community development field.

LEARNING FROM EXPERIENCE

The MacArthur Foundation has been supporting place-based community development initiatives in the United States for more than two decades. For the last decade, our community and economic development portfolio has been anchored by two large-scale community development efforts in Chicago: the New Communities Program, a comprehensive community planning and development initiative led by the Chicago office of the Local Initiatives Support Corporation (LISC Chicago), and the Plan for Transformation of Chicago's public housing.

The Foundation also has a long history of supporting information infrastructure for the social sector, both locally and nationally. The guiding assumption is that timely, accurate, and accessible information about the social and economic conditions of cities and regions is an invaluable resource that can lead to more effective programs and policies. This belief in the importance of building robust information ecosystems and capacity to use them has been shaped by investments in Chicago—in historically important players, such as Chapin Hall and the now-defunct Metro Chicago Information Center, and relative newcomers such as the Smart Chicago Collaborative—and in national partners and networks, including the Urban Institute's National Neighborhood Indicators Partnership, Harvard's Data Smart Cities initiative, the University of Pennsylvania's Actionable Intelligence for Social Policy network, among others.

Program evaluations of two of the Foundation's longest-term investments in Chicago—the New Communities Program, the multi-neighborhood comprehensive planning and development initiative, and Opportunity Chicago, the coordinated, multi-stakeholder workforce development initiative that resulted in more than 5,000 public housing residents placed in jobs in 5 years—yielded key insights that helped the

Foundation refine its theory of change over time.[9] Although of differe scale, scope, and intention, these two initiatives shared important features that are now becoming more common in community develop ment strategies using a "collective impact" framework that includes a focus on both people and places; a reliance on intermediaries to coor nate action among an array of partners; and a need to collect, analyz and communicate data from a wide variety of sources.

A principal finding of the interim evaluation of the New Communitie Program was that the initiative had built critical supporting infra-structure for community development work in Chicago: a network of strong organizations that collectively came to be known as "the platform." The publication of the now oft-cited article "Collective Impact"[10] advanced another framework to describe the infrastructure needs of the social sector: LISC Chicago and the lead agencies, as wel as the Partnership for New Communities, the funder collaborative th oversaw Opportunity Chicago, all acted as "backbone organizations" to undergird complex community change initiatives.

The publication of "Collective Impact" was timely because its frame-work included an element that was present in Opportunity Chicago b largely absent from the New Communities Program: a strong shared measurement system for the initiative as a whole. The formative evalu ation of Opportunity Chicago was starting to suggest that the progra design features most critical to Opportunity Chicago's successes were related to the way information was used to set an agenda, ensure alignment, and track progress. These same features were relevant to t New Communities Program model, but played out in different areas different ways and across the whole initiative. Where they were in pla for components of the New Communities Program agenda—to guide the Centers for Working Families and Elev8 programs, for example— they seemed to be working. But while LISC Chicago was establishing a field standard for high-quality process documentation and internal

---

9   See the 10-year report on the New Communities Program, "The Promise of Community Development," http://www.mdrc.org/publication/promise-comprehensive-community-developmen and the FSG case study of Opportunity Chicago http://www.fsg.org/Portals/0/Uploads/Document PDF/CI_Case_Study_Opportunity_Chicago.pdf.

10 Kania and Kramer, 2011.

measurement of their own investments in the platform, the Foundation assessment and external evaluations were not in full alignment or recognizing of the value of this interim outcome.

Reflecting on the successes and challenges of these programs, in the next phase of the New Communities Program, which LISC Chicago calls Testing the Model, LISC Chicago and the Foundation made several specific adjustments in response to these insights. We needed to pay more attention to the value of the process of building the network of organizations and people serving as "the platform." In addition, the funding strategy needed to include specific support for programs to use information to measure their progress more effectively. These included more support for LISC Chicago's internal capacity to build systems to use information more effectively and tactical, technical improvements in performance management systems. The Foundation also needed to help the entire network of organizations in the New Communities Program build the level of sophistication of data systems, technology, and organizational process that they needed to successfully perform all of the key functions of a strong community development network: organizing, planning, coordinating and implementing projects, and fundraising. But most importantly, we needed to ensure better alignment of language, expectations, and measurement processes for outcomes—whether intermediate process, outputs, or long-term community change.

In recalibrating the Foundation's work to follow through on these insights, several lessons have emerged that may be helpful to other funders and those working in partnership with them to improve their communities. They relate to various components of the information ecosystem and lifecycle: crafting useful and sensitive metrics to track progress, supporting organizations in learning to use data at all stages of a program, designing new information systems for community development, and identifying new partners to assist in the work.

Lesson #1: Organizations and funders alike benefit from aligning shared measures of progress that value both process and outcome measures.

What does progress in community development look like? What kind of change, at what scale, and over what time horizon, constitutes sufficient return on investment? These are questions that vex the social sector in general, but as has been noted elsewhere in this volume and by others expert in the evaluation of place-based community development initiatives, their complexity—not only the number of moving parts, people and organizations, but the interrelated nature of the issue being addressed—make them particularly challenging to measure. Establishing shared expectations of what progress looks like, how it will be measured, and at what scale and in what timeframe it will be achieved is critical to the sustained effort that it takes to make change neighborhoods.

At the outset of the New Communities Program, the Foundation made significant investments in collecting information and evaluating progress. In addition, LISC Chicago established a high bar for documenting its own process and tracking investments in capacity building. But what all of the stakeholders in the New Communities Program—the Foundation, LISC Chicago, its network of lead agencies, the members of the evaluation team—learned is that although we were collectively tracking and measuring many indicators of change, from housing value to crime rates to investment flows, they were not necessarily the right measures, or the sufficient measures to tell the full story. Furthermore, not all of the stakeholders were tracking the same things at the same time. Whereas the Foundation and the evaluation team were both oriented toward tracking changes in conditions at the neighborhood level, LISC Chicago and its partners in the New Communities Program were tracking both process measures and project-level metrics at a different scale—number of participants in Centers for Working Families receiving financial services, units of housing built.

Particularly in a complex initiative such as the New Communities Program, it is essential to have some common metrics, or standards of measurement, that are widely shared and understood among all participants and stakeholders. These metrics are distinct from the indicators of neighborhood change (e.g., income, housing quality, crime) that we expect will track progress and chart the trajectory and health of neighborhoods. These metrics, or "performance indicators," can track shorter-term goals and help keep all of the actors in a networked initiative, such as the New Communities Program, aligned toward common goals.

In designing new systems for collecting, analyzing, and communicating information, LISC Chicago and its partners wanted to understand a number of dimensions related to both process and outcomes. Although still in development, conversations to date suggest that a system to support complex community development work needs to accommodate:

- quantitative and qualitative measures of change;

- project-level data, both inputs (dollars in, resources on the task) and outputs (community gardens planted, murals painted, units of housing developed, people assisted);

- context-level data, information about neighborhood and individuals that is tracked, mapped, and analyzed in as close-to-real-time as is possible;

- Process or "platform" data, information about how social and organizational networks are growing, the added value of increased organization and connectivity.

Process measures are particularly important and are tied to the difficult task we all have of making the case for infrastructure investments. The lack of clear metrics and a more-than-descriptive framework to document the growth and development of the organizing, planning, and development infrastructure that LISC Chicago and its partners built meant that nobody could say for certain what it was, how it worked, what it was producing, or how it could be improved. But these platform or process outcomes *can* be measured, albeit not through observable facts about neighborhood conditions such as housing values or crime rates. Although few established measures exist for the short-term growth in "collective efficacy," "resilience," or "tensile strength," it is possible (and less difficult and costly than ever) to track the growth of social and organizational networks. To correct for this, we contracted with the evaluation firm MDRC to conduct a network study that aims to generate insights about the growth of networks and partners that LISC Chicago believes are critical to the platform building that makes community improvement efforts more effective.

Lesson #2: The network of diverse organizations involved in community change efforts often have different levels of existing capacity to use information and different infrastructure needs. All need to be met where they are; the challenge is finding ways to balance the competing demand for simplicity and precision, specificity and standardization.

In the New Communities Program, the spread and diversity of organizational capacity to execute many types of tasks is highly variable. Organizational capacity becomes its own kind of management program, and one of the principal reasons that an intermediary organization, such as LISC Chicago, is so critical for successful investment in collaborative initiatives, whether within neighborhoods or among them. When LISC Chicago conducted a scan of technical capacity in its partners, the degree to which each organization understood the needs for information in their day-to-day operations, could identify available data sources and tools for analysis and mapping, and could make an appropriate match between the need and the appropriate source or tool varied considerably. But LISC Chicago also discovered that among all of the groups there was a consistent desire to use information in more effective ways to drive their various activities.

The MacArthur Foundation's role was to fund the assessment of baseline conditions and capacity, and to meet the organizations wherever they were with flexible support to move forward in a shared direction. The Foundation then helped identify the right external, expert partners to assist with scoping information needs, identifying sources, and developing appropriate systems for ongoing tracking and analysis. The last step was the most difficult, and is still very much a work in progress. Identifying "data intermediaries" with the right blend of issue-specific expertise and ability to translate it effectively to this diverse array of community partners, working in tandem to develop and refine strong theories of change, and communicating effectively through project implementation continues to be a messy, iterative, unscientific process. But the value of such intermediaries—the cross-trained translators with technological skills and the ability to apply them to a range of community development issues—is clear and increasing. With an evaluation team in place to document the process at work in the New Communities Program, we—LISC Chicago, MDRC, and the Foundation—hope to have more specific lessons to share with the field about what makes for successful technical information partnerships in the near future.

Lesson #3: Good data and information are key inputs for all stages of a successful community development initiative: design, planning, implementation, evaluation, and stage-appropriate information infrastructure is necessary for each—but we don't have good models or tools at every stage.

We need a widespread organizational culture shift that recognizes information as one of the key building blocks of community development, as essential as money, people, bricks, and mortar. The program design changes in the next phase of the New Communities Program were in many ways only specific, information-centered tweaks to the capacity-building mindset that LISC Chicago was already building among the partners in its network. It became clear that building information capacity was as essential as organizing capacity or fundraising capacity—fundamental and useful for advancing all of the other objectives of community development.

In a complex endeavor such as community change, it is important for everyone involved in the project—from the managing intermediary to funders and evaluators—to share the same broad view of the value of information at all stages of the program life cycle. Because this broad view has been lacking, the field's technical solutions are more mature for accountability and evaluation purposes than they are for the planning and process aspects of implementation.

LISC Chicago and most organizations like it do not have information systems that are sufficiently sophisticated to manage the complex array of data that its programs generate, or to translate this data efficiently into information that can guide, in real-time, course-corrections and future program decisions. This is true for many nonprofit organizations. LISC Chicago and many others have very strong elements in place. In part, what is needed is a simple, adaptable interface to help pull all of these inputs together and allow them to be visualized and analyzed clearly, and for different audiences. However, in this niche marketplace, finding the right resources to help design and build such a solution can be difficult.

The creation of better data and information systems to support comp[...] community change work is partly a technical challenge. We believe th[...] the right skills, technologies, and inputs exist somewhere (although not necessarily in the community development field), and we only nee[...] to find the right resources and broker the right connections to build a[...] solution. However, adaptive challenges are also evident: What does th[...] move toward more data-driven development mean for organizations? For long-term funding? How will these new tools, once developed, be sustained? How will we deal with the challenge of constant evolution and adaptation to new information technologies? These challenges ar[...] not unique to the nonprofit sector, but the resource gap and widespre[...] underinvestment in information technologies keep the organizations [...] rely on to deliver social services, organize resources in neighborhood[...] and perform key planning functions in our cities from reaching highe[...] levels of effectiveness and efficiency.

Lesson #4: The rapid evolution of the information landscape demands flexible, core capacity investments that allow organizations to evolve a[...] adapt, in addition to investment in specialized intermediaries that can broker resources and stay abreast of changes.

Since the Foundation's two major place-based investments began mo[...] than a decade ago, the landscape of information consumption and production has changed rapidly and dramatically (although the ends, far as our ultimate social change objectives are concerned, remain the same). More data—and more tools to turn data into information—ar[...] available to community development practitioners and the public than ever before, and all signs suggest that the volume, diversity, and, hopefully, quality will continue to increase. In just the last year, the open data movement in the public sector has gained traction across th[...] country. Many new important data sources for community develop-ment purposes—ranging from crime, to public health, to education, t[...] transit—are suddenly free and available to the public as raw material and as building blocks for coders and application developers who kn[...] how to analyze and build things with it. The result is an explosion of new possibilities to create low-cost, adaptable, and user-friendly tool[...] aid community development practitioners in their work.

However, the availability of data does not mean that the data is useful or usable for community development practitioners. Cities and counties are increasingly pledging to make their data openly available, regularly updated, and "developer-friendly," but this means only that we now have the raw material to build meaningful applications for community development. To harness all of this potential on behalf of our cities and neighborhoods, funders will need to pay attention to the changing information needs of our communities. We will need to provide flexible dollars to meet organizations' core information needs and to broker better partnerships with the expanding cadre of civic technologists. In addition, we will need to invest in specialized organizations that form the backbone information infrastructure of our cities and regions. These issue specialists must be technology experts with broad reach among issue areas, and they must be able to develop more effective ways to use information for the benefit of the communities we care about.

It is too soon to tell how successful LISC Chicago and its partners will be in their efforts to build better information infrastructure, but the progress to date is encouraging. What is certain is that in a field in which change at scale is complex and progress can feel imperceptible in the short term, these efforts to improve and evolve must be sustained and supported over the long term.

LOOKING FORWARD: WHAT CAN FUNDERS DO?

Signs already indicate that the challenge of finding new ways to use information is invigorating and, hopefully, attracting more resources and investment from funders and other partners. As LISC Chicago's essay in this volume notes, it has been encouraging to witness the widespread demand from the diverse group of community development organizations in the New Communities Network for support, the curiosity and eagerness to learn new about new ways of working, and the openness to identifying new partners to support the process.

The MacArthur Foundation is committed to continued support for this critical area work, encouraged by the progress, and enthusiastic about all there is to learn from its grantees as it continues to search for new ideas for investment. The Foundation has sharpened its focus on specific efforts to strengthen capacity for informed decision making in all of the work it supports. In closing and looking ahead, I offer four suggestions for ways that funders could strengthen information infra structure for the community development field and build capacity to it to improve conditions in neighborhoods.

First, we can commit to becoming smarter about the information nee of the nonprofit and public sectors, and make the ongoing process of educating ourselves and our grantees about the ever-changing landsc of data sources, information technologies, and information policies t are available to support social sector activity a routine and expected part of our jobs.

Admittedly, this can feel like a daunting task, but it's not an unreaso able one. The capacity to use information to support program planni implementation, performance management, and evaluation in increa ingly sophisticated ways cuts across program interests and even fund models: It is simply a fundamental component of a high-performing organization. But engaging in conversations and grant negotiations about data and information technologies requires a baseline level of technical expertise and language to be accessible, and the rapid evolution of tools and players in the space only adds to the challenge Making an explicit commitment to stay on the learning curve ourselv (and identifying the right people to help) is an important first step that can go a long way toward strengthening our funding strategies. Fortunately, some excellent resources offer ways to think about the r of information in place-based grant making, from the Urban Institut to Living Cities to *Stanford Social Innovation Review* to Markets for Good, but it is incumbent on all of us to think deeply about how to this information to strengthen our capacity as funders. The same is tr for the organizations we support.

Second, we can embed a focus on the quality of grantee information systems and the ability of grantees to use them in routine due diligen processes. If we peek inside the big black box of "capacity" that we all use as shorthand for many elements of organizational health and effectiveness, many of us would admit we know and ask too little about the way information is used. We are trained to rigorously asses quality of leadership, financial position, and presence of strategy, but it is rare to ask systematic questions about organizations' ability to access, analyze, interpret, and communicate information outside of the context of a specific project. We need to start asking questions about the invisible information infrastructure that is so often the backbone of any project we support: the software, the technology, and the architecture of the solutions that organizations need to do their work, measure their progress, and communicate the story of their impact. By becoming more specific and precise about the types of questions we ask about information capacity in the due diligence process and throughout a funding relationship, and by establishing a shared commitment to developing a culture of learning and continual improvement, we can be more supportive partners in the complex project of community change. This could include initiating conversations with grantees about how they stay on top of new tools and trends; building low-cost, high-impact opportunities for ongoing professional development (such as LISC Chicago's excellent "Data Fridays" series) into program funding; and supporting information capacity assessments—including the information technologies and systems that organizations use and the sources of information they rely on—on an ongoing basis.

Third, all of us can become more informed about the information "ecosystems" in the places where we work, and invest in efforts to strengthen them. It is challenging to marshal coordinated information infrastructure investments because most funders are oriented towards specific programmatic objectives, defined by issues like health, education, or climate, rather than the ecosystem as a whole. Generating support for multi-purpose community improvement infrastructure—whether for specific places like LISC Chicago, the Smart Chicago Collaborative, or for the field as a whole, like the National Neighborhood Indicators Partnership—can feel like a massive collective action problem, with many benefitting but too few willing to pay. Yet these organizations are the utilities of the community development world, the essential, but too often invisible supporting infrastructure that provides information, capacity, and other important public goods that make the field work.

Place-based funders and community foundations have special responsibility and ability to support efforts to assess the functions and capacities of local information producers and consumers, and efforts to raise community-wide awareness of available information resource as several cities, most recently Chicago, have begun to do with user conferences known as "data days."[11] By identifying organizations wit expertise with and access to data on specific issues, as well as those w cross-cutting capacity (public libraries, local data intermediaries, or c technology organizations such as the Smart Chicago Collaborative), local funders can help organize the market for information that supports social good. Such place-based, whole-system focused efforts help reveal gaps where investments in data, access, or skills are neede allow foundations to be better matchmakers between project needs a information resources, and make it easier for community developmen organizations to identify partners that can help them use information strengthen their work.

Finally—and most important in our role as funders—it is our job to provide adequate financial support to those that are leading the charg to find ways to use information to do their work better. This means investing directly in community development organizations, their performance management and internal assessment capacities, their ongoing professional development opportunities in this area, and staf who focus on strengthening the use of information in all areas of wor It means supporting the local data intermediaries and civic technologi who contribute to a robust information ecosystem in places, and for national funders, identifying and supporting those organizations that do the same ecosystem-level information work for the field as a whole And looking to the future, it means investing in building a pipeline of community development professionals who have both the technical skills and content knowledge to put information technology to work for the field.[12]

---

11 Urban Institute/NNIP – Assessment of the Chicago Metropolitan Area Community Information Infrastructure, March 2013.

12 "Data Days" have emerged in cities around the country, from Boston to Charlotte. The Chicago School of Data Project is an ongoing effort to map and organize the community information ecosystem in Chicago, and included a two-day conference in September 2014. The National Neighborhood Indicators Partnership maintains documentation about these events around the country: http://www.neighborhoodindicators.org/activities/partner/charlotte-data-day-2014.

This chapter has benefitted from a robust dialogue about what works in community development that many others have been active in shaping for years. It also benefits from the keen insights of peer foundations, policymakers, nonprofit organizations, researchers, consultants, and observers of the community development field—some, but not nearly all, of whom are citied here. I hope it will contribute to that dialogue and that funders of community development initiatives in particular will learn something from the MacArthur Foundation's experience that improves their work just as the Foundation's strategies have grown out of decades of research and practice that came before.

Participating in this conversation and sharing what has not worked as candidly as what has is part of the commitment to continual improvement that we expect from our grantees, our partners, and ourselves as investors. But the project of working toward a country where no person lives in poverty, and where all of our neighborhoods increase families' chances of achieving health, safety, economic opportunity, and connection instead of diminishing them, is a collective responsibility. Each of us, regardless of our position within or outside of the field of community development, is a stakeholder. Let's do everything we can to invest in this invisible infrastructure, and to make sure that we are engaged and consistent contributors to the crowdsourced roadmap of how to build a more informed community development field, so that 50 years from now (and hopefully, sooner) the picture of progress might become even clearer.

■ ■ ■

ALAINA HARKNESS *is a program officer for the John D. and Catherine T. MacArthur Foundation. Her portfolio focuses on improving conditions in cities and strengthening the field of community development. She has a special interest in information technologies and their relationship to cities and democracy. Alaina is a Fellow of Leadership Greater Chicago and serves on the boards of Chicago Women in Philanthropy, The Funders' Network for Smart Growth and Livable Communities, and the Harris School's Alumni Advisory Council. She holds dual master's degrees from the University of Chicago and a bachelor's degree from the University of Rochester.*

6

CONCLUSION

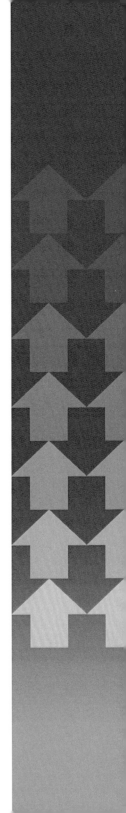

WHAT COUNTS?

Naomi Cytron
Federal Reserve Bank of San Francisco [1]

Are we making a difference? What impact do the efforts of community developers, public health officials, social service providers, and others have on the lives of children and families? The answers to these seemingly simple questions are frustratingly elusive. In part, this is because our ambitions—to make sure that the places where people live provide opportunities for all children to grow up healthy and ready to learn, and support economic stability and advancement for all residents—entail complex interactions among people, institutions, and policies. As such, getting a true grip on what is working, for whom, under which conditions, and compared to what, is far more complicated than counting numbers of houses built or programs financed. To fully comprehend the reach and impact of our efforts, we must align information from across sectors and institutions working to improve communities. And that is not easy.

The authors in this volume contend that developing better data "infrastructure"—which includes technologies, but also skills, capacities, and leadership—can help. Improving how we collect, and more critically, share data across institutions, they argue, can advance our efforts to see the connections across sectors and better understand the outcomes of our work. By linking the data of a public health clinic with attendance records at schools, or aligning housing data with information on transportation networks, for example, we can more easily spot resource gaps or opportunities for amplification of positive outcomes. This, in turn, can help us work together in joint action across sectors. Ultimately, better data infrastructure can help us be more strategic and efficient in our work, and can yield the information needed to influence policy and decisions about resource allocations.

---

1   The views expressed in this essay belong to the author and do not necessarily represent the views of the Federal Reserve Bank of San Francisco or the Federal Reserve System.

As Kathryn L.S. Pettit and G. Thomas Kinsgley noted at the outset of this volume, the community development field—broadly defined to include all who work to advance equitable outcomes for low-income communities—is at an exciting moment. We now have more data than ever, and we have the computing power to crunch it. The authors in this volume point to measurement tools, indicator systems, and visualization strategies that exponentially increase our ability to galvanize a wide array of community actors, from residents to service providers to funders to politicians, to challenge current ways of doing business, and to develop novel strategies for intervention design and implementation.

But they also point to the progress yet to be made. They outline the practices that must change to ensure that the data we collect are as representative as possible of community conditions, and that we are using it in ways that reflect community interests. They draw attention to range of capacities that must be built among funders, leaders, and front line service providers to use data meaningfully. They discuss the need to boost data transparency and to further connect the dots among various types of data to better assess the performance of programs and policies relative to diverse social and economic factors. Although it is impossible to fully capture the richness of the authors' insights, what follows is a synthesis of key themes in the volume.

IMPROVING RAW MATERIALS

It's a basic point to make, but our tools and systems for making meaning out of data are only as good as the data they harness. Although there will always be gaps, errors, and omissions in any data set, the authors point to a number of key considerations in ensuring that data assembly practices are capturing the complexity of the communities we serve as accurately and fully as we can. The first is nuance. The data that we often count on to gauge progress—poverty rates, unemployment rates, educational attainment rates—are blunt instruments at best. We must dig deeper, in both collecting and verifying data, if we are to gain thorough understanding of which programs and policies work to effect positive change.

One point that the authors stress is the importance of routinely double checking data during collection to ensure its validity. For example, Ira

Goldstein discusses the importance of "ground-truthing" data to ensure that data accurately reflect on-the-ground conditions. Validation is especially critical when data systems pull information from secondary data sets that may be flawed or outdated, or when there is some degree of automation in data assembly. Goldstein discusses how, in the case of the Market Value Analysis (MVA), which aggregates data from a variety of administrative sources, a built-in data validation process uncovers, and corrects, flaws early, before conclusions are drawn. Annie Donovan and Rick Jacobus, who discuss data systems that automatically consolidate and standardize transaction information, point out that those who are closest to real-world conditions should review the first run of charts and graphs to ensure that the data reflect reality and that analysts are drawing conclusions that make sense.

The authors also stress that we need to pay attention to data comprehensiveness, and the need to assemble data from multiple sources to decipher trends driven by multiple factors. In their discussion of the National Mortgage DataBase (NMDB), Robert Avery, Marsha Courchane, and Peter Zorn discuss how none of the current data sources about the mortgage market include all the data necessary for accurately benchmarking, tracking, and evaluating the marketplace. By bringing together myriad data, the NMDB will enable a deeper understanding of market dynamics. In a similar vein, Claudia Coulton discusses how difficult it can be—and offers solutions—to accurately gauge residential mobility and resulting neighborhood change using only one data source. Several authors discuss how community residents themselves are important sources of data and information, and make the case that qualitative data can help sort out the "why" and "how" of community change. Meredith Minkler advocates for community involvement in collecting and analyzing data, and shows how community-based participatory research can enhance data validity and yield unanticipated insights that can ultimately improve program and policy design. In a similar vein, Patricia Bowie and Moira Inkelas discuss how surveying residents about their experiences with neighborhood services and programs can help front-line providers and program leaders more fully assess whether programs are ultimately delivering on outcomes they set out to achieve.

Our authors also stress that timely data are critical, particularly if our aim is to be responsive to dynamic community conditions. Bowie and Inkelas discuss how the Magnolia Place data dashboard synthesizes monthly survey data in "real-time" so community workers can assess their ongoing roles in community change and adjust practices to better achieve goals. Likewise, David Fleming, Hilary Karasz, and Kirsten Wysen call for greater use of intermediate outcomes and rapid-cycle surveys on health and community development outcomes to more accurately determine whether mid-course corrections are needed. Ira Goldstein also underscores the point that frequently updated data are vital for understanding neighborhood dynamics, and notes that the local government administrative data in the MVA, which are more frequently updated than sources like the census, better capture how market conditions change over time. The key in all these efforts is the need for ongoing access to detailed data and trends so practitioners and leaders can quickly learn about changing conditions and adjust accordingly.

MAKING DATA MEANINGFUL ENTAILS MORE THAN COLLECTING IT

Many of the authors reinforce the point that data do not do anything on their own; it takes skill to make the information meaningful. While technical skills for manipulating data tables are important, we need to build a wide range of "softer" skills to use data effectively and appropriately on a long-term basis.

Fundamentally, to make data actionable, it must be easily digestible by a range of audiences. Maps and infographics can often help make complex information more accessible. Bridget Catlin describes how data visualization tools used by the County Health Rankings have evolved help laypeople understand the multiple factors that contribute to health outcomes and to help users with different skill levels access data in formats that are meaningful to them. Storytelling and marketing skills are no less important in bringing data to life. Raphael Bostic hammers home the point that without a compelling storyline and a method to reach key audiences, decision-makers will not fully absorb or use data and evidence, regardless of their quality and import. He proposes a central repository where data and evidence on similar topic areas can distilled and readily accessed everyone involved in data-driven decision-making. Catlin also speaks to this issue, noting that for data and evidence to ultimately influence policy and program decisions, findings must be packaged for the media. Staff at the County Health Rankings, she says, work closely with communications experts to develop messages that can be widely disseminated to multiple audiences.

Many other "translational" skills are needed to help practitioners inject data into decision-making. Victor Rubin and Michael McAfee discuss how, in PolicyLink's role as a technical assistance provider, they helped Promise Neighborhoods and Sustainable Communities grantees to understand how to use data to guide decisions and manage program performance and community relationships. Alex Karner, Jonathan London, Dana Rowangould, and Catherine Garoupa White similarly discuss how the Center for Regional Change at the University of California, Davis, supplemented its social equity mapping tools by helping groups build their capacities in navigating the political landscape and framing controversial issues. These skills have helped community partners use the data to align policy and program changes across fragmented jurisdictions.

Another key idea that runs through many of the essays in this volume is that, above and beyond technologies and staff capacities, organizational culture and leadership approach can significantly impact the quality and sustainability of data collection and use. These factors relate to the priority that is placed on data collection, analysis, and use, which in turn affects how time, money, and attention are allocated to these processes. In other words, establishing data-driven practices, whether to measure impact, adjust programs, or foster accountability among partners, takes commitment not just from data analysts, as Susana Vasquez shows, but also from funders, leadership, and other staff. Echoing the point on the importance of funder commitment to this work, Alaina Harkness calls attention to the need for foundations to boost support for expansion of data capacities among grantees. Erika Poethig speaks to how these issues play out in local government settings. She describes how strong data practices became embedded into management processes within the City of Chicago's Department of Housing, where it took strong internal leadership to implement and sustain improvements in data collection and use. Cory Fleming and Randall Reid similarly discuss how in Baltimore, sustained leadership and accountability mechanisms prompted local government agencies align around using performance assessment tools in designing program strategies and adjusting practices as needed.

Finally, the authors remind us that data are not neutral. Rather, there are values and assumptions that underlie what and who gets counted and how much one data point counts versus another. As such, we must hone our critical thinking skills and be alert to the biases embedded in our data collection and measurement frameworks. A number of authors discuss, for instance, the considerable subjectivity built into seemingly objective data platforms and systems, and how the ways that we define what counts shapes, and in some cases, limits, program and policy design. In each of their essays, J. Benjamin Warner, Bridget Catlin, and Ira Goldstein point out that analysts and planners must make an array of choices when synthesizing and distilling data into more manageable and actionable information. These include decisions about which data to assemble and analyze in the first place, which benchmarks to use in assessing progress or change, and the thresholds that separate success from failure. Warner explicitly considers how different frameworks and political orientations affect the scope of data that is used for assessing community conditions and the range of interests that are taken into account in decision-making processes. Several authors underscore that just the process of defining problems and solutions can be fraught. Bowie and Inkelas note how the scope of a logic model identifying causes for particular problem, if too narrow, limits the range of data that is collected and the questions that are asked of that data, ultimately shrinking the solution set. In a similar vein, Ian Galloway considers the ways that impact investors choose to define "impact," and how investor preferences might skew resource allocation. All of these factors, which ultimately depend on human decisions more than data, can significantly affect the design and targeting of data-driven programs and policies. As such, we need to keep our eyes open and take corrective actions when certain populations or practices are overlooked, undercounted, misrepresented by the data feeding our decisions.

BUT WHAT EXACTLY ARE WE SUPPOSED TO MEASURE?

One cannot make data actionable without first collecting it. For many communities, this basic question is the hardest: what data should we collect and analyze? Alas, there is no silver bullet. Instead, the authors raise a number of considerations that can inform how we can craft data systems to help make sense of the context of our work and to ascertain the real impact of the investments and programs we implement.

Several authors, for instance, speak to the merits of data standardization. When multiple organizations use shared metrics, they argue, it's easier to compare performance across organizations, initiatives, and communities. Paige Chapel discusses the importance of standard metrics for community development financial institutions (CDFIs), arguing that uniformity is critical for accessing capital and investments. Annie Donovan and Rick Jacobus show how standard data aggregated across organizations allows groups to compare performance and identify market conditions that all organizations may be facing. David Fleming, Hilary Karasz, and Kirsten Wysen call for uniformity and standardization in health data, which would allow for a quicker grasp of which health interventions work in various settings and the cost-effectiveness of implementing different types of approaches. Maggie Grieve speaks to the strengths of shared and standardized metrics in helping to align the actions of multiple organizations working toward the same essential goals.

A challenge with standardization is that, by definition, it does not accommodate nuance. Bridget Catlin and Ben Warner each raise this issue in discussing rankings and indices. These types of tools can help distill disparate data into standardized metrics that can grab headlines, and thus help to direct attention to important issues. But the standardization and simplification means a necessary loss of information. As a result, disparities can be masked, and conditions that are unique to particular communities or populations can be overlooked. More detailed and granular information is typically required to sort out how to design and target programs that meet diverse community needs.

Adding to this point, Bowie and Inkelas note that different actors— from community residents to front-line providers to managers to policymakers—need different types of information during design, implementation, and assessment of community interventions. Therefor data collection and reporting systems must be expansive and nimble enough to accommodate different types of data, such as data on individual actions, program performance, and community context. Alaina Harkness makes a similar argument, suggesting that a data system that aims to capture the complexity of community conditions must accommodate:

- Quantitative and qualitative measures of change;

- Both inputs (dollars in, resources on the task) and outputs (community gardens planted, murals painted, units of housing developed, people assisted);

- Contextual data—real-time information about a neighborhood and individuals;

- Process or "platform" data—information about how social and organizational networks are growing, and the added value of increased organization and connectivity.

Of course, the idea that each organization's data system must "do it a is overwhelming. Essentially, though, the authors are suggesting that some set of common standards and definitions is vital for comparing performance of programs, aligning activities among organizations working toward similar ends, and understanding large-scale trends. At the same time, we'll need to be able to weave together additional layer of data to understand the context and reach of our activities, and the process of change, across geographies and populations.

The former will most likely require organizations to relinquish some degree of control and power over decision-making, a requirement that often doesn't come naturally, to say the least. Maggie Grieve, for example, suggests that organizations participating in a shared measurement framework have to give up some degree of organizationa autonomy and learn to accommodate the approaches of partner organizations to data collection and definition. Similarly, Bill Kelly and Fre Karnas suggest that efforts to create consistent data across organizatic will require leaders to step back from "proprietary" processes, some of which likely entailed significant expense and time to establish, and consider alternatives.

The latter will necessitate enhanced access to and interoperability among data sets, regardless of whether data are being generated by a CDFI, a health department, or a school. Aligning data from various institutions and agencies operating in a given area or serving a given population will be critical for making sense of how particular programs and investments play out in concert with the full complement of community- and regional-level activities also in play. To make a more significant leap forward in understanding how to achieve holistic and lasting impact, public, private and non-profit institutions will need to consider ways to make individual stores of data more commonly available to others. The next section looks at this topic in more depth.

BOOSTING DATA ACCESS AND CONNECTING THE DOTS

We place many demands on data; we seek a mirror and a map, odometer and oracle. To achieve these ends, community-serving entities must more broadly and consistently increase data transparency and link fragmented data sets together. The authors point to many different types of data sets that can be linked: individual behavioral data, community or regional socioeconomic data, organizational performance data, government administrative data, and private, corporate data.

One problem in putting these data sets to use, though, is that many are locked behind organization walls. However, in certain corners, this is changing. Emily Shaw discusses the growth of "open data," noting that government entities are increasingly publishing administrative data for use by the public as a way to support good governance and community engagement in planning decisions. Ren Essene, along with Robert Avery, Marsha Courchane, and Peter Zorn, discuss how increased access to mortgage data can better identify market trends and performance in fair lending practices. Eric Bakken and David Kindig discuss how greater access to data on how hospitals are allocating community benefit resources can help promote coordinated action among multiple groups tackling the social determinants of health. Amias Gerety and Sophie Raseman discuss My Data, a system that allows individuals to access

their personal data from government or corporate sources and share i
third parties. They point to the possibilities of using both open data a
My Data to build smart disclosure practices, where previously unavai
able data can be aggregated in safe and secure ways to help consumer
make better decisions and push suppliers of goods and services to cha
their practices.

Data access is only one piece of the puzzle, though. The authors sugge
that a more critical component of this work is about directly or indire
linking data across domains, for example, across housing, health, and
education programs. Linking data can help us better understand and
address the interwoven nature of the factors affecting individual and
population outcomes. Encouragingly, they point to a number of tools
approaches that hold promise in this effort. Aaron Wernham, for inst
points out that Health Impact Assessments, which assemble multiple t
of quantitative and qualitative data about housing, transportation, an
the environment, can help urban planners and developers understand
building designs, redevelopment plans, and transit infrastructure can I
recalibrated to improve health outcomes. Nancy Andrews and Dan R
discuss how a "social impact calculator" can use social science resear
estimate the impact of affordable housing or early childhood educatio
health improvements and lifetime earnings.

Other authors discuss data approaches that trace how individuals inte
with multiple programs and institutions. Rebecca London and Milbre
McLaughlin discuss the use of Integrated Data Systems (IDS), which I
individual data from across agencies. These systems help combat the
and redundancies in service that spring from institutional isolation. T
speak in particular to the possibilities for IDS to better support youth
The linked data from multiple social service institutions can allow the
craft interventions that connect the dots among youths' social, cogniti
emotional, and physical development. John Petrila similarly points ou
IDS can help better diagnose problems and develop solutions by ident
how interwoven systems – from health to environment to housing – a
individuals and communities over time. Bill Kelly and Fred Karnas tac
the topic of data linkage from a different angle, noting that the Outco
Initiative prompts affordable housing developers to collect and use da
health, employment, education, and other critical facets of resident lif

uncover how service integration works and to spur policy development that supports the "whole person."

Boosting data transparency and linking across data sets that include personally identifiable information raise important questions about data privacy and confidentiality. Rebecca London and Milbrey McLaughlin consider the multiple facets of this issue. Organizations that agree to share data with one another must establish trusting relationships and develop agreements about how the data will be used and accessed. They also must determine how to share and store data such that all parties are compliant with relevant data safety and security protocols. Petrila cites resources that offer guidance on crafting these kinds of data use agreements, and considers some of the technological and method-ological advances in storing data and matching individual data across data sets that offer enhanced privacy protections.

MOVING FORWARD

It is likely apparent by now that this volume is only partially about data in and of itself. The authors ultimately focused less on metrics than on the cultural and institutional factors that enable or impede efforts to learn about what is working, or what might work better, to collectively generate positive outcomes for the communities we care about most.

In part, this is because we are at the front of a new era in the work of creating opportunities in low-income communities. Community devel-opers are beginning to work differently, employing new strategies that simultaneously engage adjacent sectors, including health, education, public safety, transportation, and others. We are making strides toward what Paul Grogan called out in our prior volume of essays, *Investing in What Works for America's Communities*:

> What then is the future of community development? It lies in turning the architecture of community development to meet urgent challenges of *human development*. How to turn a successful community organizing and real estate development system toward the goal of increasing educational outcomes, employment success, family asset building, individual and

community resilience to weather setbacks? As an industry, we need new strategies to face these challenges.[2]

The cornerstone of the new era of community strategy is data. It is th tool that allows us to set a baseline; provides us the language to speak to one another across sectors and align our work; gives us feedback s we can constantly fine tune our interventions to meet the evolving nec of communities; and ultimately helps us to communicate "wins" to the communities we serve and to government, foundations, and other funders and investors.

Our authors tell us that being data-driven goes far beyond brandishin skills with calculators and rulers. Rather, they send home the message that communities are complex systems, and that our approaches to understanding the part we play in community change must match the complexity at hand. There is no single answer for how to do this. But a minimum, we need to embrace the idea that data is for learning. To often, data collection and analysis are seen as extraneous to the "real work," important only for reporting or compliance procedures—for checking boxes and passing the test. But under a learning mindset, da become key for understanding performance, improving practice, and holding ourselves accountable to our real clients, the communities we serve. A learning mindset motivates data- and information-sharing th can yield collective knowledge and action.

But that's just the beginning. For new practices to take root, substant investment will be required. The more we invest in capacities to colle and align data, the better we will be at learning what works and wha doesn't in supporting families and communities. In turn, this will hel us use resources more wisely and generate better outcomes. This volu intentionally brings together ideas from practitioners, researchers, funders, and policy experts from multiple fields to begin the conversa tion about what will need to change, from organizational behaviors to funding patterns to regulations and accountability mechanisms, if we are to better assess and articulate the impact of our work in low-income communities. As did *Investing in What Works for America's*

---

2 Paul Grogan, "The Future of Community Development." in *Investing in What Works for Americ Communities*, edited by the Federal Reserve Bank of San Francisco and the Low Income Investme Fund. (San Francisco, CA: 2012).

Communities, we hope this volume serves as a model for continued cross-sector dialogue and action to help achieve what should not be such a lofty goal: a nation where everyone has a fair shot at living a healthy, fulfilled life.

■ ■ ■

NAOMI CYTRON *is a senior research associate in the Community Development department at the Federal Reserve Bank of San Francisco. Her primary research interests are neighborhood revitalization and regional equity, and she has authored numerous articles and reports on topics ranging from concentrated poverty to transit-oriented development. Previously, Naomi worked as a consultant in affordable housing finance and managed a fair housing testing program. She has a master's degree in city and regional planning from the University of North Carolina at Chapel Hill and a bachelor's degree in biology from Macalester College.*